Register Now for Online Access to Your Book!

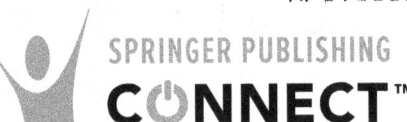

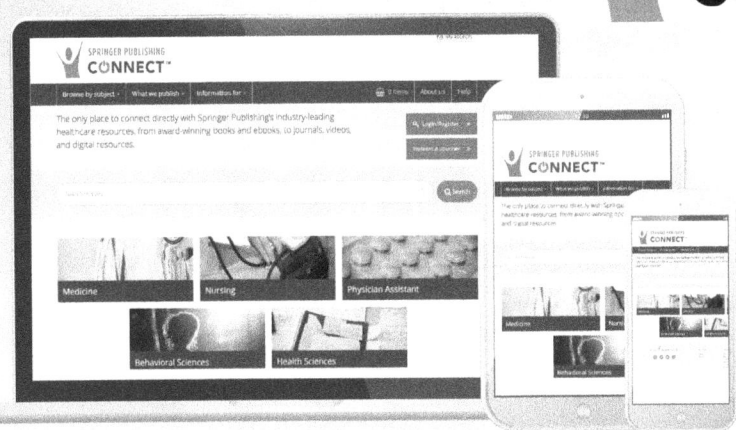

Your print purchase of *EMDR and Attachment-Focused Trauma Therapy for Adults* **includes online access to the contents of your book**—increasing accessibility, portability, and searchability!

Access today at:
http://connect.springerpub.com/content/book/978-0-8261-3689-3
or scan the QR code at the right with your smartphone. Log in or register, then click "Redeem a voucher" and use the code below.

2P7VGFD0

Scan here for quick access.

Having trouble redeeming a voucher code?
Go to https://connect.springerpub.com/redeeming-voucher-code

If you are experiencing problems accessing the digital component of this product, please contact our customer service department at cs@springerpub.com

The online access with your print purchase is available at the publisher's discretion and may be removed at any time without notice.

Publisher's Note: New and used products purchased from third-party sellers are not guaranteed for quality, authenticity, or access to any included digital components.

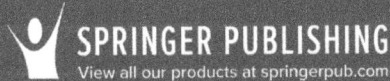

EMDR and Attachment-Focused Trauma Therapy for Adults

Ann E. Potter, PhD, has worked for over 45 years in the mental health field as a psychiatric nurse, educator, therapist, psychologist, evaluator, researcher, writer, presenter, and consultant. She has a bachelor's degree in nursing from Creighton University, a master's degree in counseling from the University of Nebraska Omaha, and a doctorate in counseling psychology from the University of Nebraska–Lincoln. She has been in private practice since 1989. Dr. Potter's areas of expertise include trauma, attachment, addictions, personality disorders, domestic violence, and sexual assault, and she has specialized training in Eye Movement Desensitization and Reprocessing (EMDR), Dialectical Behavioral Therapy (DBT), and Radically Open Dialectical Behavioral Therapy (RO DBT). She is a certified therapist and approved consultant in EMDR and a certified RO DBT therapist. She piloted outcome research related to phase-based trauma treatment (DBT/EMDR) for adults and published articles on the roles adults played as children in alcoholic families, a therapist manual and companion client workbook on trauma treatment, and articles on EMDR therapy.

Debra Wesselmann, MS, LIMHP, has specialized in treating trauma and attachment problems in adults and children for over 30 years and cofounded The Attachment and Trauma Center of Nebraska in Omaha, Nebraska. She is an Eye Movement Desensitization and Reprocessing (EMDR) Institute trainer and develops EMDR specialty child and adult attachment and trauma-focused trainings for clinicians and trains clinicians online, around the United States, and overseas. She is an EMDR International Association (EMDRIA)-approved consultant and serves on the editorial board for *The Journal of EMDR Practice and Research*. Wesselmann has coauthored articles, chapters, and books related to attachment and trauma, including two chapters that were coauthored with Francine Shapiro and the recent treatment manual for the EMDR and family therapy integrative model as well as the companion parent guide. She has been invited to give workshops and keynotes at numerous conferences nationally and internationally.

EMDR and Attachment-Focused Trauma Therapy for Adults

Reclaiming Authentic Self and Healthy Attachments

Ann E. Potter, PhD

Debra Wesselmann, MS, LIMHP

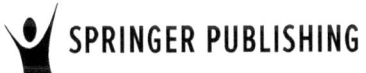

Copyright © 2023 Springer Publishing Company, LLC
All rights reserved.

No part of this publication may be reproduced, stored in a retrieval system, or transmitted in any form or by any means, electronic, mechanical, photocopying, recording, or otherwise, without the prior permission of Springer Publishing Company, LLC, or authorization through payment of the appropriate fees to the Copyright Clearance Center, Inc., 222 Rosewood Drive, Danvers, MA 01923, 978-750-8400, fax 978-646-8600, info@copyright.com or at www.copyright.com.

Springer Publishing Company, LLC
11 West 42nd Street, New York, NY 10036
www.springerpub.com
connect.springerpub.com/

Acquisitions Editor: Kate Dimock
Compositor: Transforma

ISBN: 978-0-8261-3688-6
ebook ISBN: 978-0-8261-3689-3
DOI: 10.1891/9780826136893

Printed by LSI

The author and the publisher of this Work have made every effort to use sources believed to be reliable to provide information that is accurate and compatible with the standards generally accepted at the time of publication. The author and publisher shall not be liable for any special, consequential, or exemplary damages resulting, in whole or in part, from the readers' use of, or reliance on, the information contained in this book. The publisher has no responsibility for the persistence or accuracy of URLs for external or third-party Internet websites referred to in this publication and does not guarantee that any content on such websites is, or will remain, accurate or appropriate.

Library of Congress Cataloging-in-Publication Data
Names: Potter, Ann E., author. | Wesselmann, Debra, author.
Title: EMDR and attachment-focused trauma therapy for adults : reclaiming
   authentic self and healthy attachments / Ann E. Potter, Debra
   Wesselmann.
Description: New York, NY : Springer Publishing Company, [2023] | Includes
   bibliographical references and index.
Identifiers: LCCN 2022023500 | ISBN 9780826136886 (paperback) | ISBN
   9780826136893 (ebook)
Subjects: MESH: Eye Movement Desensitization Reprocessing--methods | Object
   Attachment | Psychological Trauma--therapy
Classification: LCC RC455.4.A84 | NLM WM 425.5.D4 | DDC
   616.85/88--dc23/eng/20220711
LC record available at https://lccn.loc.gov/2022023500

Contact sales@springerpub.com to receive discount rates on bulk purchases.

Publisher's Note: New and used products purchased from third-party sellers are not guaranteed for quality, authenticity, or access to any included digital components.

Printed in the United States of America.

To those who walked before us, the pioneers of EMDR therapy and attachment, trauma, and therapy fields; and those who share expertise, kindness, encouragement, and humor with us now; thank you! To those of you who will travel after us, be brave! You have everything you need inside.

To family and cherished friends in the family of my heart, to my highly esteemed and much appreciated friends and colleagues, and to clients who continue to show me what courage, determination, and humility really mean; no words can really express how you have changed me. (AP)

Thank you to my family, my friends, and my colleagues for your support, for your laughter, and for your acceptance of me just as I am. I think the world of you. Thank you to my healers and guides; you give me just what I need when I need it, and to my clients; you never cease to amaze me with what you can do. (DW)

Contents

Foreword Marshall Lyles, LMFT-S, LPC-S   *ix*
Preface   xi
How to Use This Book   xvii
Acknowledgments   xxi

1. Introduction and Foundational Theories for Attachment-Focused Trauma Therapy for Adults   *1*

2. Therapist Mindfulness and Parallel Process in Attachment-Focused Trauma Therapy for Adults   *11*

3. Internal and External Secure/Earned Secure Attachments in Attachment-Focused Trauma Therapy for Adults   *19*

4. External and Internal Nonsecure and Disorganized Categories of Attachment in Attachment-Focused Trauma Therapy for Adults   *25*

5. Framework for Attachment-Focused Trauma Therapy for Adults: Enhanced Preparation Phase of EMDR Therapy   *39*

6. Assessment of Client Readiness and Treatment Planning for EMDR Therapy in Attachment-Focused Trauma Therapy for Adults   *53*

7. Explaining the Parent-Adult-Child (P-A-C) Diagrams in Attachment-Focused Trauma Therapy for Adults   *69*

8. Safe Place and Higher Power for Adult Part of Self in Attachment-Focused Trauma Therapy for Adults   *91*

9. Safe Place and Higher Power for Child/Adolescent Part(s) of Self in Attachment-Focused Trauma Therapy for Adults   *107*

10. Creating an Internal Resource Team in Attachment-Focused Trauma Therapy for Adults   *121*

11. Strengthening the Competent Adult Part of Self in Attachment-Focused Trauma Therapy for Adults   *141*

12. Providing Corrective Attachment Experiences Between Child/Adolescent and True Parent Parts of Self in Attachment-Focused Trauma Therapy for Adults   *153*

13. Parts' Work: Negotiating New Roles for Parent and Adult Parts of Self in Attachment-Focused Trauma Therapy for Adults   *167*

14. Parts' Work: Tucking Child/Adolescent Parts of Self Into Their Safe Places in Attachment-Focused Trauma Therapy for Adults   *183*

15. Revising the Early Bonding Contract Rules in Attachment-Focused Trauma Therapy for Adults   *205*

16. EMDR Therapeutic Story Method in Attachment-Focused Trauma Therapy for Adults   *217*

17. The Emotionally Corrective Therapeutic Relationship in Attachment-Focused Trauma Therapy for Adults   *227*

18. Getting Client Permission to Transition From Preparation Phase to Phases 3 to 8 of EMDR Therapy With Attachment-Focused Trauma Therapy for Adults   *239*

19. Client Transition From Enhanced Preparation Phase in Attachment-Focused Trauma Therapy for Adults to EMDR Phases 3 to 8   *253*

20. Adaptations for EMDR Reprocessing and Desensitization in Attachment-Focused Trauma Therapy for Adults   *265*

21. Applications of Attachment-Focused Trauma Therapy for Adults With a Dissociative Identity Disorder Diagnosis   *277*

22. Supplemental Materials for Use With Clients in Attachment-Focused Trauma Therapy for Adults   *293*

Index   329

Foreword

Marshall Lyles, LMFT-S, LPC-S

In writing *EMDR and Attachment-Focused Trauma Therapy for Adults: Reclaiming Authentic Self and Healthy Attachments*, Ann E. Potter and Debra Wesselmann have brought a much-needed resource to the world of trauma therapy. Having been trained by these wise clinicians, having met with them in soul-affirming consultation, and having voraciously read this remarkable book, I cannot wait for the clinical world to feel the impact of their voices.

Attachment-Focused Trauma Therapy for Adults (AFTT-A) provides an organized and highly relational approach to understanding the need for careful and nuanced treatment planning for adult clients impacted by attachment woundedness. By expanding and enhancing the Eye Movement Desensitization and Reprocessing (EMDR) preparation phase, Potter and Wesselmann have increased the capacity for therapist sensitivity during EMDR therapy, paving the way for clients to access the felt safety required to turn inward; thus, setting the stage for clients to bring care to their most vulnerable parts of themselves.

Potter and Wesselmann thoughtfully articulate the unique impact of attachment trauma on the developing person. The authors' Parent-Adult-Child (P-A-C) approach to parts' work is straightforward and easy to understand. Conceptualizing inner parts through the P-A-C lens normalizes client experiences and provides therapists a solid yet flexible foundation that enhances attunement to the needs of each client's inner world. Furthermore, they ask the clinical world to understand that attachment-sensitive, EMDR-based parts' work requires clinicians to maintain their own attachment self-awareness so that the therapeutic relationship remains a stable foundation for EMDR planning. This sensitivity is apparent throughout their writing as well as their protocol worksheets.

Making the case that wounded attachment parts understandably struggle to embrace safety, this book thoroughly details how to create reliable EMDR internal resources for all ages of clients' parts. The extended EMDR resourcing put forth emphasizes bringing relational elements into the preparation phase, even inviting caregiving and Higher Power figures into the work. In so doing, the authors are supporting a gentle scaffolding toward the reprocessing of attachment wounds so that narratives that began even in preverbal moments can be securely updated.

In addition to these innovative resources being delightfully relational, the clinical process is outlined with ease and organization. Since adults with attachment trauma often possess pockets of internalized disorganization, this structured, but not at all rigid, process offers a layer of grounding for both members of the therapeutic relationship. EMDR clinicians can rest into feeling held by the trustworthy process, freeing up the space to stay focused on clients' inner worlds.

Another feature outlined by Potter and Wesselmann in the AFTT-A process involves working with moments of woundedness within the context of an overall client narrative. Increasing narrative coherence and reflective functioning are hallmarks of attachment healing. EMDR clinicians will feel prepared to navigate the complex nature of healing complex trauma as the outlined treatment process continually emphasizes the benefits of returning to the overall story being reauthored. Clients' attachment wounds will be carefully and artfully witnessed, nurtured, and updated as the EMDR treatment moves forward.

Potter and Wesselmann have taken the time and effort to produce helpful EMDR clinical scripts and worksheets that bring order to complexity. These tools facilitate a disciplined understanding required for the type of client-focused EMDR treatment planning needed when working with unfolding and emerging parts of Self.

As an EMDR therapist who has worked in the area of attachment healing for many years, this book represents a point-of-view the field has desperately needed. EMDR therapists will undoubtedly benefit from the generously shared knowledge, furthering their own holding capacity for others' attachment trauma. As a result, EMDR clients will have increased access to a secure provider and safe clinical process. I can think of no worthier outcome of reading such a book! With an abundance of sincerity, I thank Deb and Ann for creating a resource that will help to shift a multitude of family trees for years to come toward attachment security.

Preface

DEVELOPMENT OF ATTACHMENT-FOCUSED TRAUMA THERAPY FOR ADULTS

Attachment-Focused Trauma Therapy for Adults (AFTT-A) has part of its foundation in the alcoholism field from the 1980s when it began to examine and bring to light the negative, lifelong impact of parental alcoholism on children (Black, 1982; Bradshaw, 1992; Potter, 1994; Whitfield, 1987; Woititz, 1983). My (AP) doctoral dissertation in the late 1980s involved development of a measure to examine the roles children from alcoholic families played that gave preliminary validation to the observations in clinical settings that children used distinct patterns and roles to cope with parental alcoholism and to function in alcoholic environments. The childhood roles correlated with levels of self-esteem and use of social support in adulthood, and similar patterns were found with children whose parents had other kinds of dysfunction, for example, mental illness (Potter & Williams, 1991).

Based on my own experiences in therapy in the late 1980s and building on Berne's Parent-Adult-Child diagrams in the Transactional Analysis model and Bradshaw's conceptualization of healing the "Inner Child," I developed the basic therapy for clients with histories of childhood trauma (what we now describe as attachment trauma) that provides parts of the underpinnings of the AFTT-A model for reconstructing the internal personality system (Potter, 1994). Even before being trained as an Eye Movement Desensitization and Reprocessing (EMDR) therapist, my practice was comprised of complex clients who were affected in many aspects of themselves and their lives by invalidating childhood environments in addition to the impact of memories of adverse childhood experiences.

Debra Wesselmann attended a presentation I gave in the late 1980s about reconstructing the internal personality system and by the mid-1990s, she and I were friends and colleagues in the same private practice. She worked with at-risk families as well as adults and children with a history of attachment disruptions and found herself drawn to the seminal works in the attachment field (Ainsworth, 1978; Bowlby, 1982; Main & Hesse, 1990) as well as to the work I was doing around restructuring the internal system. Our clinical collaboration led to our curiosity about the impact of nonsecure and disorganized attachment patterns on attachment patterns between internal parts of Self and consideration for the impact of the therapists' attachment patterns on client progress. Furthermore, we found that integrating the attachment work and the parts' work was a powerful combination.

We both became trained in EMDR therapy around the same time we started collaborating. Our early clinical experiences with EMDR therapy convinced us of its tremendous power for healing but also taught us that clients with a history of attachment trauma needed to learn emotional regulation and relationship skills, heal their sense of Self and the effects of ruptured childhood attachment relationships, and develop a Safe/Calm Place and resources through Resource Development and Installation (RDI; Korn & Leeds, 2002) to become emotionally ready for trauma reprocessing. Reconstruction of the internal personality system, skills training, internal attachment work, and the emotionally corrective therapeutic relationship evolved into the AFTT-A model.

PURPOSES AND SCOPE

Childhood attachment trauma negatively impacts adults in the development of a strong sense of Self; balanced internal personality structure and functioning; and the ability to form secure, healthy attachments in present-day relationships including partners, friends, family, and therapeutic alliances. Lack of security in close relationships interferes with clients' abilities to utilize attachments as a buffer for stress, thereby increasing their risks for mental health symptoms while decreasing their ability to benefit from the therapy process for healing.

AFTT-A applies the EMDR therapy adaptive information processing (AIP) model to conceptualize how both relationships among parts of Self (internal attachments) and relationships in adult life (external attachments) are impacted by attachment trauma. For example, the neural networks of adults with histories of childhood attachment trauma contain unprocessed traumatic memories and, as a result, the lack of information, misinformation, and mis-linked information negatively affects both clients' relationships among inner parts of Self and the overall structure and functioning of their personality system, as well as patterns in their present-day relationships.

The AFTT-A model proposes that trauma therapy with clients who experienced childhood attachment trauma needs to reconstruct their internal personality system through the transformation of the over- and underdeveloped parts of Self. Clients use the healthier new versions of parts of Self to build a strong sense of an Authentic Self.

Through a sequence of protocols, the AFTT-A process teaches therapists methods and strategies aimed at helping clients access, strengthen, and empower their Authentic Self through a process of: (a) strengthening healthy boundaries and enriching relationships among inner parts, (b) transforming and reorganizing the blended and cut-off parts within the internal personality structure, (c) developing and installing an internal system or team of inner resources and strengths, and (d) reintegrating the personality system with the Competent Adult part of Self in charge of orchestrating the internal structure as well as present-day life and relationships.

The AFTT-A steps and associated protocols are implemented within the preparation phase for EMDR therapy, readying clients to reprocess traumatic memories in phases 3 to 8 and providing tools for clients to apply during EMDR trauma work. EMDR bilateral stimulation is applied to deepen positive affective shifts made with each of the AFTT-A protocols.

AFTT-A is not designed to be a comprehensive treatment of dissociative identity disorder (DID); however, with adaptations and consideration for the increased complexity of the internal personality system, the protocols of the AFTT-A model can enhance therapy for clients with DID by helping to create a healthier internal personality system with DID clients prior to addressing traumatic memories.

The AFTT-A model details the parallel process between clients and their therapists and advocates for therapists to explore their own histories and internal personality systems in order to develop mindful attunement to clients and provide an emotionally corrective experience within the therapeutic relationship. Therapists are guided through a sequence of assignments that parallels the AFTT-A steps for clients, aimed at enhancing their own ability to self-reflect, gain insight, and adopt intentional and mindful secure-based responses to client emotions, reactions, nonsecure attachment patterns, and behaviors.

RATIONALE

Integration of Attachment and Trauma Approaches

Sixty percent of adults in the United States report abuse or other difficult circumstances during childhood according to the National Center for Mental Health Promotion and Youth Violence Prevention. According to the Centers for Disease Control and Prevention, the very large longitudinal Adverse Childhood Experiences (ACEs) study found adverse experiences in childhood to be directly linked to unhealthy behaviors in adulthood, such as substance abuse, poor job and educational functioning, and chronic health problems such as obesity, heart problems, cancer, and premature death (Felitti, 2002).

Research in the field of attachment similarly makes clear that emotional well-being is intertwined with felt security related to relationships and quality of attachments established in early childhood. Early patterns tend to become lifelong patterns without intervention or a powerful emotionally corrective experience. Nonsecure attachment patterns include nonsecure patterns related to insensitive parenting and unresolved/disorganized patterns with respect to unresolved childhood abuse or unresolved losses. Nonsecure and disorganized attachment patterns are not diagnoses; they are present in 30% to 40% of the nonclinical population. However, they are associated with risk for emotional and relationship instability (Ainsworth, 1978).

The EMDR AIP model helps explain the tenacity of our early-life attachment patterns. The AIP model hypothesizes that adverse childhood experiences such as rejection, invalidation, neglect, and abuse are stored in unprocessed form in separate neural networks. The unprocessed material, including perceptions, sensations, and emotions can be activated by conscious or subconscious present-day reminders. Gestalt therapy, Transactional Analysis, Psychodynamic, and Ego State models of psychotherapy add to our understanding of lifelong struggles rooted in early experiences through conceptualization of stored childhood perceptions and feelings as "parts of Self," sometimes referred to as "ego states" or "affect states." In adulthood, a Child part of Self or child affect state can be triggered and impact the adult's thoughts, feelings, and actions.

The AFTT-A model uses a multimodal, step-by-step approach to restructuring the internal personality system by differentiating Child parts of Self from unhelpful versions of Parent and Adult parts, orienting all parts to the present moment in which unmet childhood needs for nurturing and protection can be met within clients themselves, strengthening the Competent Adult part to be in charge of inner and external attachments, and transforming parts into healthier versions that play more helpful roles; thus enabling clients to move toward the secure end of the attachment continuum and choose healthier patterns in relationships. The model espouses some unique basic assumptions, including a core concept that every client retains a "Spiritual Essence," a core of goodness, present from birth and the unshakeable belief that clients have within themselves all the resources and strengths needed for health and healing.

Therapist Use of Self

Research indicates that an emotionally corrective relationship improves the quality of external attachment patterns in adults (Cohen, 2005; Saunders et al., 2011). In therapy, clients' nonsecure attachment patterns can interfere with utilization of the therapy due to mistrust, reactivity, and avoidance. Additionally, therapists' own unresolved issues can create barriers to understanding and helping clients in their therapy process and prevent the formation of the essential experience of a corrective attachment relationship for clients. Challenging clients are often ones who bring to the surface therapists' blind spots, prejudices, nonsecure attachment tendencies, and trauma triggers. The AFTT-A model recognizes that resolution of the therapist's unhealed trauma enhances their capacity to provide a secure-based, emotionally corrective experience for their clients.

CONTENTS

EMDR and Attachment-Focused Trauma Therapy for Adults: Reclaiming Authentic Self and Healthy Attachments describes a strength-based, attachment-focused model that moves clients toward healthier internal and external functioning and attachment patterns. A scripted sequence of protocols develops and deepens access to the client's own strengths through creation of an internal system of resources. The protocols build healthy boundaries and a nurturing relationship with inner Child parts of Self, strengthens the Competent Adult part of Self, and reworks under- or overdeveloped Parent parts of Self into healthier versions capable of playing more nurturing and protective roles. Clients examine their "early bonding rules" (adaptive behaviors they adopted as young children that are not relevant, and even detrimental, to adult life) and then choose and adopt a new set of healthy relationship rules with permission from younger Child parts of Self. Clients create a Therapeutic Story that makes sense of the childhood experiences and incorporates present-day, adaptive information and choices. Finally, creative and powerful elements and tools from the internal restructuring work are utilized to enhance and deepen clients' capability to reprocess traumatic material in phases 3 through 7 of EMDR therapy.

Throughout the book, the authors encourage therapists to reflect on their own attachment patterns brought to the surface in therapy sessions, implement activities to help themselves move toward healthier attachment functioning, and resolve their own trauma history if needed. Therapists are guided to provide secure-based responses to their clients' nonsecure behaviors, reactions, and statements that act as the foundation for an emotionally corrective experience within the therapeutic relationship, helping clients move toward greater attachment security.

USE IN INTENDED MARKET

Audience

AFTT-A is a therapist manual primarily intended for EMDR therapists, master's level or higher, who work with adults with a history of attachment trauma having difficulty improving mental health and relationship issues through therapy. Although the primary target audience will be the population of more than 100,000 EMDR-trained therapists worldwide, therapists using other trauma therapies will find the model easy to integrate with other non-EMDR modalities. Therapists who are trained in other modalities such as Dialectical Behavioral Therapy, Radically Open Dialectical Behavioral Therapy, psychodynamic therapies, Trauma-Focused Cognitive Behavioral Therapy, and other trauma therapies can easily integrate this model with the other approaches utilized in their practices.

EMDR and Attachment-Focused Trauma Therapy for Adults: Reclaiming Authentic Self and Healthy Attachments helps therapists conceptualize and treat mental health and relationship instability using both the attachment and trauma lenses. Dr. Potter and Ms. Wesselmann teach the AFTT-A model in workshops and presentations, and feedback from participants describes the model as a roadmap. The model organizes trauma treatment into a step-by-step process giving therapists clear directions to help the many complex clients they previously struggled to understand and treat. After Dr. Potter and Ms. Wesselmann spoke at the 2019 EMDR International Association preconference, one participant stated, "Even if I don't go to any other workshops, I got exactly what I needed from the two of you."

Uniqueness Among Competitors

EMDR and Attachment-Focused Trauma Therapy for Adults: Reclaiming Authentic Self and Healthy Attachments joins a wealth of trauma therapy books, distinguishing itself from other books with emphases on reconstruction of the internal personality system as a stand-alone therapy that improves and enriches external attachments; integration with EMDR therapy resourcing and reprocessing phases to deepen affective shifts and bring stored attachment trauma to adaptive resolution; recognition of nonsecure attachment patterns in clients and therapists; use of therapist Self in mindful attunement to clients; and provision of corrective attachment experiences within the therapeutic relationship through therapist secure responses to nonsecure client reactions, patterns, and behaviors. The AFTT-A book organizes and details the sequence of therapeutic interventions in a practical, step-wise manner, guiding therapists to learn and utilize scripted protocols while, at the same time, encouraging them to view difficulties with clients as opportunities to explore and resolve their own issues.

REFERENCES

Ainsworth, M. D. S., Blehar, M., Waters, E., & Wall, S. (1978). *Patterns of attachment: A psychological study of the strange situation.* Erlbaum.

Black, C. (1982). *It will never happen to me.* Central Recovery Press.

Bowlby, J. (1982). *Attachment* (2nd ed.). Basic Books.

Bradshaw, J. (1990). *Homecoming: Reclaiming and healing your inner child.* Bantam Publishing.

Cohen, D. L. (2005, August). *Exploring the role of secondary attachment relationships in the development of attachment security.* (Publication No. 67292299) [Doctoral dissertation, University of North Texas]. UNT Digital Library. http://digital.library.unt.edu/ark:/67531/metadc4891/

Felitti, V. J. (2002). The relation between adverse childhood experiences and adult health: Turning gold into lead. *The Permanente Journal, 6*(1), 44–47. https://doi.org/10.7812/tpp/02.994

Korn, D. L., & Leeds, A. M. (2002). Preliminary evidence of efficacy for EMDR resource development and installation in the stabilization phase of treatment of complex posttraumatic stress disorder. *Journal of Clinical Psychology, 58*(12), 1465–1487. https://doi.org/10.1002/jclp.10099

Main, M., & Hesse, E. (1990). Parents' unresolved traumatic experiences are related to infant disorganized attachment status: Is frightened/frightening parental behavior the linking mechanism? In M. T. Greenberg, D. Cicchetti, & E. M. Cummings (Eds.), *Attachment in the preschool years: Theory, research, and intervention* (pp. 161–182). University of Chicago Press.

Potter, A. E. (1994). *Inside out: Rebuilding self and personality through inner child therapy* (therapist manual). Accelerated Development, Inc.

Potter, A. E., & Williams, D. E. (1991). Development of a measure examining children's roles in alcoholic families. *Journal of Alcohol Studies, 52*(1), 70–77. https://doi.org/10.15288/jsa.1991.52.70

Saunders, R., Jacobvitz, D., Zaccagnino, M., Beverung, L. M., & Hazen, M. (2011). Pathways to earned-security: The role of alternative support figures. *Attachment & Human Development, 13*(4), 403–420. https://doi.org/10.1080/14616734.2011.584405

Whitfield, C. (1987). *Healing the child within: Discovery and recovery for adult children of dysfunctional families.* Health Communications, Inc.

Woititz, J. (1983). *Adult children of alcoholics.* Health Communications, Inc.

HOW TO USE THIS BOOK

STEP-BY-STEP THERAPY PROCESS

EMDR and Attachment-Focused Trauma Therapy for Adults: Reclaiming Authentic Self and Healthy Attachments outlines a set of sequential, practical, easy-to-use protocol scripts that organize and enhance trauma therapy. The Attachment-Focused Trauma Therapy for Adults (AFTT-A) process can be utilized as a stand-alone therapy that improves and enriches both internal and external attachments. Integrating AFTT-A with Eye Movement Desensitization and Reprocessing (EMDR) resourcing and reprocessing phases deepens affective shifts and brings stored attachment trauma to adaptive resolution.

PROTOCOLS AND PROTOCOL SCRIPTS

This AFTT-A book contains protocols and protocol scripts for each step of the therapy process. The authors explain the steps and protocols within associated chapters.

SUPPLEMENTAL MATERIALS FOR USE WITH CLIENTS

EMDR and Attachment-Focused Trauma Therapy for Adults: Reclaiming Authentic Self and Healthy Attachments offers therapists assessment templates, checklists, and outlines in formats conducive for use in client sessions. Digital versions are available for download through Springer Publishing Connect: Use the code on the opening page of this book to access the digital product and select Chapter 22.

PARENT-ADULT-CHILD DIAGRAMS

The AFTT-A model provides therapists with a way of conceptualizing and teaching clients about the personality system and parts of Self that simplify and normalize their inner experiences related to the impact of attachment trauma.

IN-DEPTH UNDERSTANDING OF CLIENT BEHAVIORS THROUGH ATTACHMENT AND TRAUMA MODELS

The AFTT-A therapist model provides therapists with a method for hypothesizing attachment patterns through clients' words and behaviors. The patterns are viewed as a natural response to trauma in early attachment relationships. Adaptive information processing (AIP) is the foundational model for EMDR therapy that explains unprocessed disturbing attachment memories as underlying unhealthy attachment patterns and beliefs.

EMOTIONALLY CORRECTIVE EXPERIENCE WITHIN THE CONTEXT OF THE THERAPEUTIC RELATIONSHIP

The AFTT-A model emphasizes mindful attunement to both therapist Self and client, allowing secure-based interactions and an emotionally corrective therapist–client relationship.

CLIENT EXAMPLES

The authors share short vignettes about aspects of client treatment and excerpts from client sessions throughout the book to illustrate the application of AFTT-A steps and protocols.

POINTS TO REMEMBER

EMDR and Attachment-Focused Trauma Therapy for Adults: Reclaiming Authentic Self and Healthy Attachments summarizes important information at the end of each chapter.

TROUBLESHOOTING TIPS

In Chapters 5 through 21, the authors note common challenges with clients in each step of the AFTT-A process and recommend therapist interventions to overcome problematic situations.

KINTSUGI ANALOGY

The Kintsugi process of transforming broken pottery into works of art is analogous to the healing process in AFTT-A. As with Kintsugi, AFTT-A does not intend to return clients to earlier versions of themselves prior to adverse childhood experiences and attachment relationship ruptures but, instead, recognizes that past experiences cannot be undone. AFTT-A aims to go beyond the repair of broken parts of Self by reconnecting clients to their Spiritual Essence and transforming the emotional scars in a way that reveals clients' true nature of resilience, strength, and beauty.

PAUSE AND REFLECT FOR THERAPISTS

In each chapter of *EMDR and Attachment-Focused Trauma Therapy for Adults: Reclaiming Authentic Self and Healthy Attachments,* therapists are offered the opportunity to develop awareness of their own barriers to being present in the moment with clients, recognize the impact of the therapist Self on clients in sessions, and resolve their own unfinished pasts. Exercises and activities encourage therapists to observe their own emotions and reactions to challenging clients to strengthen mindfulness and capacity for attunement to clients in the present moment during sessions.

AUTHORS' STORIES

The authors share experiences of their own barriers to being mindfully attuned and present in therapy sessions, their awareness of what triggered their reactions, the ways in which their own issues impacted client therapy, and how client difficulties or "stuck points" often resolved when the authors were able to work out those issues.

ACKNOWLEDGMENTS

Francine Shapiro, PhD

Andrew Leeds, PhD, and Deborah Korn, PsyD

Deany Laliotis, MS

Kate Dimock, former Director, Behavioral Science, Springer Publishing, for asking us to write this book and for championing the book to be published.

Mindy Okura-Marszycki, Senior Acquisitions Editor, Behavioral Science; Kirsten Elmer, Assistant Editor, Behavioral Science; and Rachel Haines, Senior Production Editor at Springer Publishing, and M Mythili, Project Manager, Transforma Pvt Ltd. for transforming our manuscript into a book worthy of publication. Leigh Montville, Director, Special Sales and Business Development, Springer Publishing, for your ideas and positive energy about our book reaching as many readers as possible.

Joan Lovett, MD, for your suggestions regarding the Therapeutic Story.

Myriam Greff of Atelier Kintsugi for the photos of the process of creating the Kintsugi vase on the book cover and in Chapter 5.

Morty Bachar of Lakeside Pottery Studio for the photos of the process of creating the Kintsugi vase in Chapter 17.

Sandra Wendel, Editor, Write On, Inc., for your generosity with time and help finding someone to create keywords and the book index.

Ann Baker, Manager, Editorial, Design, and Production Department, University of Nebraska Press, for initial guidance with APA style and format.

Shelby Janke, BA, Technical Services Librarian, Papillion Public Library, for your accuracy and efficiency in developing keywords and the index for the book.

Tim Potter, MA, graphic design consultant and artist extraordinaire, for your generosity, time, patience, expertise, focus, persistence, and humor. You are the best brother and friend ever!

Gail Little-Osberg, Office Administrator with our clinical practice, The Attachment and Trauma Center of Nebraska, for helping us with creating the editable downloadable forms.

CHAPTER 1

Introduction and Foundational Theories for Attachment-Focused Trauma Therapy for Adults

INTRODUCTION

Self and Attachment Trauma

Thagard (2007) explains that people's sense of themselves or their "Self" (sometimes called the True, Real, or Essential Self) integrates multiple levels of neurobiology, genetics, psychology, emotions, beliefs, sociability, and spirituality. He noted that people's minds are intended to develop a Self as a foundation for their self-esteem and sense of well-being. People have intrinsic needs for both a sense of themselves as unique and separate from others as well as for acceptance and bonding in relationships with others. The concept of Self is often equated with identity and includes the "perception of one's own traits, memories, and experiences which then inform self-beliefs and guide behavior" (Thagard, 2007, p. 1).

The Self integrates memories of the past with the present moment and with future possibilities. Fundamental to the development of a healthy or positive sense of Self is the experience of early attachment relationships comprised of consistency, love, and a sense of protection. Relationships with early attachment figures initiate people's beliefs about themselves and others and their expectations about how they will be treated by others in relationships and society in general. The Self "only survives to the extent" it is "nourished in relationships" (Talaifar & Swann, 2018, p. 2).

Adults who were raised by parents who were sensitive and responsive to their needs developed a sense of security regarding their relationship with others and with themselves. As the attuned, sensitive parent responds to their children's emotions, they interpret their children's emotions and needs. As a result, the children develop into adults who can reflect upon their own internal state and attune to the emotions in their own children.

Adults who were raised by parents who lacked capacity for emotional attunement are unable to find a sense of security in their relationship with others or within themselves. Due to growing up without anyone to help them with their emotions, they now lack capacity to understand themselves and may feel shame related to their internal state. The Attachment-Focused Trauma Therapy for Adults (AFTT-A) model leads to new, internal, healthy attachments, the experience of a secure-based therapeutic relationship, and a newfound capacity for self-reflection.

The AFTT-A model adopts the foundational belief that clients have a Spiritual Essence at the core of their Authentic Self. Attachment trauma may cause clients to lose sight of their basic goodness, but their Spiritual Essence is never lost or damaged. The AFTT-A model also assumes that clients have the inner wisdom and all of the internal resources (such as courage, persistence, and self-compassion) they need to heal their damaged parts of Self and transform their internal personality structure into an Authentic Self that is capable of resolving traumatic memories, learning and using necessary skills, and forming healthy and satisfying relationships in their adult lives.

Attachment Trauma Versus Single-Event Trauma

AFTT-A has part of its foundation in the alcoholism field from the 1980s when it was used to examine and bring to light the negative, lifelong impact of parental alcoholism on children (Black, 1982; Bradshaw, 1990; Potter, 1994a, 1994b; Potter & Willimas, 1991; Whitfield, 1987; Woititz, 1983). The concept of attachment trauma has evolved from the clinical work in the alcoholism and mental health fields to encompass the experiences of emotional, verbal, physical, and sexual abuse and/or neglect within the context of childhood relationships with attachment figures such as parents or other parent figures. Attachment loss includes separation from or loss of an attachment figure in childhood due to medical procedures or hospitalization, physical or mental illness, death, divorce, or adoption. Attachment trauma, sometimes called developmental or complex trauma, is distinct from single-event trauma in several ways: Traumatic or neglectful experiences in childhood and/or adolescence are often ongoing, disrupt optimal development, leave unmet needs and skills deficits, create unresolved traumatic memories with associated negative cognitions and affect, and cause a rupture of the trust and sense of protection in the attachment relationship itself.

Abuse by attachment figures may lead to an unresolved/disorganized attachment pattern in adulthood. Mental disorientation and disorganization can be observed when the adult attempts to discuss the traumatic events. The pattern of disorganization most likely began in childhood and is associated with ongoing experiences of dissociation. Attachment trauma and loss have long-term negative consequences for adults in developing a strong sense of Self, affect regulation and expressions, personality structure and functioning, the ability to form healthy attachments in present-day relationships (including the therapy relationship), and the capacity to benefit from Eye Movement Desensitization and Reprocessing (EMDR) therapy. Present-day relationships and circumstances reflect and repeat what these adults observed and experienced in childhood:

- nonsecure attachment patterns,
- dysfunctional intra- and interpersonal boundaries,
- life skills deficits, and
- the search to resolve childhood trauma and meet unmet childhood needs for love, acceptance, trust, and connection through adult relationships.

As a result, the therapy needed to help clients effectively resolve attachment trauma requires more complex and comprehensive approaches than therapy that resolved single-event trauma. EMDR therapy was originally designed to resolve single-event trauma (Shapiro, 2018). As EMDR therapists began to see adults with histories of attachment trauma, they encountered unexpected reactions and barriers to and difficulties with EMDR therapy's trauma desensitization and reprocessing phases. It became clear that without appropriate preparation and modifications, clients with a complex presentation could be flooded with multiple traumatic memories and related negative affect or unable to access traumatic memories or the affect associated with those memories. Additionally, their real-life relationships were complicated, sometimes chaotic with intense cycles of emotional interactions or characterized by emotional distance and detachment. Clients presented with symptoms and behaviors that could be ascribed to any number of psychiatric diagnoses such as mood and anxiety disorders, posttraumatic stress disorder (PTSD), personality disorders, and addictions. Some clients even had chronic and/or multiple medical problems.

Felitti and Anda studied the negative impact of adverse childhood experiences on physical and mental health and on the social, legal, and economic aspects of adult life. Findings showed that traumatic events and/or unstable circumstances in childhood were highly correlated with adulthood issues such as chronic health and mental health problems, substance abuse, challenges in attaining and maintaining positive and secure relationships, and even increased vulnerability to further victimization (Felitti, 2002).

Kintsugi: Analogy for Healing From Attachment Trauma

Kintsugi or "golden joinery" is the Japanese process of transforming broken pottery or ceramics into unique works of art that reflect strength and resilience, "each with its own story and beauty" (Carnazzi, 2016). Underlying the Kintsugi process is the belief that broken objects are not discarded; just because an object is broken doesn't mean it no longer has value or use.

The goal of Kintsugi is not to return a pottery piece to its original state or hide the damage done to it but to highlight, accent, and even celebrate and show pride in the "scars" of the piece's history. The repair is not only visible but emphasized by highlighting it with gold. The object's past is taken into consideration, thus transforming it into a "unique, precious, and irreplaceable object" (Santini, 2019, p. 38). Through Kintsugi reconstruction, the true essence of the broken pottery is revealed and strengthened. Kitty (2020) interprets Kintsugi as the "art of defiance" through which the fate of a broken object is not predetermined by circumstances but is chosen by creating a "new beginning … from the rubble of the past" (p. 9).

Past experiences of abuse and neglect cannot be undone. The impact of attachment trauma can only be temporarily hidden or avoided. Clients with histories of attachment trauma who resolve distressing past experiences aren't the same person they were prior to traumatic events. They won't be the person they might or could have been if they hadn't been abused or neglected. One of the most powerful lessons from Kintsugi is that clients who face their brokenness do not stay broken. They choose the healing process of therapy to move beyond the search for a former version of themselves or the repair of broken pieces; they transform themselves into persons who are connected to their essence of goodness and their spiritual core, who have reconstructed their inner Self, and who are capable of living their present-day lives through their most Authentic Self.

AFTT-A and Attachment Trauma

To address the complex nature of clients' therapy issues related to their experiences of attachment trauma, the AFTT-A model incorporates EMDR therapy with an extended period of EMDR's preparation phase prior to initiating trauma work (phases 3–8). Based on decades of clinical experience with adults with histories of attachment trauma, AFTT-A expands and enhances standard EMDR therapy protocols, adds other protocols to EMDR's preparation phase, and integrates the outcomes of the extended preparation into subsequent trauma reprocessing and desensitization. The extended preparation phase in AFTT-A allows therapists to help clients

- restore the foundation of their sense of Self by accessing and strengthening their connections to their Spiritual Essence and other internal resources;
- develop balanced internal and external boundaries and attachments;
- transform the internal structure of enmeshed and dissociated parts into a strong, Authentic Self;
- differentiate between "back then" when their needs weren't met through their primary attachments and they were in danger from abuse and neglect and "now" in the present moment when their adulthood needs are met, their self-beliefs are positive, and they have the skills they need to self-regulate as well as develop close, healthy relationships; and
- heal traumatic memories using their Competent Adult part of Self by accessing memories from the neuro-network clusters in their "Kid Brain" held by the Child/Adolescent parts of Self and connecting them to the adaptive information processing (AIP) system in the "Adult Brain."

Therapist Use of Self

A strong, therapeutic bond between therapist and client is essential to working with adults with histories of attachment trauma. The healthy therapy relationship not only holds a safe space for clients to reconstruct their inner Self and resolve past traumas, it also provides clients with a corrective emotional experience in the present moment. Therapists' use of their own Authentic Self in therapeutic relationships with clients is central to the underlying philosophy of the AFTT-A model.

We, as therapists, expect clients to be brave and vulnerable; to face and resolve early traumatic experiences and relationships; and to share with us their most core self-beliefs and painful emotions. Yet, when there are "stuck" points in the therapy during which clients don't seem to be making progress, therapists often look solely at clients as the source of the problem instead of broadening the scope of their reflection to include their own similar but unresolved issues that have impact on the therapeutic relationship. Therapists' own internal structure, self-beliefs, emotions, social and cultural prejudices, and patterns often create blind spots or biases that impede clients' progress in therapy. Thus, AFTT-A emphasizes therapists' self-awareness and willingness to do their own emotional work and to face their own biases, which is essential for promoting the clients' healing process as well as for providing a corrective emotional experience within the therapeutic relationship.

FRAMEWORK OF THE AFTT-A MODEL

The AFTT-A model for adults is based on a framework that addresses the issues of under- and overdeveloped parts of Self and enmeshed and partially dissociated types of attachments among internal parts and relationships with others: (a) differentiation, (b) protection, (c) nurturing and strengthening, (d) reconnection, and (e) integration. One of the underlying assumptions of AFTT-A about adults with a history of attachment trauma is that the boundaries, roles, and communication taught and modeled during childhood are reflected in both the inner attachments among their parts of Self and in their relationships in adult life. When clients learn healthy boundaries in relationships with attachment figures, they are encouraged to develop a strong sense of Self separate from others as well as a sense of safety and security in relationship with others. As a result, their inner parts are separate yet connected, and their adult relationships mirror a balance between individuality and interconnectedness.

Adults raised in relatively healthy or optimal families have well-developed parts of Self that assist them in the coping with varying circumstances in their lives. Parts of Self perform a range of roles depending on what is required in certain situations, so clients successfully manage their adult lives and navigate healthy adult relationships. For example, the Child/Adolescent part of Self provides emotions, playfulness, fun, humor, the ability to be absorbed in the present moment, passion for ideals, intuition or innate wisdom, and the ability to read situations and respond in adaptive ways. The parts of Self formed by internalizing messages from real-life adults during childhood and adolescence become the Parent part of Self that contributes needed encouragement and reassurance; reminders of morals, principles, and conscience; and alerts to the need for self-protection. The Adult part of Self regulates affect and emotions and acts as mediator among the other parts.

In addition to having unique roles, clients' inner parts form attachments or relationships among themselves to establish the cooperation and coordination often needed to respond effectively to the complex aspects of adult life. The Adult part of Self primarily mediates among inner parts and balances both clients' internal responses as well as assesses and coordinates clients' reactions to and behaviors in real-life events and situations.

Adults with a history of attachment trauma often have a poorly developed sense of Self and the internal aspects of themselves may be either underdeveloped or overdeveloped and have formed either overly close (blended/enmeshed) or overly distant (detached or dissociated) internal relationships. Clients may come to therapy with Child/Adolescent parts of Self or "Kid Brain" instead of the client's Competent Adult part of Self or "Adult Brain" in charge of their lives and relationships. They often present as overly emotional and impulsive and engage in intense and sometimes chaotic relationships. In such an instance, the Child/Adolescent part is overly developed and the Parent and Adult parts of Self are underdeveloped. The Child/Adolescent part tends to be blended or enmeshed with the Adult aspect of Self and directly connected to the overly critical Parent part. As a result, the Child/Adolescent part does the internal Adult part's job of directing clients' behaviors and reactions with only the child-like cognitive resources and without the ability to reason or problem-solve or the benefit of parental guidance or wisdom. Meanwhile, the Adult and Parent parts of Self abdicate their roles of moral compass, protector, regulator, mediator, and director.

Clients may also present in an opposite manner: They may overcontrol emotions and behavior, lack spontaneity, come across as controlling and/or critical, and keep others at a distance. In this case, the Adult and Parent parts of Self are overdeveloped and closely connected while the Child/Adolescent part remains underdeveloped and cut off from the other parts of Self. Such clients tend to be rigid about following rules, hypervigilant to avoid emotional vulnerability, overly focused on achievement, and value control in relationships.

Differentiation

Differentiation among parts of Self is essential to clients' sense of themselves as uniquely special and to their capacity for forming satisfying, long-lasting relationships. The AFTT-A model addresses the creation of healthy inner boundaries among parts of Self. Firm and flexible boundaries are created and replace the weak, overly close type of boundary indicative of enmeshment as well as the too tough, overly distant kind of boundary involved in detached or dissociated parts of Self. Emotional space is introduced into overly close internal attachments while compassion, communication, and acceptance are proposed for relationships with parts of Self that have been denied.

Protection

Clients who have a history of attachment trauma suffer abuse and/or neglect in relationships with attachment figures and thus experience a violation of their personal boundaries. They learn that they are vulnerable and unable to protect themselves from harm, even by the very people who were tasked with keeping them safe. In relationship to the outside world, clients may have overdeveloped boundaries that distance them from others, or they may have underdeveloped boundaries through which they lose a sense of themselves as separate from others. They were not taught while growing up how to discern between people who are safe and trustworthy and those who are not. They have a deficit in the emotional and social skills necessary for developing healthy relationships and for a healthy level of self-protection.

The AFTT-A process assists clients with developing a sense of safety and healthy relationships internally. The internalization of a sense of safety and healthy inner relationships instills clients with confidence and competence to navigate closeness in their adult relationships.

Nurturing and Strengthening

Children need attachment figures in their lives who believe that, no matter what, they are special, unique, and loved. Children's self-worth is dependent upon adults' regard for them.

Young children's thinking is egocentric. They believe they somehow are involved in everything that happens around them. They think they cause both the good and bad that occur in their families. Their perceptions impact how they feel about themselves. If good things happen, they are good. If bad things happen, they must be bad. They have not yet developed more advanced reasoning skills. They aren't yet able to take into consideration a variety of more abstract factors before drawing their conclusions. Rather, they interpret what happens through the normal and immature lens of their child-like brains. Piaget (1969) posited that children think they are the center of their universe and can't be expected to understand differently Consequently, the quality of attachment relationships in childhood affects how positive or negative the foundation of children's self-image will be. The beginnings of negative cognitions such as "I'm bad" or "I'm unlovable" originate from the early attachment experiences in which children's needs for love and appreciation are not met and, as a result, haunt them into adulthood.

The AFTT-A model assumes that clients have a spiritual core or an essence of goodness that is not damaged by adverse experiences with attachment figures. Therapists believe that clients have all the inner strengths they need to heal and grow into their most Authentic Self. The AFTT-A process helps clients transform their view of themselves. Positive beliefs replace negative cognitions and are reinforced through the AFTT-A sequence of protocols.

AFTT-A enhances clients' sense of inner nurturing and acceptance by introducing healthy attachment figures such as Higher Powers for Adult and Child/Adolescent parts of Self and Resource Team members and connecting the True Parent part and Child/Adolescent parts of Self through healthy internal attachment experiences. Internal attachment figures offer consistent unconditional love and acceptance within the context of safe and stable boundaries and serve as models for healthy real-life relationships.

Reconnection

Once internal parts are separated out from each other and from the Competent Adult part of Self and there are firm and flexible boundaries within the client's system, each part is strengthened and encouraged to play the roles they were originally intended to fulfill. Parts of Self reconnect to their Spiritual Essence and each other in ways that balance individuality with connection, separateness with wholeness. The internal system reclaims its individual parts as well as its ability to function as a whole through new, healthy, internal attachments among the parts and between the parts and the Competent Adult part of Self. As a result, the Child/Adolescent parts again offer emotions, playfulness, curiosity, innate wisdom; the Team of inner resources is easily accessed to guide and mentor clients' Competent Adult part; the newly revitalized True Parent part supports with love and provides protection with healthy boundaries; and the Emotion Controller-Regulator modulates emotions as appropriate for real-life situations. The newly reconstructed system with its healthy attachment relationships among parts reflects clients' strengths for forming strong attachments in their current lives.

Integration

Children raised in optimal environments develop a cohesive internal structure that is intended to provide a lifetime of self-worth, belief in inherent goodness, realistic views of both strengths and limitations, and the abilities and skills essential to successfully navigate life and relationships. The internal configuration is formed and encouraged by supportive and protective attachment relationships during childhood.

If relationships with attachment figures are not healthy and the needs for nurturing, acceptance, safety, and security are not met, children's development is negatively impacted, their inner system is fragmented, and inner resources and skills are absent or immature. The AFTT-A model helps clients differentiate and create healthy boundaries and healthy relationships among parts of Self, strengthens parts' sense of being separate and unique, reinforces time orientation, re-orders and reassigns parts' roles, and empowers their Competent Adult part of Self to be in charge of inner and external relationships. Once clients' inner systems are reconstructed to include healthy individual parts that are reconnected to their spiritual source and capable of working together, the relationships in their adult lives reflect the more balanced and integrated inner structure.

SOCIAL AND CULTURAL CONSIDERATIONS

EMDR therapy is successfully utilized across a wide range of social, cultural, and gender (identity and affection) contexts and addresses socially and culturally based trauma and adversity such as social exclusion and discrimination experiences. EMDR therapy is culturally responsive due to the following aspects (Nickerson, 2017, pp. 10–11):

- decreased need for extensive verbalization and use of nonverbal modalities
- memories can be kept private
- group options
- flexible memory points
- attunement to cultural, religious, and gender identity resources and beliefs

AFTT-A takes into account the familial, social, and cultural aspects of clients' lives in assessing and treating the impact of attachment trauma and advocates for the use of Nickerson's ASK (Attitude, Skills, Knowledge) model in working with diverse groups (Nickerson, 2017; Sperry, 2010).

POINTS TO REMEMBER

- The AFTT-A model integrates multiple theoretical backgrounds including Self psychology, Transactional Analysis, attachment, attachment or complex trauma, EMDR therapy, structural dissociation, ego states or parts of Self, and mindfulness.
- The AFTT-A process is analogous to the Kintsugi art of transforming broken pottery or ceramics into works of art that emphasize the object's resilience, strength, and beauty.
- The structure of the AFTT-A model encompasses the four elements of differentiation, nurturing and strengthening, reconnection, and integration.
- The focus of AFTT-A is the reconstruction of the internal personality system, the corrective emotional experience within the context of the therapeutic relationship, and healing of relationships in clients' adult lives.

- The AFTT-A process strengthens positive aspects of and reprocesses traumatic material from clients' familial, social, and cultural experiences.

PAUSE AND REFLECT FOR THE THERAPIST

We invite you to reflect on your clinical work and begin to identify clients with whom you have some challenges. Perhaps, you feel anxious at times or have the urge to "fix" a client in session. Or possibly you are frustrated with a client and feel like you are doing more work than they are in therapy. As you work with the challenging clients in the next week, become aware of emotions, cognitions, and body sensations that come up for you in sessions. We will ask you throughout the book to consider how your own history and experiences may impact your therapeutic work with clients and to begin to identify and explore those issues so you can be more mindfully attuned to clients in therapy. We encourage you to find a consultation group or an EMDR International Association- (EMDRIA-) approved consultant with whom you can share your process and a therapist with whom you can do your personal therapy if needed. Be brave! We have an unshakable belief that you already have the inner strengths and support you need to become more aware of your own reactions and heal any parts of your past that might get in the way of your therapeutic relationships.

USEFUL TERMS AND DEFINITIONS

ACES: Adverse Childhood Experiences Study

"Adult Brain": The parts of the brain that house EMDR's AIP system and include higher cognitive processes such as learning, problem-solving, decision-making, language, understanding of emotions, and narrative memory.

AFTT-A: Attachment-Focused Trauma Therapy for Adults

EMDR: Eye Movement Desensitization and Reprocessing

"Kid Brain": The neural network clusters in the emotional/social part of the brain that store unprocessed memories of adverse events and are disconnected from a sense of time and from the parts of the brain capable of processing memories and transferring them into narrative memory. AFTT-A views the neural networks as encapsulating more than memories of adverse events and includes the experiences, cognitive development, and learning during a particular client age.

EMDRIA: EMDR International Association

REFERENCES

Black, C. (1982). *It will never happen to me*. Central Recovery Press.
Bradshaw, J. (1990). *Homecoming: Reclaiming and healing your inner child*. Bantam Publishing.
Carnazzi, S. (2016, January 30). *Kintsugi: The art of precious scars*. Lifegate. https://www.lifegate.com/kintsugi

Felitti, V. J. (2002, Winter). The relation between adverse childhood experiences and adult health: Turning gold into lead. *The Permanente Journal, 6*(1), 44–47. https://doi.org/10.7812/tpp/02.994

Kitty, A. (2020). *The art of Kintsugi: Learning the Japanese craft of beautiful repair*. Schiffer Publishing.

Nickerson, M. (Ed.) (2017). *Cultural competence and healing culturally based trauma with EMDR therapy*. Springer Publishing Company.

Piaget, J., & Inhelder, B. (1969). *The psychology of the child*. Basic Books, Inc.

Potter, A. E. (1994a). *Inside out: Rebuilding self and personality through inner child therapy* (therapist manual). Accelerated Development, Inc.

Potter, A. E. (1994b). *Inside out: Rebuilding self and personality through inner child therapy* (client workbook). Accelerated Development, Inc.

Potter, A. E., & Williams, D. E. (1991). Development of a measure examining children's roles in alcoholic families. *Journal of Alcohol Studies, 52*(1), 70–77. https://doi.org/10.15288/jsa.1991.52.70

Santini, C. (2019). *Kinstsugi: Finding strength in imperfection*. Andrews McMeel Publishing.

Shapiro, F. (2018). *Eye movement desensitization and reprocessing (EMDR) therapy: Basic principles, protocols, and procedures* (2nd ed.). Guilford Press.

Sperry, L. (2010). *Core competencies in counseling and psychotherapy: Becoming a highly competent and effective therapist*. Taylor & Francis Group, LLC.

Talaifar, S., & Swann, W. (2018, March 28). *Self and identity*. Oxford Research Encyclopedia.

Thagard, P. (2007). *Mind: Introduction to cognitive science* (2nd ed.). MIT Press.

Whitfield, C. (1987). *Healing the child within: Discovery and recovery for adult children of dysfunctional families*. Health Communications, Inc.

Woititz, J. (1983). *Adult children of alcoholics*. Health Communications, Inc.

CHAPTER 2

Therapist Mindfulness and Parallel Process in Attachment-Focused Trauma Therapy for Adults

INTRODUCTION

The Attachment-Focused Trauma Therapy for Adults (AFTT-A) model recognizes that therapists are human and experience their own emotional and physiological responses to interactions within the therapy office. The therapist's own emotions can be a powerful force enhancing the client's progress or impeding it. The AFTT-A model posits that by practicing mindful awareness, the therapist can stay conscious of their personal triggers and automatic responses in the therapy office. While mindful, the therapist can use their self-observations for personal growth and to gain information about the client's relationship functioning. Finally, mindfulness allows the therapist to respond to the client with emotional attunement and a therapeutic perspective. This attuned connection calms the client's nervous system, increases therapeutic trust, and increases the client's receptivity to the therapist's interventions (Wesselmann & Potter, 2019).

SYMPATHETIC AROUSAL IN THE AUTONOMIC NERVOUS SYSTEM

It's helpful to understand affect dysregulation in our clients and in ourselves through the lens of the polyvagal system (Lynch, 2018; Porges & Dana, 2018). Beneath conscious awareness, our senses are always at work, detecting cues from the environment to determine level of danger versus safety. These processes, termed *neuroception*, determine whether the sympathetic or parasympathetic sides of the autonomic nervous system (ANS) are activated and the extent to which we feel safe, open, relaxed, and free to engage with others (Figure 2.1). Our bodies are directed by the ventral vagal aspect of the parasympathetic ANS when we have a sense of ease and safety. When our body detects cues of danger, the sympathetic part of our ANS is activated and heart rate and respiration kick into high gear. We experience tension and anxiety and are in survival mode, braced to fight or flee. Our ability to take in external cues becomes more limited and, in our need to recognize potential danger, we tend to perceive others as possible sources of danger. When a sense of danger overwhelms our sympathetic nervous system, the dorsal vagal part of the parasympathetic ANS steps in. Heart rate and respiration slow. Mentally and emotionally, we become numb, detached, or dissociated, and we're disconnected from others.

When children experience a frightening or hurtful event with nowhere to go for safety, the fight/flight/freeze reaction of their ANS is stored in an unprocessed form within a disparate memory network that is isolated from any stored, adaptive information. The stored fight/flight/freeze state, ready to be activated with any environmental danger cues, is a survival mechanism. Any perceived signs of danger later in adulthood activate the vigilant child state. Figure 2.1 illustrates the impact of attachment trauma on the client's sense of safety and their ANS.

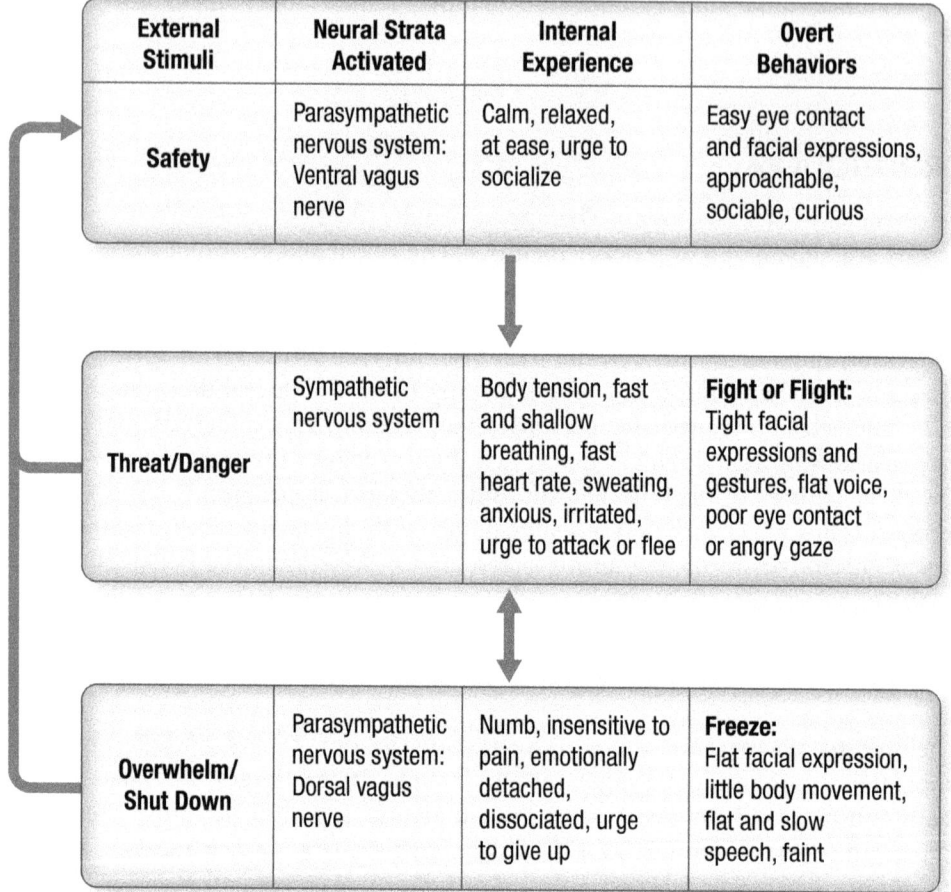

FIGURE 2.1 Impact of attachment trauma on client's sense of safety.

Source: Adapted from Lynch, T. (2018). *The skills training manual for radically open dialectical behavior therapy: A clinician's guide for treating disorders of overcontrol.* Context Press.

THE PARALLEL PROCESS

The client with a history of attachment trauma needs safety, trust, and connection with the therapist as part of preparation before addressing painful attachment memories with Eye Movement Desensitization and Reprocessing (EMDR) therapy. However, clients who associate relationships with painful emotions may have high needs for connection while simultaneously assuming negative intent on the part of others. The clients' nervous system reads danger when there is none, activating the sympathetic state and defense mechanisms.

The therapeutic relationship is vital to helping the client's ANS shift to perceptions of safety and protection. The mindful therapist who attunes to the client's experience while staying regulated can build a trusting connection over time. Trust and connection with their therapist allow the client to calm through the therapist's calm state. Co-regulation from the therapist can provide an emotional life raft for the client during subsequent trauma work.

If the therapist is not adequately mindful and intentional about staying attuned and calm, the therapist can become dysregulated in parallel to the client's dysregulation. If the therapist's sympathetic nervous system becomes activated, the client will detect danger cues in the therapist's expression, body posture, or voice tone that leave the client vigilant to any perceived signs of disapproval, rejection, fear, or anger on the part of the therapist.

Parallel processing involves staying self-reflective regarding our own state while helping clients become aware of their thoughts and feelings. Intentionally processing what is happening inside of ourselves in tandem with our clients' process is one of the best ways we can evolve personally and become more effective professionally. The AFTT-A therapist specifically focuses on awareness of the parts within the therapist that may become activated throughout the work of therapy. When we take our self-observations to professional consultation or peer consultation, we can gain an objective understanding of our triggers and vulnerabilities. When we can stay conscious of the processes of neuroception happening within ourselves, we can better manage our ANS and stay in the "social safety zone." Only within the social safety zone can we listen, communicate, and connect. In the social safety zone of the ventral vagal part of the ANS we can engage and co-regulate our client so they can more effectively engage in the work.

Therapeutic trust and co-regulation activate ventral vagal and social safety for our clients, which provides a good secure base for preparation phase parts' work and eventually the work of EMDR reprocessing. With a calm brain and nervous system, clients can more readily work with their internal system as well as the traumatic material, lessening the power of their danger circuits and increasing access to the ventral vagal state.

COUNTERTRANSFERENCE AND TRANSFERENCE

When the therapist is genuinely engaged in assisting clients with the healing process, clients are likely to grow in feelings of trust and connection with the therapist and share more openly over time. This condition is optimal for emotional growth, but also leaves clients vulnerable to the phenomenon of transference, confusing the relationship with the therapist with their other most significant relationships. For example, consider the client who was rejected by their parents while growing up. As the client's feelings of connection to the therapist become stronger, their vigilance regarding potential rejection is heightened. The emotional stakes may become so high that when the therapist fails to respond to a phone call in a timely manner or cancels an appointment due to personal reasons, the client's Child/Adolescent parts of Self may become activated, causing hurt and anger carried forward from childhood into the therapeutic relationship. To clarify the meaning of this sentence, this sentenceshould say: In turn, the therapist may respond with "countertransference," projecting traits of their own significant others onto the client and activating the therapist's Child/Adolescent parts of Self.

If our sympathetic nervous system is activated and we behave in a way that creates a rupture in the therapeutic relationship, self-awareness allows us to self-regulate and facilitate a relationship repair. Repairing a breach in the relationship with a client can be invaluable for rebuilding trust and role-modeling healthy relationship behaviors.

When we stay mindful of emotions, sensations, thoughts, or images that surface during a therapy session, we can manage our countertransference responses. When we stay curious, without assigning blame, we are in a place to ponder both our own state and our client's state simultaneously. With mindful intention, we can bring ourselves back to emotional and social safety and process what is happening in tandem with our client's processing.

THERAPIST TRIGGERS

Following is an example of a clinical scenario in which a client is triggered in session, subsequently triggering the therapist who responds from a dysregulated state.

> **BOX 2.1 CLIENT EXAMPLE: THERAPIST IS TRIGGERED, LEADING TO A DEFENSIVE RESPONSE AND A BREACH IN THE THERAPEUTIC RELATIONSHIP**
>
> A client admits to becoming angry and aggressive with their voice tone and words when their partner made a critical remark about the way they loaded the dishwasher. The therapist knows that the client was criticized strongly as a young child and points out that the client's reaction may have been stronger than the situation warranted due to memories of criticism as a child. The client's voice, face, and posture show immediate irritation. The client states, "I was upset because my partner was mean to me. You're minimizing and invalidating my feelings by blaming my feelings on my childhood. Now you're the one letting me down. I didn't need this from you today."
>
> The therapist becomes anxious (moving into sympathetic nervous system arousal). The therapist leans forward in their chair and says with an intense voice tone, "I have nothing but positive intentions, here. I shared my observation because I thought it might be something we could explore. But clearly, you need to calm down first."
>
> The client says, "Now, you're shaming me." The therapist feels suddenly helpless and is unable to respond any further. The client shuts down for the remainder of the session.

Have you ever experienced a clinical situation in which you became triggered and dysregulated or immobilized in response to a client's words or behaviors? Were you aware as it was happening, or did you become aware later? Were you able to self-regulate and repair the breach? Or did you become overwhelmed by anxiety or frustration?

Even with the best of intentions, we all occasionally say or do things that are received poorly. Our timing might be off, we might miss a cue regarding our client's emotional state, or the client has a transference response that we couldn't have predicted. How we respond to the problem makes all the difference for moving forward. In the client example, the therapist may have been able to make a repair by staying mindful of their own internal shift into sympathetic activation, breathing deeply, down-shifting back into the social safety zone, dropping their shoulders and saying with a calm voice tone, "I clearly was not well-attuned just now. When I told you to calm down, I added another layer of hurt to what you were already feeling. Thanks for letting me know. Can we try this again? I'd like to start by listening to what you're going through." The therapist's relaxed body and attuned response might go a long way toward getting the session back on track.

The parallel process here would involve the therapist getting curious about their initial emotional response. After the session, the therapist might ponder the interaction, journal, take the case to supervision or peer consultation, or take the situation to their own therapy session. Using situations like this to delve a little deeper can take us right where we need to go for important insight and growth.

Another common trigger for therapists who treat trauma is the client's description of their experiences. If a client describes a trauma that is reminiscent of an unprocessed trauma stored in the therapist's memory network, the therapist's sympathetic state can become activated. If the therapist's nervous system mirrors the client's nervous system, there is no way to lead the client safely through their own work.

Client behaviors such as lateness, missed appointments, unpaid bills, or excessive demands for between-therapy contact can trigger feelings of frustration or overwhelm for the therapist. The feelings can show on the therapist's face, in their body posture, or in their words or tone of voice, leading to heightened defensive reactions in the client and stalling the therapeutic progress.

Although the client's therapy-interfering behaviors are frustrating and inappropriate, they likely reflect patterns developed for getting needs met early in life. When we can stay mindful, we can hold our boundaries without activating the client's defenses. When we stay regulated, we can explore some hypotheses about the origin of the behaviors and gain insight into our client's history by asking ourselves, "How might this behavior have been helpful for getting their needs met or protecting themselves while growing up?" "When are these behaviors triggered in therapy?" "When do they ease up?" The answers to these questions can help us let go of judgments and add important information to case conceptualization. With a non-shaming, mindful approach, we can invite our client to ponder these questions and gain insight into the conditions that created the defenses.

BALANCING THE PUSH FOR CHANGE WITH ACCEPTANCE

Many therapists tend to over-function. We enter the therapy profession because we like to help. We have strong values around working hard and solving problems. When we're successful, we feel competent and in control. When things don't go the way we'd hoped, we may become anxious or frustrated. When we lose our footing, our first response may become our worst response.

To better manage our personal and clinical responses when things are not progressing the way we would like, the Dialectical Behavioral Therapy (DBT) approach (Linehan, 1993) recommends balancing the push for change with acceptance. The DBT term "radical acceptance" translates to, "I don't love it, but I can make a choice to accept where my client is in this moment and let it be." This balancing act can reduce over-functioning and increase attunement. Pressure is lessened for both client and therapist. When the time feels right, the therapist can provide another push toward change.

POINTS TO REMEMBER

- Mindful therapists seek consultation or join a peer consultation group, or they become part of a community through professional organizations or through collaboration with other therapists.
- Mindful therapists may self-reflect through journaling, through sharing personal feelings in close relationships, and/or through personal therapy.
- Mindful therapists look at their own emotional reactions in the therapy office as an opportunity for self-reflection and growth.
- Mindful therapists become acquainted with their triggers, parts of Self, and the emotions, sensations, and perceptions associated with changes in autonomic state or activated Child/Adolescent parts.
- When struggling with judgments regarding a client's behaviors, mindful therapists examine the behaviors through a trauma lens and reflect on how the client's behaviors were helpful at an earlier time in the client's life.
- Mindful therapists stay aware of activated child states in the client and in themselves.
- Mindful therapists balance the push for change in the therapy office with acceptance.

PAUSE AND REFLECT FOR THE THERAPIST

BOX 2.2 ANN'S STORY: GETTING UNSTUCK WITH ASSISTANCE FROM A PEER CONSULTATION GROUP

I (A.P.) felt emotionally "stuck" with a specific client, so I brought the client's case to my peer consultation group. The client's progress had stalled in the therapy. I realized I was having judgments about the way my client was talking about their partner. After I shared the case with my peer consultation group and really examined the judgments I was having, I was able to go back to session with the client and be much more present. Through mindfulness, I was able to get back in touch with my compassion for the client and the client started to make progress again. I realized that the real obstacle to my client's progress was my judgmental thinking.

BOX 2.3 DEB'S STORY: LOSS OF THERAPEUTIC RAPPORT DUE TO THERAPIST OVER-FUNCTIONING

I (D.W.) was working with a client who had suffered from depression for most of his life and was resistant to trying any of my suggestions for addressing the symptoms. My response was to hit the accelerator. I went into hyper-drive in an attempt to push the client toward change in various ways. During one session, the client turned to me and said, "I liked you much better the other way."

"What other way?" I asked in surprise.

"I really liked it when you were more present. You were genuine and kind, and I felt cared for. Now you're not happy with my progress and you're pushing me too much."

(continued)

BOX 2.3 DEB'S STORY: LOSS OF THERAPEUTIC RAPPORT DUE TO THERAPIST OVER-FUNCTIONING (*continued*)

I realized that my client was correct. The situation had kicked in my over-functioning self—the part of me who hates feeling helpless and needs to find answers in order to feel in control and successful. I was on a quest to prove to myself that I could fix this client, and our relationship had suffered the consequences. I shifted my focus on staying emotionally present. Our therapeutic relationship was re-established. This client most needed to feel seen and heard to feel worthy. I'm grateful they were able to express what they were feeling in that moment.

Jot down two or three specific clients who activated vulnerable, defensive, or over-functioning responses in you. Consider what it was about their behaviors or situations that were most triggering. Take those situations into account as you estimate your past distress (0 to 10) when you have found yourself in the following situations:

My client appears to be ...

1. Critical toward me _____
2. Demanding toward me _____
3. Disrespectful toward me _____
4. Uncooperative with me _____
5. Defensive with me _____
6. Making no progress _____
7. Avoiding addressing real issues _____
8. Power struggling with me _____
9. Shut down with me _____

Next, think about your responses to challenging therapeutic situations.

Do I get ...

1. Direct and forceful? Never __ Sometimes __ Often __
2. Defensive? Never __ Sometimes __ Often __
3. Distant and shut down? Never __ Sometimes __ Often __
4. Anxious and confused? Never __ Sometimes __ Often __
5. Tense in my body? Never __ Sometimes __ Often __
6. Disorganized and disoriented? Never __ Sometimes __ Often __
7. Sleepy? Never __ Sometimes __ Often __
8. Frozen? Never __ Sometimes __ Often __

Consider bringing your responses to your personal therapy and utilizing the EMDR "float back" method, starting with the situations that are triggering, the associated feeling, and letting your mind "float back" to associated memories to find targets for your personal EMDR therapy work.

USEFUL TERMS AND DEFINITIONS

AFTT-A: Attachment-Focused Trauma Therapy for Adults

ANS: autonomic nervous system

DBT: Dialectical Behavioral Therapy

REFERENCES

Linehan, M. M. (1993). *Cognitive behavioral treatment of borderline personality disorder*. W. W. Norton.

Lynch, T. (2018). *The skills training manual for radically open dialectical behavior therapy: A clinician's guide for treating disorders of overcontrol*. Context Press.

Porges, S. W., & Dana, D. (2018). *Clinical applications of the polyvagal theory: The emergence of polyvagal-informed therapies*. W. W. Norton.

Wesselmann, D., & Potter, A. E. (2019, September). *Attachment through the lifespan*. EMDRIA Preconference Presentation, Orange County, California.

CHAPTER 3

Internal and External Secure/Earned Secure Attachments in Attachment-Focused Trauma Therapy for Adults

INTRODUCTION

Early research by Ainsworth (1967), a student of Bowlby's, provided a more in-depth understanding of the differences in the quality of attachment relationships between mother/infant dyads through the development of the Strange Situation assessment. During the assessment, Ainsworth observed the behaviors of a mother and infant in a situation in which the mother and a stranger move in and out of the room, creating a stressful situation for the toddler. Ainsworth discovered that the reaction of the mother and child upon reunification was most significant. When the mothers returned, about two thirds of the toddlers went straight to their mothers and were easily soothed by them. The mothers of those toddlers were especially sensitive and responsive to their toddlers' emotional needs. The toddlers had learned to trust their mothers and were developing a secure attachment pattern.

Approximately one third of the toddlers were not among the secure group. The nonsecure toddlers either did not seek their mothers' comfort or were not receptive to their mothers' attempts to soothe them.

LATER OBSERVATIONS REGARDING ATTACHMENT SECURITY

In a major longitudinal study (Sroufe et al., 2005) it was found that children with a secure history were viewed by teachers as more sociable, more positive, more empathic, and more friendly. The children with secure histories appeared to maintain attachment security as they grew older. They were lower risk for behavioral disorders and major mental health disorders.

Attachment Security on the Adult Attachment Interview (Hesse, 1999)

The Adult Attachment Interview (AAI; Main et al., 2005) identifies attachment patterns in adulthood through a structured interview that assesses the subject's state of mind with respect to attachment relationships. The interview does not depend upon the subject's self-report regarding their state of mind, nor does it categorize attachment designation based on the subject's report of experiences with attachment figures in childhood. The AAI scorer detects clues to attachment functioning that are unconscious to the subjects by examining transcripts of the interview and looking for specific features in the discourse that are associated with each of the attachment designations (Main et al., 2002).

In general, individuals with a secure attachment pattern can recount positive memories and negative memories in an organized manner and without either hyperbole or avoidance and denial. If a secure individual states that early experiences included nurturing and protection, they can recount specific examples as evidence. When they describe early negative experiences, they can recount those experiences with organized dialogue and with an appropriate level of emotions.

Secure Attachment Through Bowlby's Internal Working Model

British psychiatrist Bowlby (1988) first recognized the importance of early attachment experiences for healthy development of infants and young children when he and his colleagues observed children who were separated from parents during World War II and during hospitalizations during the 1940s and 1950s. There appeared to be a long-term negative impact on the children's emotional well-being and capacity for trust and closeness, even after reunification. However, the attachment relationship of children who experienced consistent and loving care with their parents became a secure base and a positive template for other relationships as they grew older and moved out into the world. He hypothesized that early attachment experiences impact the internal working model (IWM) for individuals lifelong. The IWM consists of beliefs about self, others, and the world. Positive attachment experiences led to an overall positive IWM—positive expectations for the individuals themselves as well as others, and positive choices and behaviors in relationships. Specifically, positive beliefs may include, "I'm good and others are good and trustworthy, too," "I deserve love," "I belong," and "Overall, I am safe in the world and safe with people."

Secure Attachment Viewed Through the Adaptive Information Processing Model

Attachment security can be viewed through the lens of the adaptive information processing (AIP) model developed by Shapiro (2018). The model theorizes that we all have some memory networks that hold adaptive, positive images, affect, and perceptions and some memory networks that hold negative images, affect, and perceptions. Adults who have secure attachment patterns hold more positive memory networks of trust, connection, significance, and comfort than negative memory networks. The positive memory networks are well integrated and have tremendous influence on adulthood relationship choices and interactions.

Secure Attachment Through the Lens of Attachment-Focused Trauma Therapy for Adults

Within the internal personality system of secure adults, the Child parts of Self hold emotions, sensations, and memories related to safety, trust, and security. The adaptive information and memory networks are integrated and accessible within the system, allowing the Adult Self to access needed information, make positive relationship choices, and provide responses to others that come from a place of security. In a healthy, integrated, internal personality system in which the Adult part of Self has access to adaptive information, Child/Adolescent parts of Self stay settled, relaxed, and secure, even when memories are triggered. The Adult part of Self accesses what is needed from the memories and handles current adult tasks while, at the same time, Child/Adolescent parts of Self are differentiated from and unconcerned with present-day life.

Balance and Attachment Security

Early seminal studies found that adults with secure attachment status as determined by the AAI desire closeness but have a balanced desire for autonomy (Feeney, 1998). They hold expectations for positive characteristics of kindness, fairness, and sensitivity. They are able to reflect upon their inner state and express their feelings and listen and attune to the feelings of others. Furthermore, secure individuals tend to have a balanced view of responsibility. They are not overly blaming of themselves or others. They hold themselves to the same expectations they have for others and give others the same grace they would want for themselves. They look for the best in others and assume positive intentions until proven otherwise.

Attachment Security and Parenthood

As parents, secure adults are able to reflect upon their own emotional state and reflect upon the emotions and needs of their children (Fonagy et al., 1991; Hesse, 1999). Secure parents make mistakes, but overall, they respond with attunement and sensitivity. For example, they are able to provide comfort when comfort is needed and stand back when the child needs to feel independent. The child's needs override their own. When they recognize a breech in the relationship with their child, they initiate a repair. Seventy to 80% of the time, the children of securely attached adults follow suit and exhibit secure attachment behaviors.

Attachment Security on a Continuum

Attachment security is not all-or-nothing; it is on a continuum. Most subjects identified as secure on the AAI have some nonsecure indicators and many have enough that they are assigned a secondary nonsecure classification. Nonsecure individuals also exhibit some secure indicators and may have enough secure indicators that a secondary secure designation is warranted (Main et al., 2002).

For example, consider a client who has a primarily secure attachment pattern in most circumstances due to a positive, affirming relationship with a secure mother while growing up. However, the client had a secondary preoccupied pattern developed within their relationship with their father, who struggled with managing symptoms of anxiety and depression for several years. Presently, the client has a relationship with a partner that is mutually supportive overall and usually a source of satisfaction. Recently, however, the partner has developed mild depressive symptoms, which have triggered feelings of anxiety and hypervigilant behaviors that are not typical for this client. Through the lens of Attachment-Focused Trauma Therapy for Adults (AFTT-A), a previously settled Child/Adolescent part of Self is activated due to the more triggering partner situation.

Earned Secure Attachment

The individual who experienced childhood rejection, neglect, abuse, or significant losses at any age may receive a secure designation on the AAI structured interview.

The events and situations do not determine the score on the AAI. Instead, the scorer examines the transcript for tells in the language used by the subject when describing events and situations. In fact, individuals who started life with poor quality attachment experiences or major losses are able to "earn" a secure attachment designation on the AAI through the experience of an "emotionally corrective relationship" with a supportive other (Saunders et al., 2011).

From the AIP perspective, the disturbing emotions and perceptions related to early attachment experiences likely remain unprocessed, affecting adulthood responses and expectations. A later significant experience with a trustworthy, secure, and supportive other enriches the adaptive memory network. Furthermore, co-regulation with a reflective, secure other may allow the nonsecure individual to reflect upon their early experiences and gain an adaptive perspective on their difficult circumstances. Considering this, a positive therapeutic relationship with an Eye Movement Desensitization and Reprocessing (EMDR) therapist can provide an emotionally corrective experience and adaptive resolution for traumatic attachment memories.

ATTACHMENT STATUS IN THERAPY

Secure individuals vary in their ability to self-reflect, communicate, and learn, but in general, secure individuals who attend therapy for life problems or mental health symptoms will utilize therapy effectively (Fonagy & Allison, 2014). In the therapeutic environment, the secure client tends to be self-reflective and open to assistance. Generally, they can communicate their thoughts, feelings, and sensations. The secure client is usually trusting of the therapist's intentions and interprets the therapist's words in the most positive way, allowing for insights and positive emotional shifts. Individuals who are more trusting, self-reflective, and open to assistance are readily able to utilize EMDR therapy effectively to reprocess traumatic experiences. They associate to positive, adaptive ideas and associations to make sense of the traumatic events. Individuals who already have a secure or earned secure attachment status are better able to tolerate feelings during EMDR trauma reprocessing. They're able to tolerate their feelings during EMDR therapy, look at memories from various points of view, integrate and generalize insights, and assign appropriate responsibility.

Most clients with serious attachment trauma do not begin therapy in a secure state, although some may have an earned secure status. Establishing an emotionally corrective therapeutic relationship is foundational to the AFTT-A model.

The Therapist With Secure/Earned Secure Status

The therapist with secure or "earned secure" attachment (through therapy or emotionally corrective relationships) can more readily reflect and self-reflect regarding their emotional and physical responses to interactions in the therapy office. The capacity to self-reflect brings the capacity to step back from an automatic personal, emotional reaction to a client's challenging words or behaviors to view the situation through the lens of the AIP model. The secure therapist can respond to nonsecure client interactions with secure-based responses, co-regulating the dysregulated client (Wesselmann & Potter, 2019). The therapist with secure or earned secure attachment is able to balance the push for change with acceptance, thus attuning to the client's struggle. In this way, the therapeutic relationship becomes a powerful force by building a foundation of emotional support and trust prior to addressing the difficult memories and emotions.

The therapist with a secure or earned secure status may have some underlying tendencies toward a nonsecure or disorganized pattern in relationships. Consultation or supervision, peer consultation, and personal therapy can all help the therapist operate from an adaptive perspective, that is, their most present-day "Adult Brain." The therapist who suspects they are not in secure or earned secure status will want to participate in their own personal EMDR therapy for reprocessing early disturbing events to move toward an earned secure status and increase their capacity for personal reflection and co-regulation.

POINTS TO REMEMBER

- Secure attachment in adulthood is associated with positive expectations and choices in relationships.
- Secure individuals have the capacity to self-reflect, self-regulate, attune, and respond with sensitivity and care to their children, partners, and others.
- Relationships are a source of satisfaction and a buffer toward stress in individuals with secure attachment status.
- Attachment security is not all-or-nothing. Adults may be primarily secure with a secondary classification or underlying tendency toward a nonsecure status.
- For adults with secure patterns, the Child parts of Self holding affect and perceptions related to trust and self-worth tend to remain in a state of healthy integration within the personality system. The Child parts of Self for the most part remain content and settled. Adaptive information is integrated and accessible to the Adult Self, who manages adult life without activation of Child parts.
- Individuals with secure patterns can readily seek assistance and utilize therapy to work through difficulties related to stress and traumatic events.
- Emotional support from secure others in adulthood can provide individuals who suffered rejection, neglect, or abuse in childhood with an emotionally corrective experience and a new, "earned secure" attachment status.
- The emotionally corrective therapeutic relationship provides clients with co-regulation and a good foundation for managing emotions and sensations during trauma work.
- The therapist with attachment security or earned attachment security is likely capable of reflecting upon their own internal responses and shifts and managing their internal state in order to stay grounded, supportive, and attuned with clients for optimal trust-building and co-regulation.

PAUSE AND REFLECT FOR THE THERAPIST

- Consider your present-day relationships. List the present-day relationships that nourish you and mitigate the effects of stress in your life.

- List any present-day relationships that have become a source of stress for you.
- Journal your plan for increasing positive, supportive connections that can strengthen your sense of security, self-worth, and trust.

USEFUL TERMS AND DEFINITIONS

AAI: Adult Attachment Interview

AFTT-A: Attachment-Focused Trauma Therapy for Adults

AIP: adaptive information processing model

EMDR: Eye Movement Desensitization and Reprocessing

IWM: internal working model

REFERENCES

Ainsworth, M. D. S. (1967). *Infancy in Uganda: Infant care and the growth of love.* Johns Hopkins University Press.

Bowlby, J. (1988). *A secure base: Parent-child attachment and healthy human development.* Routledge.

Feeney, J. A. (1998). Adult romantic attachment and couple relationships. In J. Cassidy & P. R. Shaver (Eds.), *Handbook of attachment: Theory, research, and clinical applications* (pp. 552–598). Guilford Press.

Fonagy, P., & Allison, E. (2014). The role of mentalizing and epistemic trust in the therapeutic relationship. *Psychotherapy, 51*(3), 372–380. https://doi.org/10.1037/a0036505

Fonagy, P., Steele, M., Steele, H., Moran, G. S., & Higgitt, A. C. (1991). The capacity for understanding mental states: The reflective self in parent and child and its significance for security of attachment. *Infant Mental Health Journal, 12*(3), 201–218. https://doi.org/10.1002/1097-0355(199123)12:3<201::AID-IMHJ2280120307>3.0.CO;2-7

Hesse, E. (1999). The Adult Attachment Interview protocol, method of analysis, and empirical studies. In J. Cassidy & P. R. Shaver (Eds.), *Handbook of attachment: Theory, research, and clinical applications.* (pp. 552–598). The Guilford Press.

Main, M., Goldwyn, R., & Hesse, E. (2002). *Adult attachment scoring and classification systems* (Manual in draft: version 7.2). Regents of the University of California.

Main, M., Hesse, E., & Kaplan, N. (2005). Predictability of attachment behavior and representational processes at 1, 6, and 19 years of age: The Berkeley Longitudinal Study. In K. E. Grossmann, K. Grossmann & E. Waters (Eds.), *Attachment from infancy to adulthood: The major longitudinal studies* (pp. 245–304). Guilford Press.

Saunders, R., Jacobvitz, D., Zaccagnino, M., Beverung, L. M., & Hazen, N. (2011). Pathways to earned-security: The role of alternative support figures. *Attachment & Human Development, 13*(4), 403–420. https://doi.org/10.1080/14616734.2011.584405

Shapiro, F. (2018). *Eye Movement Desensitization and Reprocessing (EMDR) Therapy: Basic principles, protocols, and procedures* (3rd ed.). Guilford Press.

Sroufe, L. A., Egeland, B., Carlson, E. A., & Collins, W. A. (2005). *The development of the person: The Minnesota study of risk and adaptation from birth to adulthood.* Guilford Publications.

Wesselmann, D., & Potter, A. E. (2019, September). *Attachment through the lifespan.* EMDRIA Preconference Presentation, Orange County, CA.

CHAPTER 4

External and Internal Nonsecure and Disorganized Categories of Attachment in Attachment-Focused Trauma Therapy for Adults

INTRODUCTION

Children and Attachment Loss

John Bowlby, the founder of attachment theory, recognized the significance of the mother/child relationship. He founded the Separation Research Unit at the Tavistock Clinic in London in 1948 and, along with colleagues, observed that children who endured long separations from their parents experienced three stages of grief, sequentially (Bowlby, 1982).

The first stage of grief involves "protest" behaviors, which begin almost immediately. When children see their parent leaving, they cry out with anger in an attempt to bring them back. Every parent has witnessed the protest stage at various times.

If the separation continues for a lengthy period of time, the protest stage gives way to the second stage, "despair." Anyone who has lost a loved one knows this type of emotional pain. Children who are separated from a beloved parent experience these intense emotions for a very long time.

If the separation continues, children move into the final stage, "detachment." They become emotionally shut down, "flat" in affect, interacting with others more superficially. Sadly, if reunification with their parents is finally achieved after they have reached the stage of detachment, many children continue to interact more superficially with their parents and others. The ongoing detachment is self-protective, in that it prevents the depth of despair that would ensue if the child reconnected and then went through another loss.

Symptoms and behaviors of adults as well as children can often be conceptualized through the lens of Bowlby's identified stages of protest, despair, and detachment. If an adult experienced childhood losses due to death, separations, abandonment, or rejection, escalated demands or complaints in present-day relationships and in therapy may be viewed as a Child/Adolescent part of Self stuck in protest. Depression, self-harming, or suicidal gestures may be conceptualized as a Child/Adolescent part who is frozen in time with old feelings of despair. Guardedness and superficiality may be viewed as a Child/Adolescent part holding onto detachment out of self-protection.

Childhood Attachment Qualities

Following Bowlby's initial discoveries around the phenomenon of children's attachment to their parents, Bowlby's student, Mary Ainsworth, examined the behaviors of toddlers with their mothers during the Strange Situation, a structured assessment to determine the quality of attachment between children and their parents (Ainsworth, 1978). During the assessment, Ainsworth placed a toddler and their mother in a room together. The interactions between the mother and child were observed while the mother and a stranger were moved in and out of the room. The children's behaviors when reunified with their mothers were found to determine the quality of the child's attachment.

About two thirds of children in the general population have a secure pattern. In the Strange Situation, the secure toddlers go to their parent for comfort and are receptive to their parents' comforting behaviors.

About one third of children are avoidant or ambivalent/resistant, the two nonsecure but "organized" categories. A much smaller number of children are designated "disorganized." Disorganized children are also provided with a secondary secure, avoidant, or ambivalent/resistant designation.

Avoidant toddlers show very little emotion when their parents leave or return to the room during the Strange Situation. However, avoidant toddlers have high levels of the stress hormone, cortisol, during the procedures, evidence that they are not relaxed. They have only learned to repress outward evidence of their distress. The parents of avoidant toddlers are generally found to have a negative response to their toddlers' strong emotions, pulling away from them instead of moving toward them when their toddlers show that they are upset. The toddlers therefore learn to suppress their distress in order to prevent their parent from rejecting them.

Toddlers classified as ambivalent/resistant are upset when their parent leaves and are angry and tearful when their parent returns during the Strange Situation. The parent may attempt to calm their toddlers, but ambivalent/resistant toddlers are quite difficult to soothe. In general, the parents of ambivalent/resistant toddlers have strong emotions themselves. They can be close and affectionate with their toddlers at times, but they are poorly attuned to their toddlers when they themselves are dysregulated. They are more responsive when their toddlers demand it, so the intensity with which the toddlers seek their parent's attention is protective. It helps them get their needs met with more consistency.

The disorganized children initially puzzled the researchers. They made up a small percentage of the children observed in the early studies, and their behaviors didn't match the behaviors of any of the other three groups. When their mothers returned to the room during the Strange Situation assessment, the toddlers covered their face or their heads with their hands, flapped their arms, twirled, or crawled backward toward the mother. It was determined that their strange behaviors reflected a disorganized mental state. It was eventually discovered that the mothers sometimes exhibited facial expressions or had voice tones that were frightening to the children (Lyons-Ruth et al., 1999). The mothers had unresolved trauma that was triggered by their toddlers, creating intense emotions of fear or anger.

MENTAL HEALTH AND ATTACHMENT THROUGH THE LIFE STAGES

Attachment Patterns Through the Lens of the Internal Working Model

Bowlby recognized through the ground-breaking attachment studies at the Tavistock Clinic that early attachment experiences, positive or negative, inform our deepest belief system, the internal working model (IWM; Bretherton, 1987). The IWM includes beliefs about self, others, and the world that impact our expectations and trust in our relationships with others, our confidence to move out into the world, and our emotional stability lifelong.

Bowlby hypothesized that early attachment experiences impact our developing IWM and posited that later life events or relationships are interpreted through the lens of the IWM (Bretherton, 1987). The IWM can be lifelong without profound intervening experiences. When our IWM includes a positive view of self and others, we approach others with positive intentions and an open heart. Parenthood is approached with the same positive expectations, allowing us to enjoy positive moments in the parent/child relationship.

When our IWM includes negative perceptions of self and others, our chance of developing fulfilling relationships is lower. We approach others with our defenses in place, interpreting their behaviors through a lens of mistrust. Even our relationships with our children can be negatively impacted by skewed negative perceptions and expectations. Our adulthood relationships can become a source of anxiety instead of a source of pleasure or a buffer to stress.

Attachment Through the Lens of the Adaptive Information Processing Model

Shapiro's adaptive information processing (AIP) model (Shapiro, 2018) provides a neurobiological perspective on the IWM. The AIP posits that positive childhood attachment experiences that are processed, integrated, and stored adaptively in neural networks in the brain promote healthy, adaptive functioning in adulthood relationships. However, distressing attachment memories and related affect and perceptions remain in an unprocessed form, stored in memory networks without access to adaptive information. The stored affect and perceptions can be triggered by present-day relationships, leading to self-protective, defensive behaviors, destabilizing present-day relationships.

Through the lens of the Attachment-Focused Trauma Therapy for Adults (AFTT-A) model, the triggered memory networks can interrupt continuity of Self by activating the Child/Adolescent part of Self—the perceptions, emotions, and sensations experienced in childhood. The activation can cause a "blend" of "Adult Brain" and "Kid Brain," impairing functioning. In the case of more severe dissociation, consciousness may shift completely to the activated Child part.

ADULTHOOD ATTACHMENT PATTERNS

The Adult Attachment Interview (AAI) assesses adult attachment patterns through a structured interview in which the adult is asked to describe specific memories regarding their relationship with their parents in childhood (Hesse, 1999). The transcript of the interview is scored in terms of the language and organization of the narrative. The adulthood categories of secure, dismissive, preoccupied, and unresolved/disorganized attachment correspond to the childhood categories of secure, avoidant, ambivalent/resistant, and disorganized.

Table 4.1 demonstrates the equivalent attachment categories for children and adults and describes important characteristics associated with each category.

Table 4.1 Equivalent Attachment Categories for Children and Adults

Childhood Attachment Categories	Adulthood Attachment Categories
Secure—Positive expectations in relationship with parent(s). Comforted by closeness with parent(s). Able to feel and express emotions.	**Secure**—Positive expectations from relationships. Relationships are a buffer to anxiety. Enjoys closeness. Able to feel and express emotions.
Nonsecure/Avoidant—Manages anxiety through avoidance of feelings and closeness.	**Nonsecure/Dismissive**—Manages anxiety through avoidance of feelings and closeness.
Nonsecure/Ambivalent/Resistant—Manages anxiety by control/demands with parent(s). Intense expression of emotions.	**Nonsecure/Preoccupied**—Manages anxiety by control and seeking to get needs met in adulthood relationships. Fears rejection. Often overwhelmed by emotions.
Disorganized—Wants closeness with parent(s) but fearful of parent(s). Mental/behavioral disorganization. At risk for dissociative disorder in adolescence or adulthood.	**Disorganized/Unresolved**—Mental disorganization/disorientation with respect to loss or abuse memories. At risk for dissociative disorder.

Source: Adapted from Hesse, E. (1999). The Adult Attachment Interview protocol, method of analysis, and empirical studies. In J. Cassidy & P. R. Shaver (Eds.), *Handbook of attachment: Theory, research, and clinical applications* (pp. 552–598). Guilford Press; and Main, M., Kaplan, N., & Cassidy, J. (1985). Security in infancy, childhood, and adulthood: A move to the level of representation. *Monographs of the Society for Research in Child Development, 50*(1/2), 66–104. https://doi.org/10.2307/3333827.

Dismissive Attachment Pattern in Adults

The adult with a dismissive attachment pattern, like the avoidant child, reduces relationship anxiety by repressing emotions and limiting emotional closeness, thus avoiding vulnerability to rejection or abandonment (Hesse, 1999; Main et al., 2005). In the AAI transcript, signs of a dismissive pattern include short answers and a lack of emotions. Self-insight into the avoidance tendencies is minimal or completely absent. Unfortunately, the strategy that many adults use to keep themselves protected simultaneously keeps them from feeling connected or from having stable relationships. They lack insight into the deeper feelings they are suppressing and into the emotions of their significant others, thus reducing their capacity for empathy.

There are two subcategories associated with dismissive attachment in adulthood. The derogatory subtype is associated with derogation toward at least one significant relationship. Derogatory comments about others can often be heard from adults with the dismissive derogatory pattern. The derogation prevents vulnerability to possible rejection or criticism.

The dismissive attached adult with an idealizing subtype denies difficulties in childhood and idealizes parents to avoid feelings of hurt, rejection, or abandonment. They also repress emotions and avoid closeness to self-protect.

Dismissive clients are naturally avoidant of the process of therapy, as it includes the experiencing of vulnerable emotions. Dismissive clients are frequently in therapy due to demands by a significant other, and they are at risk for leaving therapy prematurely. Mindfulness and attunement to clients' tendencies toward the dismissive pattern can assist therapists with adjusting their approach to reduce triggering clients' anxiety. For example, therapists can slow to a manageable pace; use a matter-of-fact, casual approach; and acknowledge clients' strengths to reduce triggering vulnerable emotions. For example, after the client has described a disturbing memory, instead of saying, "That must have been very hurtful to you," the therapist can say, "You had to have a great deal of strength to have coped with that experience."

Negative cognitions (NCs) stored within the unprocessed memory networks of dismissive adults may include: "Emotions are unsafe," "Memories are unsafe," "Closeness is unsafe," and "I can't trust." Dismissive clients lack insight regarding these beliefs. Through the AFTT-A preparation phase and the Eye Movement Desensitization and Reprocessing (EMDR) reprocessing of traumatic memories, dismissive clients can restructure their internal system, process and integrate their memories, and increase their sense of security. Desired positive cognitions (PCs) may include: "I can have emotions and be okay," "I can be close and I'm okay," and "It's safe to trust."

Preoccupied Attachment Patterns in Adults

The preoccupied attachment pattern indicates an overall tendency to lose perspective and become overwhelmed with strong emotions. During the AAI, subjects who are rated as preoccupied may sound either angry or fearful when discussing childhood memories. Their stories may be quite long, and they become overinvolved in their stories, falling into dialogue in which they address one or both parents directly, as if the parent were present in the interview. For example, the subject might say, "My dad's alcoholism was so bad that he died of it before he was 45 years old. I couldn't stand it when my dad drank. He was always, you know, geeze, Dad, what were you thinking? You know, I couldn't even bring friends home, you were so falling down drunk all the time. I guess it didn't matter to you how your behavior affected me, though, did it, Dad?" In this example, the subject becomes so lost in the narrative that they berate their father as if he were there in the therapy office. As with the dismissive adult, the preoccupied adult is unaware that there is anything unusual about their narrative. They typically will show few signs of self-reflection, as they are too overwhelmed by the childhood emotions, perceptions, and self-protective behaviors.

Preoccupied adults with a tendency toward anger may be intense and demanding about their needs in their relationships, including their relationship with the therapist. The demandingness may have helped get needs met in childhood, but in adult life leads to problems with partners and others. In therapy, the intensity of their emotions can trigger the therapist's anxiety and get in the way of attunement. With therapeutic mindfulness, it's possible to maintain attunement, address the client's anxiety, and maintain appropriate boundaries.

Preoccupied adults may tend toward feelings of fear instead of anger. Adults who view others through the lens of fear are hypervigilant and sometimes over-accommodating for self-protection. Although fearful preoccupation made sense in the family-of-origin, the pattern can prevent the establishment of happy, healthy relationships in adult life. Therapist mindfulness, attunement, and patience are necessary for building therapeutic trust.

Adults with a preoccupied attachment pattern hold negative beliefs associated with stored disturbing memories that continue to underly problems in partner or other relationships. As an example, preoccupied adults may hold NCs such as: "I'm unworthy," "I'm unsafe," "Others don't care about my needs," and "I have to find a way to persuade others/accommodate others to give me the attention/affection that I need."

Conceptualized through the AFTT-A model, adults with distressing childhood memories may have Child/Adolescent parts of Self holding strong emotions that are frequently activated by triggers in adult life. Child/Adolescent parts tend to be hypervigilant in adulthood relationships, protecting themselves by managing adulthood relationships and seeking to get earlier unmet needs met. The internal personality system of the preoccupied adult includes anxious Child/Adolescent parts that are activated by attachments, leading to frequent blending of "Kid Brain" and "Adult Brain" during adulthood interactions.

Through AFTT-A and EMDR therapy, clients can restructure their internal system and process and integrate their memories. The goal is to shift their beliefs to PCs such as: "I'm worthy," "I'm safe," and "I can find relationships with others that are mutually satisfying."

Unresolved/Disorganized Attachment Patterns in Adults

Adults with an unresolved/disorganized attachment designation exhibit mental disorganization in their language or behavior, but not consistently. The disorganization and disorientation are observed when memories involving unresolved loss or unresolved childhood abuse are triggered. According to the AIP model, the trauma or loss is stored in an unprocessed, unintegrated form within memory networks. When the maladaptively stored neural networks are activated, clients experience the same mental disorganization and disorientation that was experienced at the time of the traumatic events. The unresolved/disorganized attachment pattern is associated with symptoms of dissociation (Liotti, 2004). On the AAI, the disorganization is apparent in the subject's confusion of pronouns related to self and other, in misassignment of responsibility for abuse, and in evidence of time disorientation (Main et al., 2002).

When memory networks holding unprocessed memories of loss or childhood abuse are activated for unresolved/disorganized adults, NCs related to perceptions at the time of the trauma may be activated, such as: "I'm unsafe," "I'm helpless," "I'm defective," "I'm responsible for what happened," and "I don't belong." Over time, through AFTT-A and EMDR therapy, unresolved/disorganized clients can restructure their internal system and integrate unprocessed memories, shifting beliefs to PCs such as: "I'm safe now," "I have choices now," "I'm okay as I am," and "I belong."

Attachment Patterns on a Continuum

Most people think of attachment categories as an all-or-nothing designation. However, the AAI interview transcript is scored for each category on a scale with a rating from 1 to 9. Therefore, each classification is actually on a continuum with a score of 9 indicating full consistency with the designated pattern to a score of 1 indicating no indicators for the attachment pattern (Main et al., 2002).

Subjects can be given more than one designation. For example, a secure subject may have a moderate score and secondary designation in one of the nonsecure categories. Alternatively, a subject may achieve a secure designation on the AAI with no secondary designation, but they may still have a few minor indicators in a nonsecure category. The unresolved/disorganized adult attachment designation with respect to the subject's state of mind when past abuse or loss memories are activated in some way is always assigned as the first category when the score is a 6 or higher, but one of the organized patterns (secure, dismissive, or preoccupied) is assigned in addition to the unresolved/disorganized designation (Main et al., 2002).

Longitudinal Data

In a seminal longitudinal study that began in the mid-1970s, a group of infants were assessed via the Strange Situation and followed into adulthood (Sroufe, 2005). The longitudinal data confirmed the general continuity of attachment patterns from childhood into adulthood and supported the hypothesis that secure attachment through life lowers the risk factor for later mental health problems. Nonsecure and disorganized attachment in childhood is associated with the highest mental health risk. Throughout childhood and adolescence, nonsecure and disorganized children overall exhibit more behavioral and mood problems. Ambivalent/resistant adolescents appear to be at highest risk for anxiety disorders. Avoidant adolescents are at highest risk for behavioral disorders. All nonsecure and disorganized children are at higher risk for depression than secure children. Disorganized adolescents are at far greater risk of psychiatric problems, dissociative disorders, and self-harming behaviors. In adulthood, attachment security is associated with social competency, positive expectations and perceptions in relationships, and increased emotional resilience. Adults with nonsecure or disorganized patterns exhibit lower social competency, more negative expectations and perceptions related to relationships, and more vulnerability to stress.

Generational Transmission of Attachment Patterns

Early studies with the AAI found approximately 80% correlation for secure versus nonsecure attachment patterns from parents to their children (Van IJzendoorn & Bakermans-Kranenburg, 1997). It's easy to understand the generational transmission of attachment patterns when you think about the self-protective behaviors that developed in early childhood.

For example, the dismissive parent most likely was avoidant as a child, suppressing emotions and needs for closeness to keep their own dismissive parent from becoming overwhelmed and retreating. Their dismissive behaviors are likely activated in their present relationships and by parenthood, leading them to distance and avoid closeness with their own children. Because they move away from their children when their children are emotional, their children also learn to suppress their feelings and needs in avoidant fashion.

The preoccupied parent was likely ambivalent/resistant as a child, actively demanding their parent to meet their needs as a way of achieving more consistent caregiving from their parent. In their present-day relationships, they likely continue to self-protect by actively demanding what they need from others. Although they're able to be affectionate with their children, their fear of not getting their needs met reduces their emotional presence and attunement. Their children learn to demand to get their needs met more consistently; thus, the ambivalent/resistant pattern is developed.

Unresolved/disorganized mothers perceive danger when memories of abuse or loss are triggered, and their own infants and young children are likely triggers for memories of their own youth. They can't control the activation of the neural networks holding unresolved abuse or loss memories during moments of closeness with their child. Their faces may exhibit brief expressions of fear, anger, or dissociation that are frightening and disorganizing to the nervous system of their children, leading to attachment disorganization.

In seminal studies related to the self-reflective function, Fonagy et al. (1991) observed that nonsecure and disorganized parents are typically lacking in the reflective function, the capacity to think about their own thoughts and feelings and the reasons for them, as well as the capacity for reflecting upon the inner worlds of their children. Without intervention, their children grow up with no one to help them understand their own thoughts and emotions or empathize with the inner state of others.

Secure parents attune and respond with sensitivity to their children's emotions, thus assisting their children with attunement to their own emotional state (Fonagy et al., 1991). This "reflective function" allows them to reflect upon the inner state of others and respond to others with sensitivity and empathy.

Hypothesizing Adult Attachment Patterns

There exist two "gold standard" attachment assessments: the AAI (Hesse, 1999) and the Adult Attachment Projective (AAP; George & West, 2004). Both assessments involve extensive training, and both are time-intensive for the therapist and subject in session and outside of session. However, paper-and-pencil measures that rely on self-report do not provide reliable and valid attachment designations equivalent to the AAI and AAP secure, preoccupied, dismissive, and unresolved/disorganized categories. This is not surprising, given the fact that the defensive processes involved in patterns of attachment are unconscious for all of us.

Although abbreviated versions of the gold standard assessments have been used for clinical purposes, AFTT-A therapists can effectively look for patterns and attitudes within the therapy sessions and the therapeutic relationship to make reasonable hypotheses regarding attachment tendencies for clinical purposes.

Attachment Patterns and Tendencies in Therapy

Differing attachment patterns are associated with the ease with which clients utilize therapy (Levy & Johnson, 2019). Secure individuals can develop a trusting relationship with the therapist and reflect upon and discuss their experiences, thoughts, and feelings. They're able to process the words of the therapist and assume positive intent in response to the therapist's feedback. During EMDR therapy, secure individuals are capable of self-reflection, insights, and reaching adaptive resolution (Wesselmann & Potter, 2019).

Nonsecure individuals sometimes have difficulty perceiving the therapist as a reassuring or safe presence. During EMDR therapy, nonsecure individuals may have more difficulty with self-reflection and making associations to adaptive information (Wesselmann & Potter, 2019).

Clients with a dismissive pattern may appear detached and have difficulty recognizing and verbalizing emotions in therapy. Dismissive clients may miss appointments, come late, minimize feelings, say very little, or respond flippantly to the therapist's interventions. Clients with dismissive derogatory tendencies may say something negative regarding the therapy or the therapist. Clients who are dismissive with an idealizing subtype may minimize problems, deny their emotions, and avoid distressing memories.

Preoccupied clients who tend toward anger may make unrealistic demands, mistrust the therapist's interventions, or use words that are critical. Preoccupied clients who tend toward fear may be quietly mistrusting.

Signs of disorganization in therapy may surface during discussion of trauma. Clients may confuse their pronouns when describing a loss or early abuse, confuse the sequence of events, become disorientated regarding present-day versus past, and confuse who was responsible in the case of abuse.

Table 4.2 provides examples of common statements heard during therapy sessions associated with nonsecure and disorganized attachment patterns.

Table 4.2 Sample Client Statements Associated With Adult Nonsecure and Disorganized Attachment Patterns

Client Attachment Patterns	Sample Client Statements
Preoccupied	"I need more time with you." "You're not listening to me. I don't feel heard." "I'll never get better."
Dismissive	"I don't remember my childhood, but it was fine." "I'm only here because I was told I had to come." "I don't think there's anything you can offer me."
Disorganized	"I feel like I'm only half here." "I don't know." (With nonverbal signs of fear.) "You must hate me after hearing my story."

Source: Adapted from Hesse, E. (1999). The Adult Attachment Interview protocol, method of analysis, and empirical studies. In J. Cassidy & P. R. Shaver (Eds.), *Handbook of attachment: Theory, research, and clinical applications* (pp. 552–598). Guilford Press; and Main, M., Kaplan, N., & Cassidy, J. (1985). Security in infancy, childhood, and adulthood: A move to the level of representation. *Monographs of the Society for Research in Child Development, 50*(1/2), 66–104. https://doi.org/10.2307/3333827.

A hypothesized attachment designation can assist the therapist with responding to clients' words and behaviors from a place of attunement. Attunement allows the therapist to be intentional with their own words and body language and adjust their approach to be as effective as possible.

For example, when the therapist hypothesizes a dismissive pattern, they can stay mindful regarding a tolerable pace and depth of exploration. When therapeutic trust allows, the therapist may be able to offer nonjudgmental observations of avoidance and invite exploration of its childhood purpose.

In the case of preoccupied clients, when the timing is appropriate, the therapist may be able to explore with the client how preoccupation was self-protective in early life. In the case of both dismissive and preoccupied defenses, the therapist's attunement and sensitive exploration can enhance the client's capacity for self-reflection.

Awareness of attachment disorganization raises the possibility of a dissociative disorder, cuing the therapist to provide adequate time for and modifications in preparation phase interventions such as the AFTT-A protocols prior to the EMDR reprocessing phases (see Chapter 21 for application of AFTT-A to dissociative identity disorder). Awareness of disorganization highlights the importance of paying attention to when the client needs time orientation, grounding, or other interventions related to an activated Child/Adolescent part of Self.

Individuals can move down the attachment continuum toward greater security through the development of therapeutic trust and effective interventions. An emotionally corrective therapeutic relationship (described in more detail in Chapter 17) in addition to AFTT-A protocols and EMDR therapy can shift stuck emotions and beliefs and provide healing and restructuring of the internal personality system. The therapist's use of Self and mindfulness is critical to responding therapeutically to clients' nonsecure and disorganized words and behaviors and moving clients toward "earned secure" patterns. Clients with earned attachment security will demonstrate greater self-reflective capacity, empathy for others, healthier partner relationships, and more sensitive parenting. Following restructuring of the internal system and the development of therapeutic trust and self-reflective capacity, the client's internal resources can be accessed for effective EMDR reprocessing to desensitize and integrate memories of childhood attachment trauma (Wesselmann & Potter, 2009).

POINTS TO REMEMBER

- Bowlby's IWM, beliefs about self, others, and the world, has positive or negative impact on overall functioning and interpersonal relationships that tend to persist through life without significant intervening experiences.

- The AIP model conceptualizes nonsecure and disorganized attachment patterns as related to unprocessed negative memory networks holding negative emotions, perceptions, and sensations carried into present-day relationships.

- The AFTT-A model views activated Child/Adolescent parts of Self as holding negative perceptions, emotions, and sensations related to childhood attachment relationships. The hypervigilance of the Child/Adolescent part leads to frequent activation of the Child/Adolescent part within present-day attachment relationships.

- Attachment security and non-security are on a continuum. An adult with a secure attachment designation may have a nonsecure secondary classification or a mild tendency toward a nonsecure pattern.
- Attachment patterns in children tend to persist through life unless they have emotionally impactful relationships and/or effective therapeutic interventions.
- Parents transmit their secure or nonsecure designation to their children approximately 80% of the time.
- Nonsecure adults may have difficulty with trust and assume negative instead of positive intent on the part of others.
- Nonsecure clients have challenges with utilizing therapy and developing therapeutic trust due to their natural defensive patterns and lack of self-reflective capacity.
- The unresolved/disorganized attachment pattern is activated when abuse or loss memories are triggered by adulthood relationships.
- A primary or secondary organized adulthood attachment pattern is always assigned in addition to an unresolved/disorganized pattern.
- Hypothesizing attachment patterns through clients' behaviors and words in therapy can provide the therapist with insight to provide more effective therapeutic responses.
- Adults may be unconscious to their defensive behaviors and activation of disturbing memory networks or Child/Adolescent parts of Self.

PAUSE AND REFLECT FOR THE THERAPIST

Remember that attachment security and non-security are on a continuum and that even an individual with a secure attachment pattern may have underlying tendencies toward a nonsecure pattern. It's difficult for any of us to identify our own attachment patterns or secondary and underlying tendencies due to the unconscious mechanisms that are involved. However, honest self-observation and self-reflection can help us bring some unconscious processes to conscious awareness. The more self-aware and self-reflective we are, the more we move ourselves down the attachment continuum toward greater security. A moderately secure adult can become even more secure over time.

Following are some questions to help you self-observe and self-reflect:

1. What is my comfort level with sharing my emotions with at least one other person? High ___ Fairly high ___ A little low ___ Very low ___
2. Am I more comfortable ___ less comfortable ___ with sharing my emotions today than when I was younger? ___ Or is my comfort level about the same? ___
3. How often do I have conflict with a significant other because I feel they're not doing enough to meet my needs? Very often ___ Fairly often ___ Not too often ___ Rarely ___

4. Do I feel more secure ___ less secure ___ about my relationships today than I did when I was younger? Or is my level of security about the same? ___

5. Do I have memories that I avoid because they can overwhelm me to a point that I feel ungrounded or a little disoriented? ___

Many of the "pause and reflect" activities throughout this therapist guide can help you move towards greater attachment security through self-awareness, self-nurturing, time orientation, and restructuring of your internal system. Additionally, you might consider finding another EMDR therapist to assist you with the steps in this guide and with reprocessing and integrating your childhood attachment memories.

USEFUL TERMS AND DEFINITIONS

AAI: Adult Attachment Interview

AFTT-A: Attachment-Focused Trauma Therapy for Adults

AIP: adaptive information processing

EMDR: Eye Movement Desensitization and Reprocessing

IWM: internal working model

REFERENCES

Ainsworth, M. D. S. (1978). *Patterns of attachment: A psychological study of the strange situation.* Lawrence Erlbaum Associates.

Bowlby, J. (1982). *Attachment* (2nd ed.). Basic Books.

Bretherton, I. (1987). New perspectives on attachment relations: Security, communication, and internal working models. In J. Osofsky (Ed.), *Handbook of infant development* (pp. 1061–1100). Wiley.

Fonagy, P., Steele, M., Steele, H., Moran, G. S., & Higgitt, A. C. (1991). The capacity for understanding mental states: The reflective self in parent and child and its significance for security of attachment. *Infant Mental Health Journal, 12*(3), 201–218. https://doi.org/10.1002/1097-0355(199123)12:3<201::AID-IMHJ2280120307>3.0.CO;2-7

George, C., & West, M. (2004). The Adult Attachment Projective: Measuring individual differences in attachment security using projective methodology. In M. J. Hilsenroth & D. L. Segal (Eds.), *Comprehensive handbook of psychological assessment, Vol. 2. Personality assessment* (pp. 431–447). John Wiley & Sons, Inc.

Hesse, E. (1999). The Adult Attachment Interview protocol, method of analysis, and empirical studies. In J. Cassidy & P. R. Shaver (Eds.), *Handbook of attachment: Theory, research, and clinical applications* (pp. 552–598). Guilford Press.

Levy, K. N., & Johnson, B. N. (2019). Attachment and psychotherapy: Implications from empirical research. *Canadian Psychology/Psychologie Canadienne, 60*(3), 178–193. https://doi.org/10.1037/cap0000162

Liotti, G. (2004). Trauma, dissociation, and disorganized attachment: Three strands of a single braid. *Psychotherapy: Theory, Research, Practice, Training, 41*(4), 472–486. https://doi.org/10.1037/0033-3204.41.4.472

Lyons-Ruth, K., Bronfman, E., & Parsons, E. (1999). Maternal disrupted affective communication, maternal frightened or frightening behavior, and disorganized infant attachment strategies. In

J. Vondra & D. Barnett (Eds.), *Atypical patterns of infant attachment: Theory, research and current directions. Monographs of the Society for Research in Child Development* (pp. 67–96). Wiley.

Main, M., Goldwyn, R., & Hesse, E. (2002). *Adult attachment scoring and classification systems* (Manual in draft: version 7.2). Regents of the University of California.

Main, M., Hesse, E., & Kaplan, N. (2005). Predictability of attachment behavior and representational processes at 1, 6, and 19 years of age. In K. E. Grossmann, K. Grossmann, & E. Waters (Eds.), *The Berkeley Longitudinal Study attachment from infancy to adulthood: The major longitudinal studies* (pp. 245–304). Guilford Press.

Main, M., Kaplan, N., & Cassidy, J. (1985). Security in infancy, childhood, and adulthood: A move to the level of representation. *Monographs of the Society for Research in Child Development*, 50(1/2), 66–104. https://doi.org/10.2307/3333827.JSTOR 3333827

Shapiro, F. (2018). *Eye Movement Desensitization and Reprocessing (EMDR) Therapy: Basic principles, protocols, and procedures* (3rd ed.). Guilford Press.

Sroufe, L. A. (2005). Attachment and development: A prospective, longitudinal study from birth to adulthood. *Attachment and Human Development*, 7(4), 349–367. https://doi.org/10.1080/14616730500365928

Van IJzendoorn, M. H., & Bakermans-Kranenburg, M. J. (1997). Intergenerational transmission of attachment: A move to the contextual level. In I. Atkinson & K. J. Zucker (Eds.), *Attachment and psychopathology* (pp. 135–170). Guilford Press.

Wesselmann, D., & Potter, A. E. (2009). Change in adult attachment status following treatment with EMDR: Three case studies. *Journal of EMDR Practice and Research*, 3(3), 178–191. https://doi.org/10.1891/1933-3196.3.3.178

Wesselmann, D., & Potter, A. E. (2019, September). *Attachment through the lifespan.* EMDRIA Preconference Presentation, Orange County, California.

CHAPTER 5

Framework for Attachment-Focused Trauma Therapy for Adults: Enhanced Preparation Phase of EMDR Therapy

INTRODUCTION

Shapiro regarded phase 2 of Eye Movement Desensitization and Reprocessing (EMDR) therapy as "setting the stage" for reprocessing traumatic memories (2018, p. 113). She described the preparation phase of EMDR therapy as the stage of therapy in which therapists:

- Develop therapeutic alliance with clients;
- Educate clients about all aspects and components of posttraumatic stress disorder (PTSD) and EMDR therapy, especially expectations about possible levels of disturbance during and between therapy sessions;
- Assess clients' readiness for EMDR therapy; and
- Teach clients affect regulation techniques as needed; for example, relaxation, guided imagery, Safe/Calm Place or State protocol to ready them for phases 3 to 8 (Shapiro, 2018, pp. 66, 113–123, 246–248, 251–252).

Clients with a history of attachment trauma often initiate outpatient therapy related to a combination of past and present-day issues and challenges. Such clients have complex presentations related to the adverse impact of past trauma and/or loss on all aspects of their lives; inner development; self-concept and self-esteem; effectiveness of coping and self-regulation skills; and quality of family, social, and work relationships. Attachment trauma also negatively impacts clients' tolerance for the intense affect related to resolving traumatic memories and, thus, their ability to participate fully in the trauma therapy process.

The Attachment-Focused Trauma Therapy for Adults (AFTT-A) model addresses multiple issues of clients with a history of attachment trauma by expanding the scope and enhancing and adding to the protocols of the EMDR preparation phase to address the complexities of attachment trauma. AFTT-A aims to heal the impact of attachment trauma by helping clients rebuild their internal personality structure, increase healthy interactions in significant attachment relationships, and prepare for the subsequent steps of reprocessing traumatic memories in EMDR therapy.

Cultural and Social Considerations

EMDR therapy is successfully utilized across a wide range of social, cultural, and gender (identity and affection) contexts and has addressed socially and culturally based trauma and adversity such as social exclusion and discrimination experiences. Aspects of EMDR therapy are culturally responsive (Nickerson, 2017, pp. 10–11). AFTT-A takes into account the familial, social, and cultural aspects of clients' lives in assessing and treating the impact of attachment trauma and advocates for the use of Nickerson's Attitudes, Skills, Knowledge (ASK) model in working with diverse groups (Nickerson, 2017; Sperry, 2010).

RATIONALE FOR THE AFTT-A MODEL

Attachment trauma encompasses the experiences of emotional, verbal, physical, and sexual, social, and cultural abuse and/or neglect within the context of relationships with attachment figures such as parents or other parent figures. Attachment loss includes separation from or loss of an attachment figure in childhood due to medical procedures or hospitalization, physical or mental illness, death, divorce, or adoption. Attachment trauma, also called developmental or complex trauma, is distinct from single-event trauma in several ways: Traumatic or neglectful experiences in childhood and/or adolescence are repeated over time, disrupt optimal development, lead to unmet needs and skills deficits, create unresolved traumatic memories with associated negative cognitions and affect, and cause a rupture in the trust and sense of protection in the attachment relationship itself. As a result, the impact of attachment trauma is complex and requires the EMDR preparation phase to be extended as well as augmented by strategies that address the multiple consequences to clients' internal and external lives.

The Kintsugi process of transforming broken pottery or ceramics into unique works of art that reflect strength and resilience is analogous to the AFTT-A process, offering hope and encouragement to clients with histories of attachment trauma. As shown in Figure 5.1, broken objects still have use and value even though they will not be restored to their original state nor can the damage done to them be hidden or disguised. Instead, the evidence of repair is accentuated and emphasized by highlighting it with golden resin. The parallels between the Kintsugi method and the AFTT-A model teach clients that their own True Essence is not determined by past events but instead is revealed and strengthened, thus, experiencing a "new beginning … from the rubble of the past" (Kitty, 2020, p. 9).

Past experiences of attachment trauma cannot be undone. The impact is only temporarily covered over or avoided without corrective emotional experiences such as therapeutic relationships. Clients with histories of attachment trauma are not the same persons they were prior to traumatic events. They won't be the person they might or could have been if they had not experienced childhood attachment trauma. They choose the healing process of therapy to move beyond a search for a former version of themselves or the repair of broken pieces; they transform themselves into someone who is connected to their Essence of goodness and their spiritual core, has reconstructed their internal system, and is capable of living fully their present-day lives through their Authentic Self.

UNDERLYING ASSUMPTIONS GUIDING AFTT-A THERAPISTS

Like the Kintsugi process of transforming broken pottery into unique works of art that embrace their history, the primary purpose of the preparation phase in the AFTT-A

5. FRAMEWORK FOR ATTACHMENT-FOCUSED TRAUMA THERAPY FOR ADULTS 41

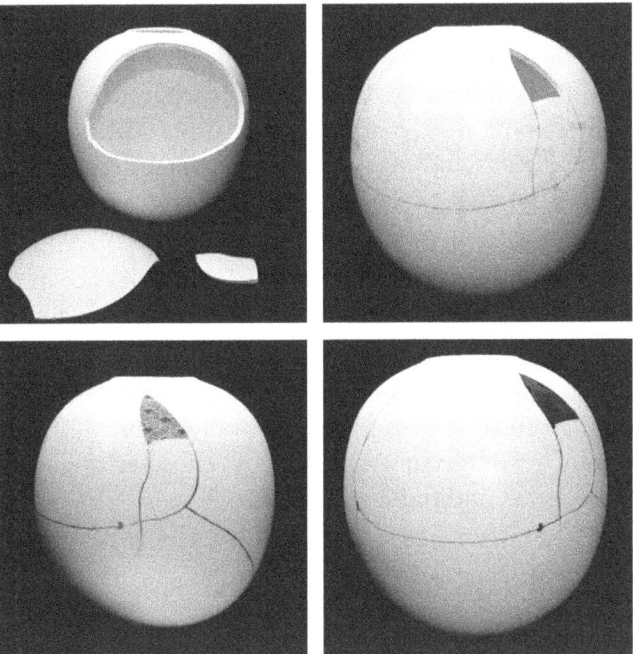

FIGURE 5.1 Client transformation process through AFTT-A: A Kintsugi analogy.
Source: Courtesy of Kintsugi by Myriam Greff.

model is to rebuild clients' personalities or internal systems into healthy, strong structures with the Competent Adult part of Self mediating and regulating internal functioning, taking charge of present-day life and relationships, and participating in all aspects of trauma therapy (Figure 5.1). The AFTT-A model holds underlying assumptions about both clients and therapists that guide therapists in their approach to working with clients who experienced attachment trauma.

Underlying assumptions about therapists emphasize how essential their self-awareness and willingness to do their own emotional work is to clients' healing process. When therapists have their own unresolved issues, their clarity, intuitive knowing, and ability to form healthy attachments with clients are hindered. Since therapists hold a sacred space for clients' emotions, beliefs, and experiences in sessions, they must be free of their own unresolved memories and associated beliefs, emotions, and sensations so they can attune to clients and the therapy process in the present moment. Thus, they create the corrective emotional relationships with clients that are crucial to their transformative therapeutic experience.

In addition to the importance of therapists' self-awareness and mindful attunement to the therapy process, the AFTT-A model also has several underlying beliefs about clients themselves that therapists use as guidelines for therapeutic interventions:

- The impact of attachment trauma goes beyond symptoms of posttraumatic stress caused by discrete adverse childhood events so the scope of the AFTT-A model extends to address and heal the ways in which experiences with attachment figures and within a social and cultural context negatively affected the structure and maturing of the internal personality system, formation of healthy and balanced external attachment relationships, and development of life skills.

- Time disorientation of internal parts that cannot separate present-day situations or circumstances from past traumatic events or unsafe attachment relationships underlies much of clients' challenges in adult life and relationships so the condition of clients' internal personality structure and functioning is reflected in the state of their present-day relationships.
- Although attachment trauma causes clients to feel an absence of or a disconnection from their Spiritual Essence or their sense of core Goodness, their Essence is not lost or damaged.
- All clients have the parts of Self, resources, and inner wisdom they need to heal themselves and their relationships as well as resolve traumatic memories and the development of a Competent Adult part of Self is key to clients' sense of competence, confidence, and self-compassion.

FRAMEWORK FOR THE AFTT-A MODEL

The AFTT-A process includes the five segments of differentiation, protection. nurturing and strengthening, reconnection, and integration. Some of the elements are integrated throughout all steps and protocols while other elements are central to one or two parts of the AFTT-A model. *Differentiation* is part of the initial stages of the AFTT-A process and refers to the individuation of inner enmeshed or blended individual parts of Self with firm and flexible boundaries, distinguishing between the past and present through time orientation, containing negative thoughts and affect during therapy tasks, and creating firm and flexible boundaries in relationships in adult life. In addition to providing an essential sense of individuation among internal parts and between clients and people in their adult lives, firm and flexible boundaries also provide a sense of protection and safety. *Protection* in the AFTT-A model refers to parts of the internal personality system attaining and maintaining time orientation and clients developing a sense of inner safety in challenging present-day situations.

Nurturing and strengthening describe the aspect of the AFTT-A protocols that enhance and deepen positive affective shifts through the use of slow, short sets of bilateral stimulation (BLS). Elements of nurturing and acceptance augment qualities of safety and protection through protocols that create internal spaces and attachment experiences, form new Bonding Contract rules, transform negative cognitions into messages of encouragement and unshakable beliefs about inherent worth and value, and foster client competence and confidence in healthy present-day relationships. *Reconnection* denotes the next segment in the AFTT-A model in which parts of Self re-form healthy and balanced internal attachments to their Spiritual Essence and to each other as well as the inner personality system as a whole.

The final building block in the AFTT-A process is *Integration*. Clients ultimately develop a cohesive internal system that empowers them to form and enjoy healthy adult attachments. The positive affective shifts in both their inner system and their present-day life builds confidence and stability prior to the reprocessing phases of EMDR therapy.

GOALS

The purposes of the AFTT-A preparation phase are three-fold: (a) rebuilding clients' internal personality structure, (b) increasing healthy interactions in significant attachment relationships, and (c) preparing clients for the subsequent EMDR therapy steps of reprocessing traumatic memories. To achieve the purposes of the AFTT-A preparation phase, two main goals address both therapist- and client-related issues.

Therapist Use of Self and the Corrective Emotional Relationship

Working with clients with histories of attachment trauma can be challenging. Those of us who have our own histories of attachment trauma have the added responsibility to recognize our own unfinished business and how it could negatively impact therapy with clients.

As therapists, we utilize mindful attunement to clients. To create corrective emotional experiences with clients within the therapy relationship, we demonstrate a compassionate presence, openness, and nonjudgmental perspective in therapy sessions to help clients accomplish their therapy goals. Clients experience, perhaps for the first time, what it is like to have someone else attuned to what they feel and who they are without judgment within a safe and nurturing environment. Through this experience, over time, clients grow in their ability to reflect upon their own inner state and to acknowledge their emotions without judgment, decreasing automatic defenses and increasing their ability to ride out their emotions in a healthy way.

To be present and attuned to clients, we pay attention to our own reactions, emotions, and self-beliefs in sessions. AFTT-A invites us to examine challenging client relationships and stuck-points in therapy as opportunities to become aware of and resolve our own unfinished business with the past so that we don't have to divide our attention between our issues and the clients' issues in therapy sessions. We ask clients to be brave; to face perhaps the most difficult situations, relationships, and memories of their lives. We owe it to our clients to be willing to show the same level of courage in resolving our own issues. When we do our work in our own therapy, we are freed to be present in the moment in sessions and to use our perceptions, experiences, and intuitions in ways that attune to clients on a deep, emotional level and foster the creation of a safe and nurturing attachment relationship.

Therapists who are willing to look at themselves and do work in their own therapy open the way for clients to make progress in therapy unimpeded by the impact of their therapists' blind spots, triggers, and/or nonsecure ways of interacting in therapy. Clients benefit from mindful therapists who are willing to clear out their own issues and the associated negative cognitions and affect and, as a result, who have more capacity to be present and attuned in therapy sessions.

Culturally competent therapists develop what Nickerson calls "cultural humility," a mindset of openness and curiosity about, respect for, and responsiveness to the social and cultural diversity in clients' lives and the impact on clients' experience in therapy. AFTT-A therapists do more than assess clients' social and cultural influences. They initiate discussions about social and cultural issues within the trusting therapeutic relationship; convey respect for cultural perspectives and values; acknowledge the impact of exclusion, discrimination, and stigma; and adopt socially and culturally sensitive strategies and techniques. As a result, they actively create a sense of acceptance, safety, and comfort in which clients can share social and cultural identities and experiences as a part of the corrective emotional relationship (Nickerson, 2017, pp. 7–12).

Reclaiming the Authentic Self

Clients work through the AFTT-A protocols aimed at reclaiming and empowering their Authentic Self. They access and strengthen their Competent Adult part of Self through a step-wise series of protocols in AFTT-A that enables them to reconstruct their inner personality system, redefine roles and functions for inner parts, and create healthy internal and external attachment relationships. The AFTT-A protocols assist clients to reclaim their Authentic Self by

- accessing and strengthening the Competent Adult part of Self to orchestrate the internal personality system and manage adult life;
- creating an inner team of resources to connect clients to their own strengths;
- nurturing and protecting Child parts internally to establish time orientation and decrease Child parts' need to meet unmet childhood needs in adult life;
- developing a True Parent part of Self to create an internal network of healthy attachment relationships;
- transforming negative cognitions into unshakable beliefs of "I'm okay," "I am lovable," "No matter what, I have what I need," and "I am not alone anymore";
- integrating reconstructed parts of Self into an internal system that acts as a functioning whole;
- strengthening positive experiences related to cultural and social identity; and
- exploring and healing negative aspects of social and cultural identity and adverse experiences.

STEPS

Assessment

AFTT-A therapists conduct a detailed and comprehensive initial assessment which provides them with: (a) an overall estimation of clients' past and current physical and mental health status, level of present-day functioning, cultural and social strengths and support, family history, experiences of abuse and/or neglect, and past and present issues, and (b) information needed to develop a treatment plan, including clients' readiness to start EMDR therapy. Such an assessment offers therapists the context in which clients will be participating in EMDR therapy.

A thorough evaluation of the presence and extent of client dissociation is essential before employing any technique that aims to differentiate personality parts, since clients with a more extensive level of dissociation already have distinct parts (see Chapter 6). Therapists also need to assess their therapeutic techniques for the potential to exacerbate dissociation.

Therapists also utilize the assessment process to begin identifying unmet childhood needs, patterns in adult life learned in childhood, extent of emotion regulation skills (including but not limited to containment and mindfulness), and individual parts of personality as well as the overall functioning of their internal system.

Psychosocial Education

Providing psychosocial education in early therapy sessions is essential for clients to have a clear understanding of the therapeutic process they're undertaking, such as what to expect from the therapy including AFTT-A process and procedures. AFTT-A psychosocial education also contains information about

- personality development and attachment patterns in both optimal/validating and nonoptimal/invalidating environments;
- cultural and social identities and influences;
- impact of attachment trauma on adult abilities, skills, behaviors, and relationships; and
- purposes, goals, and steps of AFTT-A–enhanced EMDR preparation phase.

Psychosocial education builds a cognitive foundation upon which clients accomplish the deeply emotional work of reconstructing their internal system as well as resolving the impact of traumatic childhood events and damaged attachment relationships. Psychosocial education also helps clients remain on a cognitive level when first discussing emotionally charged and potentially dysregulating material.

To reprocess and apply cognitive information, clients need to engage what we call their Competent Adult part of Self, "Adult Brain," or "Thinking Brain;" the parts of the brain that include abstract reasoning, self-reflection, and the competencies to modify clients' self-beliefs and self-perception as well as modulate emotions and behaviors. The AFTT-A model views EMDR therapy's adaptive information processing (AIP) system as a part of clients' "Adult Brain" or "Thinking Brain." Learning new information early in the therapy process stimulates the Adult part of the brain AFTT-A wants to strengthen and opens the possibility of challenging and transforming long-held or well-ingrained cognitions formed through attachment trauma.

Sequence of AFTT-A Protocols

The AFTT-A model consists of a sequence of protocols that serve as building blocks for clients to

- reconnect to the core of their Spiritual Essence;
- transform their internal personality structure;
- access and activate inner resources composed as a supportive team;
- form healthy boundaries among internal parts and in present-day relationships;
- separate the present moment ("now") from the past ("back then") so all parts of Self are oriented to time;
- develop and strengthen Competent Adult and True Parent parts of Self for improved self-nurturing, self-acceptance, confidence, and inner sense of safety and protection;

- replace old Bonding Contract rules with new rules for present-day relationships;
- create a cohesive and organized narrative about past events and present-day life in the form of a Therapeutic Story;
- learn skills needed in present-day life and relationships; and
- integrate new inner structure, resources, skills, beliefs, and sense of Self into tasks of EMDR therapy phases 3 to 8.

The *Checklist for AFTT-A Steps* assists therapists to monitor a client's progress through the AFTT-A process as well as completion of individual protocols and assignments. The checklist also reminds therapists of the sequence and details included in AFTT-A steps and protocols (see Exhibit 22.1 in Chapter 22 or access the form online through Springer Publishing Connect: Use the code on the opening page of this book to access the digital product and select Chapter 22).

Explain the P-A-C (Parent-Adult-Child) Diagrams for Validating and Invalidating Childhood Environments

The first three protocols are comprised of psychosocial education about the personality model utilized in AFTT-A. Therapists help clients understand how personality is developed through childhood into adulthood and how personality development is negatively impacted by attachment trauma, both by experiencing traumatic and/or neglectful incidents and the rupture in their primary attachment relationship(s). Clients take time to explore their own personal, social, and cultural histories in light of new information and, at the same time, begin the process of engaging their Competent Adult part of Self in the therapy process.

Create a Safe Place With a Higher Power for the Adult Part of Self

In order to meet the needs of the Adult part of Self for nurturing and safety and to offer clients a sense of respite and calm both in their present-day life and in the therapy process, AFTT-A enhances EMDR's Safe/Calm Place/State protocol by adding a relational element to the place in the form of a Higher Power. The Higher Power figure also embodies the same qualities of acceptance and protectiveness as the Safe Place, thus strengthening clients' sense of inner support and security. The first protocol also initiates the separation between the Adult part and other parts of Self; in particular, Child parts.

Design the Safe Place With a Higher Power for Enmeshed/Blended/Cut-Off Child Parts of Self

Clients with a history of attachment trauma often have under- and overdeveloped inner parts of Self and a personality system that had not been given the tools to function as a whole. Since personality parts were developed in childhood and clients were not afforded the experiences essential to grow and mature, they were not fully formed and tend to utilize child-like thinking and repeat behaviors modeled for them by others to get their needs met even in their adult lives where the patterns are no longer helpful or useful.

The second step in separating the Competent Adult part from Child parts of Self is to create a similar but age-appropriate place for Child parts where they get their needs for caring and security met within the context of a healthy attachment relationship with an age-appropriate Higher Power figure. Therapists assist clients to reassure inner Child parts that, in the present moment, all their needs are being met and that as long as they stay in their Safe Place with their Higher Power, their needs will continue to be met. As a result, Child parts no longer need to attempt to get their unmet childhood needs met in the clients' adult lives. Clients create firm and flexible boundaries between their Adult and Child parts of Self so their younger parts realize and begin to accept that they cannot redo their childhoods through the wishful, magical thinking of "If only" or "Maybe this time" in the clients' adult lives and relationships.

Build a Team of Inner Resources for the Adult Part of Self

Clients with a history of attachment trauma have many negative beliefs about themselves, others, and the world. They often see themselves with many faults and few strengths. The AIP model explains that traumatic memories are stored in separate memory networks in unprocessed form, along with associated affect and negative perceptions or beliefs. Clients with stored trauma view the world through the lens of negative perceptions that fall into four categories: (a) personal defectiveness or feeling at fault things for which they weren't responsible; (b) powerlessness, helplessness, or lack of control; (c) lack of safety; and (d) lack of connection or belonging. Trauma-based perceptions have a negative impact on relationships and general functioning in the world.

AFTT-A therapists have an unshakable belief that clients have all the inner resources and strengths they need to complete the therapy process and to have healthy and satisfying relationships. Through the next protocol in the AFTT-A model, clients access and strengthen the positive qualities they need to transform themselves on the inside, learn life skills, resolve past trauma, and develop healthy present-day relationships. As with the Safe Place protocols, the Resource Team protocol enhances EMDR therapy's Resource Development and Installation (RDI; Korn & Leeds, 2002; Leeds, 2016; Luber, 2016; Parnell, 2007; Shapiro, 2018) by adding a relational aspect to resource development in the form of a team. Clients experience corrective attachment relationships between themselves and their Resource Team members.

Strengthen the Competent Adult Part of Self

After Child parts of Self are differentiated from the Competent Adult part of Self and provided protection, the Competent Adult part of Self is strengthened. Utilizing EMDR therapy's RDI model (Leeds, 2016; Shapiro, 2018), AFTT-A clinicians invite clients to access memories in which they experienced feelings of competence, paying special attention to the posture, facial expression, and voice tone associated with their Competent Adult part of Self. A slow, short set of BLS is utilized to deepen the positive state with a cue word to represent the positive memory. AFTT-A clinicians invite clients to imaginally rehearse bringing their Competent Adult part of Self to a future challenging situation as part of the RDI procedure and to practice accessing the Competent Adult part of Self regularly between sessions to increase healthy functioning and differentiation from Child parts of Self.

Create an Attachment Experience for the True Parent and Child Parts of Self

Clients with a history of attachment trauma often experienced rejection and criticism during their childhood years and had no opportunity to experience real nurturing for themselves. Without adequate nurturing while growing up, they may struggle with providing nurturing to others. The *Corrective Attachment Experiences Between the Child/ Adolescent and True Parent Parts of Self* protocol promotes development of a nurturing True Parent part of Self and facilitates the development of a healthy attachment between the differentiated Adult and Child parts of Self. The protocol is conducted as a guided imagery that provides options and invites clients to make adjustments so the process is as comfortable as possible for the client. The True Parent part of Self is invited to enter the Safe Place developed for the Child part and to make contact with the Child part through the eyes or through some type of touch, if possible. AFTT-A clinicians facilitate nurturing dialogue from the True Parent part to the Child part that conveys worth, lovability, worthiness, safety, and freedom from responsibilities or worry. Slow BLS is applied to deepen the positive affect associated with the nurturing imagery and dialogue.

Parts' Work: Negotiate New Roles With the Parent and Adult Parts of Self

Client personality structure also consists of other parts that are not fully formed, such as the underdeveloped Nurturing Parent, the overdeveloped Critical Parent, and the overdeveloped version (Emotion Controller-Regulator) or underdeveloped version (little "a") of the Adult part of Self. AFTT-A utilizes a meeting format with the client and their Resource Team so parts of Self that have unhealthy patterns and/or boundaries can work to change with team support and guidance, and the Competent Adult and True Parent parts of Self can connect to and integrate with already-integrated inner resources.

Clients meet with their Resource Team and the parts of themselves that learned through experience and example during childhood less than effective ways to give encouragement, set limits, make decisions, and regulate emotions and behavior. Much like a job interview, the team examines parts' roles, motives, and history with the client. At the same time, the Resource Team educates the client and their parts about how (even though the parts were developed to serve essential functions for the client and they had the client's best interests at heart) they were not given needed information, tools, and skills from attachment figures to do their jobs in ways that were helpful or useful.

The strengthened Competent Adult and True Parent parts of Self begin to mentor, teach, and work together with the old Emotion Controller-Regulator or the little "a" and Critical Parent parts as well as with the client Resource Team to perform the key roles of nurturing, protection, and offering leadership to the inner personality system while taking charge of present-day life.

Parts' Work: Tuck Child Parts Into Safe Places

Therapists prepare clients for the possibility that, even though they have installed Child Parts in a Safe Place with a Higher Power in a previous protocol, those younger parts may not *stay* "tucked into" their Safe Places. When Child parts are "in charge" of a client's adult life, they tend to continue to play the roles they played in childhood. They need help to understand that continuing to act as a peacekeeper, caretaker, comedian, whistleblower, or victim in clients' adult relationships will neither make up for their losses in childhood nor will be helpful to clients in getting their adulthood needs met. The Child parts need to be reassured that the only jobs they have in the present moment are to be the age that they are and get all of their needs met in their Safe Places with their Higher Powers.

Tucking Child parts of Self into their Safe Places continues the process of differentiation from the Competent Adult part of Self. The first step is identifying Child parts of Self with their associated affect and behaviors. Therapists ask clients to begin to step back and observe themselves even during assessment and psychoeducational sessions, which helps them recognize when they are in "Kid Brain" or their Child state or when their Child part of Self "sneaks out" of their Safe Place to "eavesdrop" on their adult life. Clients in their "Adult Brain" can note certain body sensations and postures, overwhelming feelings, numbing out, long-standing negative cognitions, and urges to use old patterns of behaviors—signs that their Child part is involved in their adult life and not oriented to time. Through the *Tucking the Child/Adolescent Part of Self Into the Safe Place* protocol, therapists guide clients to work with their Child part about how they were triggered to leave their Safe Place and what reassurances and boundaries they need to return their Safe Places so the Competent Adult part of Self can manage present-day relationships and situations.

Revise the Early Bonding Contract

Infants and young children raised in nonoptimal environments learn to adapt their behaviors to prevent their parents from distancing physically and emotionally. They learn the behaviors that allow their parents to bond with them in whatever way they can. Their parents' proximity ensures the infants' survival. The adaptive behaviors become the unspoken rules of the Early Bonding Contract. Later, the early rules prevent healthy functioning in relationships. The *Revising the Early Bonding Contract Rules* protocol helps clients identify the old rules and possible new rules. The protocol guides clients in releasing Child parts of Self from worry about consequences for changing behaviors in adulthood relationships. The protocol suggests imagery that allows clients to imagine living by the new rules "at some point in the future, when it feels comfortable to do so." Slow BLS is applied for enhancing and deepening affective shifts.

Create an Organized, Coherent Internal Narrative Through the Therapeutic Story

One sign of attachment disorganization is disorientation related to one's childhood narrative. The *Creating the Therapeutic Story* protocol involves creating a sequence of events and writing a third-person story that very briefly describes traumatic events and makes sense of them with the inclusion of helpful, adaptive information (Lovett, 1999, 2015). BLS is applied at a speed of the client's choosing throughout the first reading of the story as well as additional readings of the story, to assist the client with reprocessing and integrating their story as a whole. Later, the story can be read again to identify memories that retain an emotional charge for EMDR reprocessing.

Get the Client's Permission to Transition to EMDR Phases 3 to 8 and Time Orientation

Up to this point in the AFTT-A process, clients installed Safe Places and Higher Powers for their Adult and Child parts of Self as well as a Resource Team including the newly reconfigured Critical Parent and Emotion Controller-Regulator. They reconnected with their spiritual core and inner strengths. They created new Bonding Contract rules and developed a cohesive narrative about past events and present-day life. They learned life skills and healthy boundaries. They healed their internal system and empowered their authentic Adult Self to be in charge of their inner personality structure and their adult life. They have grown in their capacity to self-reflect. They are ready to move to the phase 3 of EMDR therapy.

The preparation phase's protocols focused on connecting to and strengthening positive affect; inner strengths, resources, and skills; and reconstructing clients' internal personality system. Clients will next move into EMDR phases 3 to 8 which involve protocols targeting and resolving traumatic memories and their associated negative affect. AFTT-A emphasizes the importance of gaining clients' permission to begin the transition to trauma reprocessing.

The *Getting Client's Permission to Transition to EMDR Therapy Phases 3 to 8* protocol utilizes a Resource Team meeting as one of the final steps in AFTT-A's extended and enhanced version of EMDR's preparation phase. Clients bring together all parts of Self including the True Parent and the Competent Adult with their team members to obtain approval from all parts of clients for moving ahead in the therapy process. Child parts of Self do not attend the meeting but can communicate through an assigned team member. The main purposes of the Resource Team meeting in the *Getting Client's Permission to Transition to EMDR Therapy Phases 3 to 8* protocol are to

- talk through any doubts, fears, or misconceptions among team members and parts of Self about moving into the next therapy steps;
- ensure all inner parts are oriented to time (Martin, 2018);
- brainstorm ideas for handling potential barriers or stuck points in the subsequent therapy phases; and
- confirm the team's commitment to help clients make the shift from the AFTT-A preparation phase to identifying and resolving adverse childhood events.

Integrate Learning From the AFTT-A Enhanced EMDR Preparation Phase to Phases 3 to 8/Future Rehearsal

After clients resolve issues and form a plan with their Resource Team to apply to phases 3 to 8, therapists use the *Transition From the AFTT-A Preparation Phase to EMDR Phases 3 to 8* protocol to help them visualize and connect a sense of competence and confidence to undertaking the next steps in EMDR therapy. Clients imagine potential barriers or challenges with upcoming steps or tasks in therapy and therapists assist them to envision successfully overcoming the imagined difficulties using the Future Rehearsal protocol. Clients access and strengthen positive affect related to application of their reconstructed internal personality system and skills they learned through AFTT-A preparation phase protocols to subsequent therapy tasks. Clients utilize their new Bonding Contract rules and their team of inner resources including their Competent Adult and True Parent parts of Self to foster their belief in themselves and their ability to heal whatever adversities they will face in EMDR phases 3 to 8.

POINTS TO REMEMBER

- AFTT-A enhances and extends the preparation phase of EMDR therapy to address and resolve issues specific to attachment trauma.
- AFTT-A bases its therapy model on underlying assumptions about both clients and therapists.
- AFTT-A's goals and steps go beyond preparing clients for the subsequent EMDR therapy's steps of reprocessing traumatic memories by rebuilding clients' internal personality structures, offering a corrective emotional experience in therapy, and increasing healthy interactions in significant present-day attachment relationships.
- Time orientation in all clients' parts of Self is crucial to recovery from attachment trauma and is integrated throughout the AFTT-A process.

PAUSE AND REFLECT FOR THE THERAPIST

Find some quiet time to think about your clinical training and experiences. As you read the chapter, have you already identified clients the AFTT-A process might help? Are there aspects of the AFTT-A model you find personally uncomfortable? Will you be willing to explore your own reactions, emotions, and cognitions that may be related to your own childhood history and their potential impact on your therapeutic capacities, perceptions, and attunement in therapy sessions?

USEFUL TERMS AND DEFINITIONS

"Adult Brain": The parts of the brain that house EMDR's adaptive information processing (AIP) system and include higher cognitive processes such as learning, problem-solving, decision-making, language, understanding of emotions, and narrative memory.

AFTT-A: Attachment-Focused Trauma Therapy for Adults

BLS: bilateral stimulation

"Kid Brain": The neural network clusters in the emotional/social part of the brain that store unprocessed memories of adverse events and are disconnected from a sense of time and from the parts of the brain capable of processing memories and transferring them into narrative memory. AFTT-A views the neural networks as encapsulating more than memories of adverse events and includes the experiences, cognitive development, and learning during a particular client age.

P-A-C Diagram: Parent-Adult-Child Diagram

RDI: Resource Development and Installation

REFERENCES

Kitty, A. (2020). *The art of Kintsugi: Learning the Japanese craft of beautiful repair*. Schiffer Publishing.

Korn, D. L., & Leeds, A. M. (2002). Preliminary evidence of efficacy for EMDR resource development and installation in the stabilization phase of treatment of complex posttraumatic stress disorder. *Journal of Clinical Psychology, 58*(12), 1465–1487. https://doi.org/10.1002/jclp.10099

Leeds, A. (2016). *A guide to the standard EMDR protocols for clinicians, supervisors, and consultants* (2nd ed.). Springer Publishing Company.

Lovett, J. (1999). *Small wonders: Healing childhood trauma with EMDR*. Free Press/Simon & Schuster.

Lovett, J. (2015). *Trauma-attachment tangle: Modifying EMDR to help children resolve trauma and develop loving relationships*. Routledge/Taylor & Francis Group.

Luber, M. (Ed.). (2016). *Eye Movement Desensitization and Reprocessing (EMDR) therapy scripted protocols and summary sheets: Treating trauma- and stressor-related conditions*. Springer Publishing Company.

Martin, K. (2018, April). *Mastering the treatment of complex trauma: Transforming theory into practice*. Presentation, Omaha, Nebraska.

Nickerson, M. (Ed.). (2017). *Cultural competence and healing culturally based trauma with EMDR therapy*. Springer Publishing Company.

Parnell, L. (2007). *A therapist's guide to EMDR: Tools and techniques for successful treatment*. W. W. Norton & Company.

Shapiro, F. (2018). *Eye Movement Desensitization and Reprocessing (EMDR) therapy: Basic principles, protocols, and procedures* (3rd ed.). Guilford Press.

Sperry, L. (2010). *Core competencies in counseling and psychotherapy: Becoming a highly competent and effective therapist*. Taylor & Francis Group, LLC.

CHAPTER 6

Assessment of Client Readiness and Treatment Planning for EMDR Therapy in Attachment-Focused Trauma Therapy for Adults

INTRODUCTION

Therapists offer clients a corrective emotional experience from the first contact over the phone or via email. A therapist's conveyance of unconditional acceptance, being present in the moment, and kind but firm boundaries is critical to forming a therapeutic relationship in which clients have a sense of safety. Clients experience their therapist's experience, skills, and compassion through a detailed and comprehensive initial interview. It's important for clients to know that their therapist wants to know them for who they are as persons, their past experiences as well as their current life and relationships, while still attuning to and understanding their perspective about the traumatic events that bring them to therapy.

Assessing client readiness for Eye Movement Desensitization and Reprocessing (EMDR) therapy in Attachment-Focused Trauma Therapy for Adults (AFTT-A) includes an initial assessment completed according to state standards and professional ethical guidelines. The initial client interview consists of information clients will need to give informed consent for therapy, a comprehensive review of clients in multiple areas, and a mental status examination. Clients can complete general screening and objective tests as well as measures used to evaluate impact of trauma and readiness for EMDR prior to their first session or between initial sessions and therapists may want to obtain corroborative information from safe family members or friends. Therapists utilize the assessment information to derive diagnostic impressions, therapy goals, and an initial treatment plan.

Social and cultural aspects of clients' lives are integrated throughout the assessment process. AFTT-A therapists learn about their clients' cultural, religious/nonreligious and social identities; the importance of culture to their sense of Self, resources, and strengths; the level of clients' openness to exploring their social identities as well as their own social biases and prejudices; and the relevance to clients' needs and therapy goals (Nickerson, 2017, pp. 31, 50–74).

INITIAL ASSESSMENT

Purposes

Therapists complete initial assessments with clients according to the standards of state licensure statutes and guidelines from relevant professional organizations. A detailed and comprehensive initial assessment is essential to therapists' ability to establish clients' readiness for therapy in general and specifically for EMDR therapy. The initial assessment includes evaluating clients in multiple areas in addition to the EMDR readiness criteria. Such an assessment provides therapists with an overall estimation of clients' past and current physical and mental health status, level of functioning, social support, family history, and experiences of abuse and/or neglect as well as the current life context in which clients come to EMDR therapy.

Felitti and Anda studied the negative impact of adverse childhood experiences on physical and mental health and social, legal, and economic aspects of adult life. Adverse Childhood Experiences (ACEs) studies showed that traumatic events and/or unstable circumstances in childhood were highly correlated with adulthood issues such as chronic health and mental health problems, substance abuse, challenges in attaining and maintaining positive and secure relationships, and even increased vulnerability to further victimization (Felitti, 2002).

Even in the first session while collecting information from clients, mindful therapists utilize their expertise and intuition to note how the Child, Critical Parent, and Emotion Controller-Regulator/little "a" parts of Self potentially impact clients' present-day lives. Therapists also observe client's behavior, tone of voice, and body posture and language, and begin to identify possibly enmeshed or blended Child parts, negative messages from a Critical Parent part, and emotional over- or under-control by the Emotion Controller-Regulator part of Self.

Components

As therapists, we want to create an atmosphere of ease and encouragement for clients when they first come to therapy. In a situation where clients often feel vulnerable and uncertain, we want clients to feel as much as possible that they are in charge of the process. Giving clients a choice about where they sit in the office or asking whether or not they want something to drink (if that's something you offer to clients) are simple ways to help them feel at ease and comfortable. My (A.P.) approach is to chat with clients before getting started; perhaps asking them if they had any difficulty finding the office or have any questions about or problems accessing or filling out the paperwork that was sent them to complete before the first session.

INFORMED CONSENT

Since informed consent is required for clients when signing a Consent to Treatment form, they need to know what to expect from therapy. Inclusion of a Therapist Disclosure Statement (see Exhibit 22.2 in Chapter 22*) in clients' initial paperwork is a concise and organized way is to give clients necessary information. Disclosure statements consist of

- therapists' education, licensure, and certification;
- therapy approaches that will be used including the benefits and risks of specific therapies;

---

*Access all of the forms discussed in this chapter online through Springer Publishing Connect: Use the code on the opening page of this book to access the digital product and select Chapter 22.

- clarification about the nature of the therapy relationship;
- what constitutes therapy-related emergencies between sessions and the purpose of and protocols for emergency contact;
- fees for service, late-cancellations, and no-show appointments;
- expectations about payment and insurance coverage (if applicable); and
- therapy termination either when clients have accomplished their goals or when there is need to terminate therapy prior to clients completing their goals.

Based on decades of clinical experience, I (A.P.) find it essential to educate clients at the beginning of therapy about therapy in general and specifically expectations about therapy and the therapy relationship. For example, I realized that clients who have a history of attachment trauma often ask for between-session contact with their therapist in a variety of ways, the most evident being crisis or emergency calls. I utilize the Dialectical Behavioral Therapy (DBT) phone call protocol which encourages clients to contact their therapists for coaching in between sessions with several ground rules: Contact is short in length and not meant to revisit in-depth situations or circumstances or solve long-standing problems and is focused on how clients can use skills to decrease suicidal ideation or urges to self-harm, cope effectively with crisis situations, or repair therapeutic relationship in between the time of contact and when they come for their next session. Clients agree to accept help and to feel better by the end of contact with their therapist since one of the purposes of contact is to help clients learn to ask for help effectively and to generalize coping skills in their present-day life (Linehan, 1993, pp. 190, 326–327, 497–503).

Another example of initial client education is discussing therapy termination. I want clients to know up front that even ending therapy is a process; that it's a thoughtful series of mutual decisions based on clients' improvement and is paced to maximize clients' maintaining their progress over time. On the other hand, termination might be considered when there are issues in therapy (e.g., client regularly misses appointments, comes late, or doesn't follow through with assignments), in the therapy relationship (e.g., client is consistently critical of therapy and/or therapist, therapist believes client needs are beyond their level of expertise, or there is a personality conflict that can't be resolved), or the client isn't making progress.

Sometimes, therapists are reluctant to discuss the financial side of therapy but talking about money at the beginning of therapy helps clients understand the business side of therapy and prevents future misunderstandings; that a therapy appointment is like an appointment with their primary care physician where payment is expected at the time of service. I'm not sure how the idea developed that the financial aspects of services with a mental health provider are somehow different than those with other health providers but an initial discussion about financial responsibilities at the beginning of therapy clarifies any confusion about therapist's policies and provides the opportunity to discuss exceptions and negotiate arrangements based on client need or circumstances, if needed.

As of January 1, 2022, according to the "No Surprises Act," therapists are required to provide an estimate of expected charges (called a "good faith estimate") to clients who are uninsured, who pay for healthcare bills themselves (who don't have claims submitted to their healthcare plan), or for whom the therapist services are out-of-network. The estimate must include all items and services associated with scheduled appointments and contain details of the assigned healthcare codes and expected charges. The estimate should be provided to clients within a certain time frame after an appointment for services has been scheduled and prior to client reception of services. An estimate can be explained over the phone or in-person per client request with the provision of a follow-up written (paper or electronic) estimate (Centers for Medicare & Medicaid Services, 2022).

It's also important for clients to know that, in addition to gathering clinical information, another goal of the first session is for both the client and the therapist to decide whether they'll be a good fit for working together in therapy. I learned over the years not to give clients the idea that it's a "given" we will work together. I make sure we take time at the end of the first or second session (depending on how long the initial assessment takes) to make a joint decision about starting therapy. Clients and I review my disclosure statement and introductory information about EMDR therapy. I also encourage them to ask questions and voice concerns since one of the goals of the first session is for clients to know that they can interrupt or stop the interview if they need to or postpone talking about certain areas if they feel uncomfortable.

Initial Interview

I start initial interviews by giving clients the choice about how to start our first interview; for example, "How would you like to start? I can ask my usual questions. Or you can start by telling me a little about why you've come to see me for therapy." I don't worry about how the interview starts because I know that I will eventually cover all the areas I need to complete for the initial evaluation and I would rather offer clients the opportunity to feel more secure and less vulnerable by choosing how the interview begins.

An initial interview includes multiple areas of evaluation: reasons that bring clients to therapy at a particular time; a review of client's educational, job, religious, social, current family and family of origin, legal, medical, mental health, drug and alcohol, and trauma history; and a Mental Status Examination. The initial interview might be organized with the following outline (see Exhibit 22.3 in Chapter 22):

- Reason for therapy/presenting issue
  - Major symptoms with recent examples, triggers, contributing factors, and desired future changes (Leeds, 2016; Shapiro, 2018, 2021a, 2021b)
- History-taking
  - Highest level of education
  - Job/career—Include length of jobs, reason for leaving jobs, job satisfaction
  - Religious/nonreligious preference
  - Social—Friends (past and present, close or acquaintance), group affiliations, gender identity and affection
  - Cultural—Groups that are important to identity, how they understand themselves and their issues in a cultural context. Include strong beliefs or prejudices

- Family—Significant relationships and marriages (first name, age, length of relationship), children (first names and ages)
- Family of origin—Parents or primary caregivers (first names and ages or age at death, year of death, cause of death, divorces, remarriages); siblings (first names and ages); family history of mental illness and/or problems with substances or other addictions (include parents, grandparents, aunts, uncles, siblings, and cousins, diagnosed or undiagnosed)
- Follow-up information about significant relationships and/or marriages and family of origin—Quality of relationships; parents' personalities during client's childhood/adolescence, current relationships with parents and during childhood/adolescence, description of parents' relationship/marriage, what client learned about relationships from parents, current relationships with siblings and during childhood/adolescence. Include learned stereotypical beliefs about self and others
- General history of abuse and/or neglect in childhood/adolescence—Ask yes or no questions to begin with to contain affect about emotional/verbal, physical, and sexual abuse and emotional and physical neglect. Include culturally and socially based adversity/trauma (Shapiro, 2021a, 2021b), witnessing violence, bullying, sexual abuse (family member, neighbor, teacher, coach, religious figure, stranger, older child or teen, etc.), and sexual assault by stranger or acquaintance
- Developmental deficits—Missing information or skills usually learned or acquired in childhood and adolescence
- Strengths, skills, and internal and external resources (Shapiro, 2021a, 2021b)
- General history of abuse in childhood and adulthood—Ask yes or no questions to begin with about emotional/verbal, physical, and sexual abuse and emotional and physical neglect; areas of control (financial, social, emotional, physical, sexual, time, jobs, children)
- Follow-up information about trauma history as client is comfortable talking in more detail—Single-event trauma, ongoing attachment trauma; initial identification of client's negative cognitions in areas of responsibility (defectiveness/action), safety/vulnerability, control/choice, and connection/belonging (Shapiro, 2021a, 2021b)

• Open-ended question about what else the client thinks is important for the therapist to know and is comfortable telling them

MENTAL STATUS EXAMINATION (SEE EXHIBIT 22.4 IN CHAPTER 22)

The Mental Status Examination (MSE) is a structured evaluation of clients' current level of cognitive and behavioral functioning. The MSE adds important information to therapists' assessments by including questions about past and current mental health, behavioral, and cognitive symptoms; observations by therapists of clients during the interview and exam; and oral tests that estimate specific cognitive functions (Martin, 1990). The following items give more specific information incorporated in an MSE:

- Current and past symptoms including safety issues (suicidal ideation, suicide attempts, self-harm behaviors, harm to others)
- Changes in symptoms in the last 6 months
- Medical and medications (forms completed prior to first session)—Current medical providers (names and contact information, releases of information); current medications, medications tried in the past; date of last physical examination, need for referral for complete physical; and client's self-rating of overall physical health status; food/environmental/medication allergies and sensitivities; health risks (smoking, drugs and alcohol, sexually transmitted infections); review of current and past physical symptoms; review of physical conditions (skin, eyes, ears, teeth, lungs, urinary tract, muscles/joints, neurological system, gastrointestinal tract, reproductive system/sexual issues, endocrinological system, heart/blood, and immunological problems); past injuries/surgeries (see Exhibit 22.5 and Exhibit 22.6 in Chapter 22)
- Mental health, drug and alcohol, and prior therapy—Current and past providers; helpfulness of past therapy; need for referral to medication manager; inpatient treatment; and past and current alcohol and drug use (specific substances, when started using, length of use, when/if use became a problem, and problems caused by use)
- Legal problems—Other than traffic tickets
- Therapist observations—Appearance, general behaviors, speech, motor activity, level of consciousness, mood and affect, thought processes/productivity/content, and perception
- Tests—Orientation, concentration, recall, short- and long-term memory, intellectual ability, test and social judgment, level of reasoning

SCREENING AND OBJECTIVE TESTS

Once the initial interview and an MSE are completed, therapists obtain information about clients' symptoms and issues from objective testing in addition to clients' self-reports and screening tests and therapists' observations. I think it's essential to get information for diagnoses and treatment planning from other sources in addition to clients' self-report. Clients with a history of attachment trauma often present with an array of symptoms and many psychiatric diagnoses have similar symptoms. Screening and objective tests offer a wealth of information about the extent and severity of clients' mental health symptoms and help therapists differentiate among diagnoses and identify specifiers for diagnoses. Many screening tests are available that are easy for clients to complete and therapists to score and interpret, giving therapists valuable insight into client's symptoms, level of functioning, self-regulation, areas of concern, and diagnostic indications:

- General screenings and objective tests to complete between first and second sessions; for example, Depression Checklist and Anxiety Inventory (Burns, 1980); Behavior and Symptom Identification Scale (BASIS-32; Eisen, 1996); Personality Assessment Inventory (PAI; Morey, 1991); and Psychotherapy Assessment Checklist (PAC; McCullough, 2001)

- Drug and alcohol assessment, if needed; for example, Substance Abuse Subtle Screening Inventory–3 (SASSI-3; Lazowski et al., 1998)
- Adverse Childhood Experiences (ACE) Questionnaire for Adults (Centers for Disease Control and Prevention, 2021; Felitti, 2002; see Exhibit 22.7 in Chapter 22)

CORROBORATIVE INFORMATION

Therapists who see children and adolescents do a wonderful job getting information about their clients from parents, teachers, and other health and mental health providers. Understandably, therapists who work with adults have a different set of challenges related to obtaining corroborative information from others in clients' lives. Clients need to feel comfortable and safe about giving permission to their therapist to talk to others and there are situations when requesting corroborative information is contraindicated; for example, intimate partner violence, young adult living with parent who was or is abusive, family members who don't believe client about history of abuse. Being specific and transparent about the purposes and scope of any information-gathering when getting a signed Release of Information is essential, especially stressing that therapists will not give information to others about clients or their therapy without the client's permission and that they are clear about limits clients set related to what topics or areas can and cannot be discussed with others.

Information from other sources (family members, significant others, close friends, psychiatric medication managers, and healthcare providers) that either validates or challenges clients' self-report is invaluable to therapists in understanding clients' issues; in particular, others' perception and understanding of clients and their issues, medical conditions and other factors that affect clients' ability to make changes in therapy as well as how difficulties impact clients' ability to function in work and family relationships as well as friendships.

DIAGNOSTIC IMPRESSIONS

As stated earlier in the section on *Screening and Objective Tests*, clients who have histories of attachment trauma frequently present with a myriad of symptoms; many of which can be classified under more than one diagnosis delineated in the *Diagnostic and Statisitical Manual of Mental Disorders*, Fifth Edition (*DSM-5;* American Psychiatric Association, 2013). Clients who have previous experiences with mental health professionals often have been given numerous diagnoses. Before assigning multiple diagnoses, AFTT-A therapists discern which symptoms—such as depression, anxiety, panic, phobias, problems with sleep, concentration, memory, and so forth—are unrelated to trauma and which symptoms are primarily related to triggers from complex posttraumatic stress disorder (C-PTSD), disorders of extreme stress (DES), or dissociative disorders (DD; van der Kolk et al., 2005).

Personality disorders can add complications to the process of trauma therapy, but since the AFTT-A model views such immature personality structures as parts of Self or a system of overly close or cut-off parts, the "disordered" personality can be reconstructed into a healthier, more cooperative system with strong internal attachment relationships. Personality disorders can often give clues to the ages and issues of fragmented parts of Self.

Therapists complete all five diagnostic axes rather than concentrating solely on the first axis or the first and second axes (American Psychiatric Association, 2013). I incorporate a review of test results and all fives axes with clients in a transition session between the history-taking phase (phase 1) of EMDR therapy and the beginning of preparation phase 2. I use the review conversation to continue teaching about the impact of attachment trauma on symptoms, development, and attachment (Axes I and II); physical health status (Axis III); present-day life issues and stressors (Axis IV); and level of functioning (Axis V):

- Axis I: Clinical Diagnoses
- Axis II: Personality Disorders and Mental Retardation
- Axis III: Medical or Physical Conditions
- Axis IV: Current Environmental and Psychosocial Stressors
- Axis V: Current General Assessment of Functioning (GAF) and Highest GAF in Last Year (Aas, 2011)

ASSESSMENT OF READINESS FOR EMDR

A thorough and comprehensive initial assessment provides much of the information needed for clients and their therapists to evaluate their readiness to begin EMDR therapy and allows them to explore more extensively the areas specifically related to readiness for trauma therapy. Shapiro's main criteria for clients' readiness to initiate EMDR therapy is whether clients can maintain affect regulation while accomplishing therapeutic tasks that involve significant levels of emotions (2018, pp. 85–97).

Many issues and factors impact clients' ability to regulate affect; for example, cultural, ethnic, religious, and gender considerations; long-lasting difficulties (dissociation, personality disorders, and chronic depression or anxiety); acute problems (safety concerns and impulsive behaviors); lack of developmental information and skills; the number and seriousness of negative cognitions or core beliefs; medical conditions; unstable life circumstances; and a lack of family and social support (Leeds, 2016, pp. 93–108; Shapiro, 2021a, 2021b). Therapists also find information about how client symptoms may have been reinforced over time, their ability to tolerate positive affect in addition to negative affect, and strengths and internal resources.

Therapists use their clinical judgment about the need for screening and/or objective testing. Ideally, clients complete screening and objective tests encompassing depression and other mood disorders, anxiety, PTSD, dissociation, personality disorders, problems with substances, and overall level of functioning. In addition to data from client's initial assessment, MSE, corroborative information from others, and the aforementioned test results, therapists then collect findings from the screening and objective tests specific to readiness for trauma therapy. Therapists select appropriate tests from the following list for clients to complete and to revise diagnostic impressions as needed and begin to set goals and develop a treatment plan with clients:

- EMDR Readiness Questionnaire (ERQ; Sine & Vogelmann-Sine, 1997; see Exhibit 22.8 in Chapter 22)

- Negative Cognitions Questionnaire–Initial Form (NCQ-IF; Sine & Vogelmann-Sine, 1997; see Exhibit 22.9 in Chapter 22)
- Affect regulation and coping strategies
  - Inventory of Altered Self-Concept (IASC; Briere, 1998)
  - Styles of Coping Word-Pairs (Lynch, 2018)
- PTSD
  - Trauma Symptoms Inventory–2 (TSI-2; Briere, 1995)
  - Detailed Assessment of Posttraumatic Stress (DAPS; Briere, 2001)
- Dissociation
  - Dissociative Experiences Scale (DES-II; Carlson & Putman, 1993)
  - Multiscale Dissociation Inventory (MDI; Briere et al., 2005)
  - Multidimensional Inventory of Dissociation (MID; Dell, 2006)

A thorough evaluation of the presence and extent of clients' dissociation is essential before employing any technique that aims to differentiate personality parts, since clients with a more extensive level of dissociation already have distinct parts. Therapists also need to assess their therapeutic techniques for the potential to exacerbate dissociation.

Attachment patterns are complex and challenging to assess with accuracy unless therapists are trained to administer the Adult Attachment Interview (AAI; Hesse, 1999) or Adult Attachment Projective (AAP; George & West, 2012), the gold standard assessments for identification of adult attachment patterns. However, extensive training and time are required to be able to administer and score either of the two measures. The most used paper-and-pencil, self-report questionnaire is the Experiences in Close Relationships (ECR) scale (Brennan et al., 1998). However, the dimensions of the ECR scale are not equivalent to the secure, dismissive, preoccupied, and unresolved/disorganized categories identified by the AAI and AAP. Furthermore, the AAI and AAP do not rely on self-report, which requires self-insight, as the patterns are largely unconscious for most individuals.

For clinical purposes, formal attachment measures are unnecessary and therapist awareness of the signs of nonsecure and disorganized patterns in clients provides sufficient insight for knowing when and how to provide secure-based responses to clients' nonsecure and disorganized behaviors and words (see Chapters 3, 4, and 17).

Goals and Treatment Planning

After completing clients' initial assessment and forming diagnostic impressions, therapists approach goal setting and treatment planning with clients according to standards of their state licensure statutes and ethical guidelines from relevant professional organizations. Therapists help clients set goals and develop treatment plans based on their strengths and areas of deficits. Exhibit 22.10 in Chapter 22 shows treatment planning organized around client goals and concerns, assisting clients in identification of desired behavioral, affective, cognitive, and somatic changes (Leeds, 2016, p. 365). DBT offers a hierarchy for therapy goals/targeted behaviors as a method of organize and set priorities for goal setting in AFTT-A. The hierarchy includes guidelines for the sequence of therapy interventions and provides the following order for the focus of therapy (Linehan, 1993, p. 167):

- Commitment to therapy; for example, readiness and willingness to participate in overall therapy process
- Safety issues; for example, suicidal ideation, self-harm behavior, other impulsive behaviors
- Therapy-interfering behaviors; for example, canceling or arriving late for appointments, not completing therapy assignments, not honoring payment agreement
- Quality-of-life interfering behaviors; for example, compulsive behaviors, addictions, emotion over- or under-control, developmental skills deficits, social and cultural issues, relationship challenges
- PTSD; for example, past traumatic events, rupture in childhood attachment relationships

Regardless of therapist orientation, treatment plans include issues or diagnoses and associated long- and short-term goals, therapist interventions, an evaluation of the plan's effectiveness, plan revisions and updates, and an aftercare plan to prevent relapse and maintain progress (see Exhibit 22.11 in Chapter 22).

We, as therapists, use our clinical judgment as we integrate information from clients' assessments and behaviors to determine which level of the treatment hierarchy they need to start. Moving from phase 1 assessment into phase 2 preparation, we evaluate whether clients can meet Shapiro's criteria of readiness; that is, the ability to maintain emotion/affect regulation while participating in trauma therapy that elicits strong emotions. If clients demonstrate difficulties with therapy commitment or safety issues or exhibit therapy-interfering behavior, they are not ready to move into phases 3 to 8 in EMDR therapy. If clients report problems with either emotional over- or under-control and/or inadequate skills to effectively cope with current stressors, their treatment plan will include an extended period of stabilization in the preparation phase prior to moving into EMDR therapy phases 3 to 8.

Phase-Based Trauma Treatment/Team Treatment

Phase-based trauma treatment (PBTT) is an option for clients who lack the regulation skills to move from assessment into trauma treatment. PBTT assists clients to improve symptoms of clinical diagnoses, personality disorders, and/or substance abuse as well as healing attachment trauma. PBTT addresses both the effects of developmental skills deficits on present-day functioning and the resolution of past traumas within the context of an emotionally corrective therapy relationship. PBTT includes two-steps; first, skills development for and application to psychiatric symptoms and challenges with current stressors, circumstances, and relationships, and second, reprocessing of traumatic memories. The first, skills-based stage is a component of AFTT-A's enhanced preparation phase 2 in EMDR therapy and the second stage, trauma reprocessing, is accomplished in EMDR's phases 3 to 8.

DBT and radically open DBT (RO DBT) are both PBTTs. Their therapeutic strategies address and remedy skills deficits in the preparation phase prior to the steps involving reprocessing of traumatic memories. In the AFTT-A model, clients activate their Competent Adult part of Self or "Adult Brain" to learn and apply new skills at the same time they also begin to identify other parts of Self, how those parts were wounded in childhood, and ways in which they have been involved in current symptoms and issues.

DBT targets emotion dysregulation or under-control while RO DBT focuses on emotional overcontrol. Lynch (2018) developed the *Styles of Coping Word-Pairs* checklist to provide an initial assessment of clients' tendency to utilize either an under- or overcontrol coping style with emotions and behaviors. Typically, if the client score on the right column of the *Styles of Coping Word-Pairs* checklist is higher than their score from the left column, they may be appropriate for referral to an RO DBT therapist for more in-depth evaluation and RO DBT skills training. If the client score on the left column on the *Styles of Coping Word-Pairs* checklist is higher than their score on the right column, they may be referred to a DBT therapist for further evaluation and DBT skills training (see Exhibit 22.12 in Chapter 22).

DBT (Linehan, 1993, 2014a, 2014b) is a PBTT designed for clients who demonstrate emotional and behavioral dysregulation or under-control and whose adult lives are characterized by mood swings, emotional suffering, chaotic and emotionally intense relationships, and impulsive behaviors. In AFTT-A, clients who have difficulty containing negative emotions, thoughts, and behaviors, and who tend to be more at risk for being overwhelmed by intense affect during trauma processing are referred to DBT. DBT emphasizes clients' learning and applying self-regulation skills presented in four class modules each of which are taught twice over approximately 12 months: (1) Mindfulness, (2) Distress Tolerance, (3) Emotion Regulation, and (4) Interpersonal Effectiveness.

RO DBT (Lynch, 2018; Lynch et al., 2015) is a PBTT for clients who exhibit emotional and behavioral overcontrol and whose adult lives can be described by social isolation, loneliness, rigidity, aloof and distant relationships, ultra-perfectionism, and unrealistically high expectations of themselves and others. Clients who demonstrate emotion and behavioral overcontrol and who tend to have more difficulty accessing and experiencing emotions during trauma processing are referred to RO DBT. RO DBT focuses on assisting clients to develop skills related to openness, flexibility, and social connectedness in classes that span approximately 30 weeks.

A team approach to treating clients with a history of attachment trauma can also be helpful. Clients who present with significant levels of complexity can benefit from working with therapists who form a consultation team; for example, one therapist has the client in either DBT or RO DBT classes; if the class facilitator doesn't act as the client's individual DBT/RO DBT therapist, then a second therapist sees the client in individual DBT/RO DBT therapy to assist them in applying skills learned in classes in present day issues and relationships; and a third therapist sees the client in individual therapy for trauma therapy preparation using the AFTT-A model.

POINTS TO REMEMBER

- AFTT-A utilizes both a thorough and detailed general initial client assessment as well as a specific evaluation of client readiness for EMDR therapy in EMDR phase 1.

- A comprehensive initial assessment includes history-taking, a mental status examination, review of medications, screening and objective tests, and corroborative information from family members (if safe for clients) and clients' psychiatric and medical providers.
- Goals and treatment planning incorporate assessment of clients' emotional and behavioral under- or overcontrol and of the need for skills training with either DBT or RO DBT in the EMDR preparation phase 2 prior to moving into phases 3 to 8.
- Team treatment may be helpful in addressing the high level of complexity involved in working with clients with histories of attachment trauma.

TROUBLESHOOTING

- Clients may present in early therapy sessions as high functioning in their current situations but over- or under-control emotions and have deficits in skills essential for forming healthy attachments. Therapists attune to nonverbal communication and client family, relationship, and job histories to begin to gain information about areas to be addressed in treatment planning and initial clues to the parts and overall structure of clients' internal personality.
- Clients may present as ready and willing to begin trauma therapy and may even show impatience about beginning trauma reprocessing. Use of objective tests, assessment of EMDR readiness tools, Lynch's assessment of coping styles, and Linehan's hierarchy of treatment goals offer guidance to therapists in making effective treatment decisions about timing of therapy phases.
- Treating clients with attachment trauma is often professionally and personally challenging. Therapists can find it helpful to collaborate with clients' medical and psychiatric providers as well as form or join a team or network of therapists for consultation and support.
- Clients with histories of attachment trauma often show signs and symptoms that could be assigned to a range of psychiatric diagnoses. Use of diagnostic tests are invaluable in differentiating client diagnoses.

PAUSE AND REFLECT FOR THE THERAPIST

Give yourself some quiet time and space to consider the impact of your own social and cultural identity and groups on your life and particularly, the potential influences on relationships with clients. Nickerson (2017) uses the term "cultural humility" when describing therapists who develop a mindset of openness and curiosity about, respect for, and responsiveness to the social and cultural diversity in clients' lives and the impact on clients' experience in therapy (pp. 7–12). Think about how important your social/cultural identity is to you. What are positive and negatives aspects of the groups to which you belong? How does your affiliation with groups that are important to you help you understand yourself and others? Have you been adversely affected by discrimination, social stigma, oppression, bias, or prejudice? Have you felt the need to hide your gender/social/cultural identity? Have you internalized stigmatizing messages to the extent they are a part of how you see yourself?

Do you have strong stereotypical beliefs or prejudices against a person or groups of people? How were you taught those beliefs? Have you been criticized for your beliefs or prejudices? Have you witnessed acts of prejudice, discrimination, or oppression? Have you participated in acts of prejudice, discrimination, or oppression even when it felt wrong? Have you considered how social privilege or position has afforded you benefits or given you advantages over people of different races, ethnic backgrounds, or classes (Nickerson, 2017, pp. 50–74; Shapiro, 2021a, 2021b)?

We encourage you to discuss with your peer consultation group or approved consultant ways in which your social and cultural beliefs, values, and experiences might affect your therapy relationships, especially when they differ from clients' beliefs, values, and experiences. Brainstorm ways you can create comfort and safety in therapy sessions for clients to discuss how gender, social, and cultural issues have impacted them and their lives. Consider options for further exploring your beliefs and for learning about the values and experiences of groups about which you have stereotypical perceptions. Share socially and culturally adverse experiences in your own therapy to target any unresolved material for reprocessing.

USEFUL TERMS AND DEFINITIONS

AAI: Adult Attachment Interview

AAP: Adult Attachment Projective

ACEs: Adverse Childhood Experiences

"Adult Brain": The parts of the brain that house the adaptive information processing (AIP) system and include higher cognitive processes such as learning, problem-solving, decision-making, language, understanding of emotions, and narrative memory.

AFTT-A: Attachment-Focused Trauma Therapy for Adults

BASIS-32: Behavior and Symptom Identification Scale-32

C-PTSD: complex posttraumatic stress disorder

DAPS: Detailed Assessment of Posttraumatic Stress

DBT: Dialectical Behavioral Therapy

DES: Disorders of extreme stress

DES-II: Dissociative Experiences Scale-II

DD: Dissociative Disorders

DSM-5: *Diagnostic and Statistical Manual of Mental Disorders*, Fifth Edition

ECR: Experiences in Close Relationships Scale

EMDR: Eye Movement Desensitization and Reprocessing

ERQ: EMDR Readiness Questionnaire

IASC: Inventory of Altered Self-Concept

"Kid Brain": The neural network clusters in the emotional/social part of the brain that store unprocessed memories of adverse events and are disconnected from a sense of time and from the parts of the brain capable of processing memories and transferring them into narrative memory. AFTT-A views the neural networks as encapsulating more than memories of adverse events and includes the experiences, cognitive development, learning during a particular client age.

MDI: Multiscale Dissociation Inventory

MID: Multidimensional Inventory of Dissociation

MSE: Mental Status Examination

NCQ-IF: Negative Cognitions Questionnaire–Initial Form

PAC: Psychotherapy Assessment Checklist

PAI: Personality Assessment Inventory

PBTT: phase-based trauma treatment

RO DBT: Radically Open Dialectical Behavior Therapy

SASSI-3: Substance Abuse Subtle Screening Inventory–3

TSI-2: Trauma Symptom Inventory–2

REFERENCES

Aas, I. H. (2011). Guidelines for rating Global Assessment of Functioning (GAF). *Annals of General Psychiatry, 10*, Article No. 2. https://doi.org/10.1186/1744-859X-10-2

American Psychiatric Association. (2013). *Diagnostic and statistical manual of mental disorders* (5th ed.). https://doi.org/10.1176/appi.books.9780890425596

Brennan, K. A., Clark, C. L., & Shaver, P. R. (1998). Self-report measurement of adult attachment: An integrative overview. In J. A. Simpson & W. S. Rholes (Eds.), *Attachment theory and close relationships* (pp. 46–76). Guilford Press.

Briere, J. (1995). *Trauma symptom inventory professional manual*. Psychological Assessment Resources, Inc.

Briere, J. (1998). *Inventory of altered self capacities professional manual*. Psychological Assessment Resources, Inc.

Briere, J. (2001). *Detailed assessment of posttraumatic stress (DAPS)*. Psychological Assessment Resources, Inc.

Briere, J., Weathers, F. W., & Runtz, M. (2005). Is dissociation a multidimensional construct? Data from the Multiscale Dissociation Inventory. *Journal of Traumatic Stress, 18*(3), 221–231. https://doi.org/10.1002/jts.20024

Burns, D. (1980). *Feeling good: The new mood therapy*. William Morrow and Company, Inc.

Carlson, E. B., & Putnam, F. W. (1993). An update on the Dissociative Experience Scale. *Dissociation: Progress in the Dissociative Disorders, 6*(1), 16–27.

Centers for Disease Control and Prevention. (2021, December 1). *Adverse childhood experiences*. https://www.cdc.gov/violenceprevention/aces/index.html

Centers for Medicare & Medicaid Services. (2022, January 12). *Understanding costs in advance*. https://www.cms.gov/nosurprises/consumers/understanding-costs-in-advance

Dell, P. F. (2006). A new model of dissociative identity disorder. *Psychiatric Clinics of North America, 29*(1), 1–26. https://doi.org/10.1016/j.psc.2005.10.013

Eisen, S. V. (1996). Behavior and Symptom Identification Scale (BASIS-32). In L. I. Sederer & B. Dickey (Eds.), *Outcomes assessment in clinical practice* (pp. 65–69). Williams & Wilkins.

Felitti, V. J. (2002). The relation between adverse childhood experiences and adult health: Turning gold into lead. *The Permanente Journal, 6*(1), 44–47. https://doi.org/10.7812/TPP/02.994

George, C., & West, M. L. (2012). *The Adult Attachment Projective picture system: Attachment theory and assessment in adults*. Guilford Press.

Hesse, E. (1999). The Adult Attachment Interview: Historical and current perspectives. In J. Cassidy & P. R. Shaver (Eds.), *Handbook of attachment: Theory, research and clinical applications* (pp. 395–433). Guilford Press.

Lazowski, L. E., Miller, F. G., Boye, M. W., & Miller, G. A. (1998). Efficacy of the Substance Abuse Subtle Screening Inventory-3 (SASSI-3) in identifying substance dependence disorders in clinical settings. *Journal of Personality Assessment, 71*(1), 114–128. https://doi.org/10.1207/s15327752jpa7101_8

Leeds, A. (2016). *A guide to the standard EMDR protocols for clinicians, supervisors, and consultants* (2nd ed.). Springer Publishing Company.

Linehan, M. (1993). *Cognitive-behavioral treatment of borderline personality disorder*. Guilford Press.

Linehan, M. (2014a). *DBT skills training handouts and worksheets* (2nd ed.). Guilford Press.

Linehan, M. (2014b). *DBT skills training manual* (2nd ed.). Guilford Press.

Lynch, T. (2018). *The skills training manual for radically open dialectical behavior therapy: A clinician's guide for treating disorders of overcontrol*. Context Press.

Lynch, T. R., Hempel, R. J., & Dunkley, C. (2015). Radically Open-Dialectical Behavior Therapy for disorders of over-control: Signaling matters. *American Journal of Psychotherapy, 69*(2), 141–162. https://doi.org/10.1176/appi.psychotherapy.2015.69.2.141

Martin, D. C. (1990). The mental status examination. In H. K. Walker, W. D. Hall, & J. W. Hurst (Eds.), *Clinical methods: The history, physical, and laboratory examinations* (3rd ed.). Butterworth Publishers.

McCullough, L. (2001). *Psychotherapy assessment checklist*. https://www.affectphobiatherapy.com/forms/

Morey, L. C. (1991). *Personality Assessment Inventory professional manual*. Psychological Assessment Resources.

Nickerson, M. (Ed.) (2017). *Cultural competence and healing culturally based trauma with EMDR therapy*. Springer Publishing Company.

Shapiro, F. (2018). *Eye Movement Desensitization and Reprocessing (EMDR) therapy: Basic principles, protocols, and procedures* (3rd ed.). Guilford Press.

Shapiro, F. (2021a). *Weekend 1 training manual of the two-part EMDR therapy basic training* (revised). EMDR Institute, Inc.

Shapiro, F. (2021b). *Weekend 2 training manual of the two-part EMDR therapy basic training* (revised). EMDR Institute, Inc.

Sine, L. F., & Vogelmann-Sine, S. (1997). *Assessing for EMDR readiness, intervening with deficit areas inhibiting readiness and determining EMDR targets*. Presentation at the 2nd EMDR International Association Conference, San Francisco, California.

van der Kolk, B. A., Roth, S., Pelcovitz, D., Sunday, S., & Spinazzola, J. (2005). Disorders of extreme stress: The empirical foundation of a complex adaptation to trauma. *Journal of Traumatic Stress, 18*(5), 389–399. https://doi.org/10.1002/jts.20047

CHAPTER 7

Explaining the Parent-Adult-Child (P-A-C) Diagrams in Attachment-Focused Trauma Therapy for Adults

INTRODUCTION

Everyone shows different sides of their personalities depending on situations or circumstances. Clients may demonstrate a problem-solving or analytical aspect of themselves when at work, a nurturing and loving facet while parenting a child, and a fun-loving, playful side when on vacation or out with close friends. Everyone's personality develops over time and is influenced by real-life people and events.

Childhood events and the quality of relationships with attachment figures like parents and other caregivers impact clients' personality development or the formation of their internal structure of Self. As a result, if clients experience encouragement, acceptance, and a sense of safety and consistency in childhood attachment relationships, most of their inner parts are viewed as strengths and encouraged to develop. Those healthy parts eventually become integrated into a balanced, cooperative, and well-functioning internal personality structure that can assess and respond appropriately in relationships and to events in their adult lives.

On the other hand, if clients suffered adverse childhood events—such as physical, emotional, and/or sexual abuse; emotional and/or physical neglect; witnessed family violence; faced ongoing criticism, belittling, or bullying; and/or became parental caretakers—various personality parts are seen as weaknesses or strengths and are prevented from forming and maturing in healthy ways, thus creating an inner system whose parts are over- or underdeveloped and incapable of functioning together as a whole.

The term "parts" and "ego states" have been used to describe the clusters of varied characteristics and components of clients' inner functioning by the therapy field for decades. Variations exist within the therapy field about what defines and comprises parts or ego states. Models have been based on psychoanalysis, personality development, structural dissociation, the relationship between inner adult or parent and child/adolescent parts, and family systems theory. Some theorists in the childhood trauma field see internal parts as entities or individuals while others emphasize the roles parts learned to play in early life. Some approaches view parts as fragments or components of a unifying system while others regard parts as representing a "multidimensional complex" (Schwartz, 1995, pp. 9–17). Whatever the specific theory or theories and the particular conceptualization of parts, the most recent ways of understanding the impact of childhood trauma are based on the assumption that clients' internal systems or structures are shaped through and impacted by experiences; observations; and the patterns, roles, and relationships modeled in childhood (Black, 1982; Boon et al.,

2011; Bradshaw, 1990; Bryant et al., 1992; Carvalho, 2012; Fisher, 2017; Forgash & Copely, 2008; Fraser, 1991, 2003; Gonzales & Mosquera, 2012; Harris, 1969; Holmes & Holmes, 2007; Knipe, 2015; Lanius & Paulsen, 2014; Manfield, 2010; Martin, 2012; Parnell, 1999; Paulsen, 2009; Potter, 1994a, 1994b; Satir, 1972; Schmidt, 2009, 2020; Schwartz, 1995; Shapiro, 2016; Van der Hart & Nijenhuis, 2006; Walker, 2013; Watkins & Watkins, 1997; Whitfield, 1987; Wildwind, 1992; Woititz, 1983).

History of Therapeutic Models That Include Personality Parts

The modern concept of inner personality parts largely started with Sigmund Freud's theory of psychopathology, which has as one of its foundational ideas that the human personality is comprised of three parts of Self: Superego, Ego, and Id (Brill, 1995). In the 1950s and 1960s, Berne developed transactional analysis which has its roots in psychoanalysis but instead of exploring internal experiences such as dreams and stream of consciousness, transactional analysis analyzes communication and behavior patterns in current relationships to discover clients' long-held beliefs about themselves and others and the tacit roles and patterns rooted in those beliefs (1964).

Berne (1964) diverged from traditional psychoanalysis and Self Psychology by focusing primarily on the Ego part of the personality and what he perceived as the Parent, Adult, and Child/Adolescent parts or states of the Ego. He re-imagined Freud's three personality states: The Superego became the Parent, the Ego translated into the Adult, and the Id became the Child. Berne then integrated characteristics from Freud's personality parts into the Ego state, thus bringing the Parent, Adult, and Child/Adolescent parts of Self into conscious awareness through the Ego aspect of personality.

Attachment-Focused Trauma Therapy for Adults (AFTT-A) adapts and expands Berne's model and illustrates the adaptations in the Parent-Adult-Child (P-A-C) diagrams. (See Figures 7.2 and 7.3 for P-A-C diagrams.) Therapists assess both internal experiences as well as past and current attachment relationships to identify strengths and weaknesses in clients' inner personality system. A systematic set of protocols restores internal parts to their intended state and roles. The internal attachments among the parts are repaired through corrective experiences internally and in the therapeutic relationship. The newly healed inner structure then provides the basis for clients to create healthy and satisfying relationships in their adult lives.

AFTT-A MODEL OF PERSONALITY PARTS

AFTT-A adapts the basics of Berne's Transactional Analysis model and Bradshaw's conceptualization of the "Inner Child" into the P-A-C diagrams for therapeutic interventions with clients' inner parts or ego states for a few reasons: the simplicity of the internal structure; the ease with which concepts can be understood; and the way in which labels, language, and processes normalize personality development and functioning. AFTT-A extends the model to include versions of parts or ego states that illustrate the impact of attachment trauma on personality development and relationships.

Figure 7.1 *Developing Adult Behaviors*, based on Linehan's concepts of validating and invalidating childhood environments (1993), also explains how

7. EXPLAINING THE PARENT-ADULT-CHILD DIAGRAMS 71

Spiritual Essence (True or Real Self)

OPTIMAL DEVELOPMENTAL PATHWAY:
Validating Childhood Environment

- Imperfection
- Parental accountability
- Affirmation of emotions
- Fair, firm, and flexible boundaries
- Parent or primary caregiver with secure or earned secure attachment pattern and resolved loss/trauma
- Life skills
- Balanced participation in social, cultural, or religious groups

Sense of Self

- Well-developed life skills
- Mature Parent, Adult, Child parts or states of Ego
- Collaborative relationships among parts
- Integrated inner system
- Nurturing and protective internal boundaries and boundaries in relationships
- Balanced, regulated, and situation-appropriate emotions
- Positive cognitions or core beliefs
- Competence and confidence

Adult Behaviors

- Adaptive use of life skills
- Strong sense of individuality balanced with group identity and inclusion
- Capability for authenticity, closeness, and intimacy in relationships
- Secure or earned secure attachment pattern in relationships
- Resolved trauma

NONOPTIMAL DEVELOPMENTAL PATHWAY:
Invalidating Childhood Environment

- Big "T" and/or little "t" trauma
- Emotional and/or physical neglect
- Parental over-responsibility or irresponsibility
- Denial of emotions
- Lack of or rigid rules
- Parent or primary caregiver with preoccupied or dismissive attachment pattern and/or unresolved loss/trauma
- Life skills deficits
- Under- or overidentification with social, cultural, or religious groups

Impact on Sense of Self

- Lack of or underdeveloped life skills
- Immature Parent, Adult, Child parts or states of Ego
- Blended/enmeshed and/or dissociated relationships among parts
- Fragmented inner system
- Absence of, damaged, or rigid internal boundaries and boundaries in relationships
- Over- or under-controlled emotions
- Negative cognitions or core beliefs
- Self-doubt or self-importance

Effect on Adult Behaviors

- Difficulty using skills when needed
- Struggles with sense of Self separate from others
- Enmeshed or distant relationship boundaries
- Preoccupied or dismissive attachment pattern in relationships
- Unresolved trauma

FIGURE 7.1. Developing adult behaviors.

Source: Adapted from Bradshaw, J. (1990). *Homecoming: Reclaiming and healing your inner child.* Bantam Publishing; Linehan, M. (1993). *Cognitive-behavioral treatment of borderline personality disorder.* Guilford Press; and Potter, A. E. (1994). *Inside out: Rebuilding self and personality through inner child therapy* (therapist manual and client workbook). Taylor and Francis Group.

the processes of development diverge related to the negative impact of attachment childhood. AFTT-A utilizes both the *Developing Adult Behaviors* chart and *P-A-C diagrams* to give clients an initial framework for therapy and a psychoeducational foundation for the overall therapy process and protocols which aim to reconstruct and strengthen their inner system, provide corrective attachment experiences, and provide preparation for Eye Movement Desensitization and Reprocessing (EMDR) therapy phases 3 to 8.

Once therapists have completed the assessment phase, psychoeducation provides an important foundation for clients' understanding of therapy and AFTT-A process and protocols. Additionally, clients engage their Competent Adult part of Self, "Adult Brain," or the part of the brain that reasons, understands, and integrates new information. Since EMDR therapy's adaptive information processing (AIP) system is part of clients' Competent Adult part of Self, learning new information both stimulates the part of the brain we want to strengthen and empower and begins to challenge long-held negative cognitions formed through attachment trauma. Initially approaching emotionally charged material at a cognitive level often aids clients in maintaining emotion regulation.

Therapists find it helpful to review the *Developing Adult Behaviors* chart with clients prior to the P-A-C diagram protocols to describe elements of optimal/validating and nonoptimal/invalidating childhood environments and how those types of upbringings impact the clients' sense of Self and the later development of behaviors in their adult lives. Therapists often use the discussion as an opportunity to clarify possible misconceptions that "optimal" or "validating" means a "perfect" environment; that an imperfect childhood environment can still include aspects of support, encouragement, and a sense of safety.

The left side of the *Developing Adult Behaviors* chart in Figure 7.1 shows the elements that contribute to an optimal/validating childhood environment such as parents taking responsibility for their own actions and considering their children's feelings and parents forming secure attachments with their children. They can then look at the positive effects of a validating childhood environment indicated by a balanced and secure sense of Self, a positive view and feelings about themselves, well-developed skills, mature personalities, and the ability to regulate themselves and their emotions. Lastly, clients can begin to understand the effects of a validating childhood environment in adult life; for example, skillful behavior and a strong sense of themselves as individuals balanced with forming and maintaining close relationships in familial, social, and cultural contexts.

Alternately, information from the right side of the *Developing Adult Behaviors* chart delineates components of a nonoptimal or invalidating childhood environment such as abuse, neglect, nonsecure attachment relationships, and life skills deficits. An invalidating childhood environment links to a nonsecure sense of Self with under- or overdeveloped personality parts; absent, damaged, or rigid internal and external boundaries; and under- or overregulated emotions. An invalidating environment also leads to life skills deficits, negative cognitions or core beliefs, and a significant sense of self-doubt or self-importance. Clients are taught through the *Developing Adult Behaviors* chart that being raised in an invalidating childhood environment and having unresolved attachment trauma carry consequences into adulthood such as issues with separateness, closeness, life skills deficits, and nonsecure attachment patterns in adult relationships.

As therapists, we want to make foundational information easily understood and practical as well as presented in an informal and normalizing way. AFTT-A describes and explains the *Developing Adult Behaviors* chart and *P-A-C diagrams* in a conversational manner between the therapist who gives information and examples and the client who is encouraged to interrupt, ask questions, get clarification, and talk about how the information reflects aspects of their own upbringing. The protocols also provide specific times to ask for questions, ensuring clients understand what's being taught and getting feedback from clients about the relevance to their lives. However, therapists can stop anytime they sense their clients are not understanding, are reacting to, or are struggling with the material being presented. And, again, clients are encouraged to feel comfortable speaking up or asking questions at any time.

The three *P-A-C diagrams* protocols include:

- Introduction and explanation of the P-A-C diagrams and how the inner personality system forms in the context of a validating environment;
- Illustration of how invalidating childhood environments negatively impact personality development; and
- AFTT-A's reconstruction process of personality parts and the clients' internal systems.

Dividing up psychoeducational material in the three *P-A-C diagrams* protocols affords therapists and clients ample time to explore each protocol while still having time for other topics in sessions as needed. The protocols offer clients the opportunity to reflect on the material between sessions so they have time to formulate more questions and can talk more extensively about their own experiences.

P-A-C DIAGRAMS PROTOCOL #1: STEPS FOR EXPLANATION OF VALIDATING CHILDHOOD ENVIRONMENT

For more information, see Protocol Script 1 at the end of the chapter.

1. Introduce Concepts of Personality Parts and Aspects of Self

We want clients to come away from the discussions about personality parts and the Self with a few essential understandings:

- Having parts is normal.
- Feeling weird about having parts is normal (ha!).
- It's about what happened to them, not about them. And what happened to them was not their fault. Nothing is wrong with them. As children they couldn't have known how to handle what happened to them and around them any other way than the way they did. Kids' brains do what kids' brains do.

AFTT-A uses terms like parts, aspects, sides, characteristics, facets, qualities to normalize the composition of the inner personality system, for example, wearing

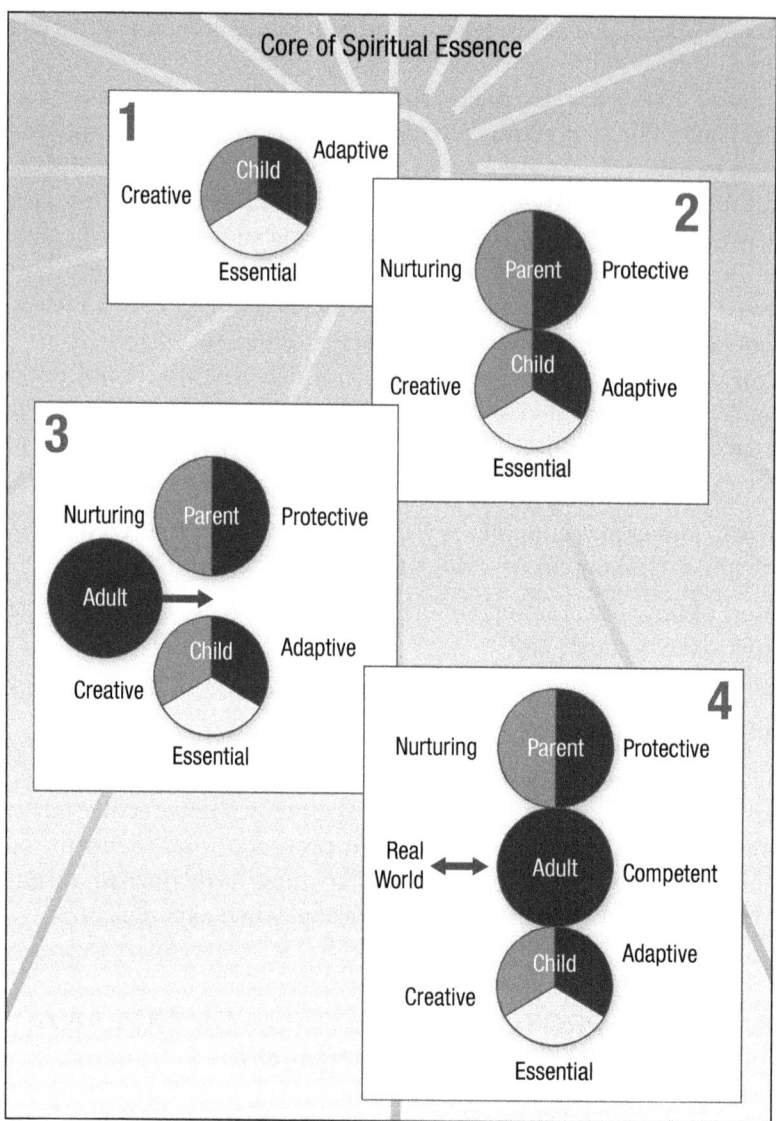

FIGURE 7.2 P-A-C diagrams: Validating childhood environment.
Source: Adapted from Berne, E. (1964). *Games people play: The basic handbook of transactional analysis*. Random House; Bradshaw, J. (1990). *Homecoming: Reclaiming and healing your inner child*. Bantam Publishing; and Potter, A. E. (1994). *Inside out: Rebuilding self and personality through inner child therapy* (therapist manual and client workbook). Taylor and Francis Group.

different "hats." Therapists in this model shy away from using terms that tend to pathologize clients' inner and real-life experiences. AFTT-A also emphasizes simplicity in the ways parts, personality, roles, and childhood development are conceptualized and translated to clients. Beyond the basic model that employs familiar and easily understood terms and relationships, clients are given the freedom and opportunity to label or even relabel and describe their own parts and functions. For example, clients may prefer to call their Child/Adolescent part of Self, "Kid Brain," "a younger me," "me at a younger age," "the child inside," or "my inner child."

In the first step, therapists provide an overview of what personality parts are and the process of personality development in a validating childhood environment by using the *P-A-C Diagrams: Validating Childhood Environment*. The *P-A-C Diagrams: Validating Childhood Environment* include illustrations of the process of personality development within the context of both a validating or optimal childhood environment (see Figure 7.2).

2. Explain the Concept of Spiritual Essence and Its Relationship to Personality Development and Integration

One of the core concepts of the AFTT-A model is Spiritual Essence. Clients' spiritual center is sometimes considered a major component of what philosophers and theorists call the "Self." One of the underlying assumptions of the AFTT-A model is that people are innately good and when connected to their core of goodness, they desire to grow in ways that benefit themselves, others, and the world as a whole. Spiritual Essence is also regarded as an energy that connects people to all living things and, as described in 12-step programs, to "a Power greater than ourselves" (Alcoholics Anonymous, 2001, p. 59). Clients who are part of religious organizations or ascribe to specific social, cultural, or religious beliefs may want to discuss how the idea of a Spiritual Essence fits (or doesn't fit) into their belief system and may rename or refine the concept to align with their convictions (Figure 7.2).

3. Describe the Process of Development

Therapists use the four sequential diagrams in Figure 7.2 *P-A-C Diagrams: Validating Childhood Environment* to illustrate personality development within a validating childhood environment. Again, the therapist reviews the concept of Spiritual Essence and explains the positive effects of a validating childhood environment on Spiritual Essence and its link to the Child/Adolescent part of the personality. Clients then learn about the three components of the Child/Adolescent part of Self: Essential, Creative, and Adaptive. The therapist then discusses the purposes of these aspects of the Child/Adolescent part of Self and how clients benefit from those characteristics and purposes.

The link between the Child/Adolescent part and real-life attachment figures such a parents, grandparents, or other primary caregivers, is the Adaptive portion of the inner Child whose job is to respond to and deal with nurturing and protective messages, rules, standards, and expectations from those real-life people. Actual messages are then internalized into and become the beginnings of the Nurturing and Protective portions of the Parent part of the personality. When raised in an optimal childhood environment, messages from attachment figures match up with and enhance the positive beliefs inherent in the Spiritual Essence, so the Adaptive Child/Adolescent part easily adjusts to communications that mirror already instilled messages. The Parent and Child/Adolescent parts of Self interact in ways that help clients solidify a sense of worthiness, esteem, safety, and protection and begin to modify behaviors in ways that reflect those inner beliefs.

As clients mature into adolescence and adulthood, they develop the parts of their brain that reason, think abstractly, set and follow through with goals, and problem-solve. The "Thinking Brain" or "Adult Brain" also contains the AIP needed to reprocess traumatic memories. Clients' Competent Adult part of Self is positioned in between the Parent and Child/Adolescent parts to mediate between the parts and make sound decisions about what is needed from which parts to appropriately respond with competence and confidence to real-life situations and in adult relationships.

4. Discuss What Aspects of Discussion Apply and/or Don't Apply to the Client
The therapist offers clients an opportunity to pause and ask questions as well as reflect on ways the information can be applied to their lives. At this point, clients often say that they don't relate to the description of a "validating" childhood environment or may be able to identify many positive aspects of their own experiences.

P-A-C DIAGRAMS PROTOCOL #2: STEPS FOR EXPLANATION OF INVALIDATING CHILDHOOD ENVIRONMENT

For more information, see Protocol Script 2 at the end of the chapter.

1. Describe How the Process of Personality Development Is Altered by Attachment Trauma
Therapists use the three, sequential diagrams included in Figure 7.3 *P-A-C Diagrams: Invalidating Childhood Environment* to illustrate personality development within an invalidating childhood environment. Again, the therapist reviews the concept of Spiritual Essence and explains how the Child/Adolescent part still has an initial connection to the Spiritual Essence. The therapist emphasizes that the problems are not inherent in clients; rather, the negative messages are external and originate with attachment figures in their life. A lack of nurturing messages, conditional nurturing messages, an excess of hurtful, critical messages, and adverse experiences such as abuse and/or neglect negatively impact personality development. Overall, the personality parts remain immature and don't learn what they need to work effectively as an internal system. Negative, external messages disconnect clients from the loving and encouraging messages of their Spiritual Essence and are internalized into negative cognitions or core beliefs. A distorted version of each personality part is created based on clients' negative cognitions. The explanation to clients includes how the negative messages alter personality development by

- shaping the Nurturing Parent to underdevelop and the Protective Parent part to morph into an overdeveloped Critical Parent;
- hindering the Essential and Creative aspects of the Child/Adolescent part of Self from developing and forcing the Adaptive Child/Adolescent part to overdevelop in attempts to align clients' behaviors with unattainable parental expectations as the Broken-Hearted Child/Adolescent part;
- preventing the Adult parts of the brain to mature and triggering either an overdeveloped Emotion Controller-Regulator or an underdeveloped little "a" to be in charge of the internal system without the necessary parental guidance, skills, and age-appropriate learning experiences; and
- creating damaged boundaries between personality parts with absent or weak boundaries causing blending or enmeshment of parts and rigid boundaries causing parts to be cut off or dissociated from each other.

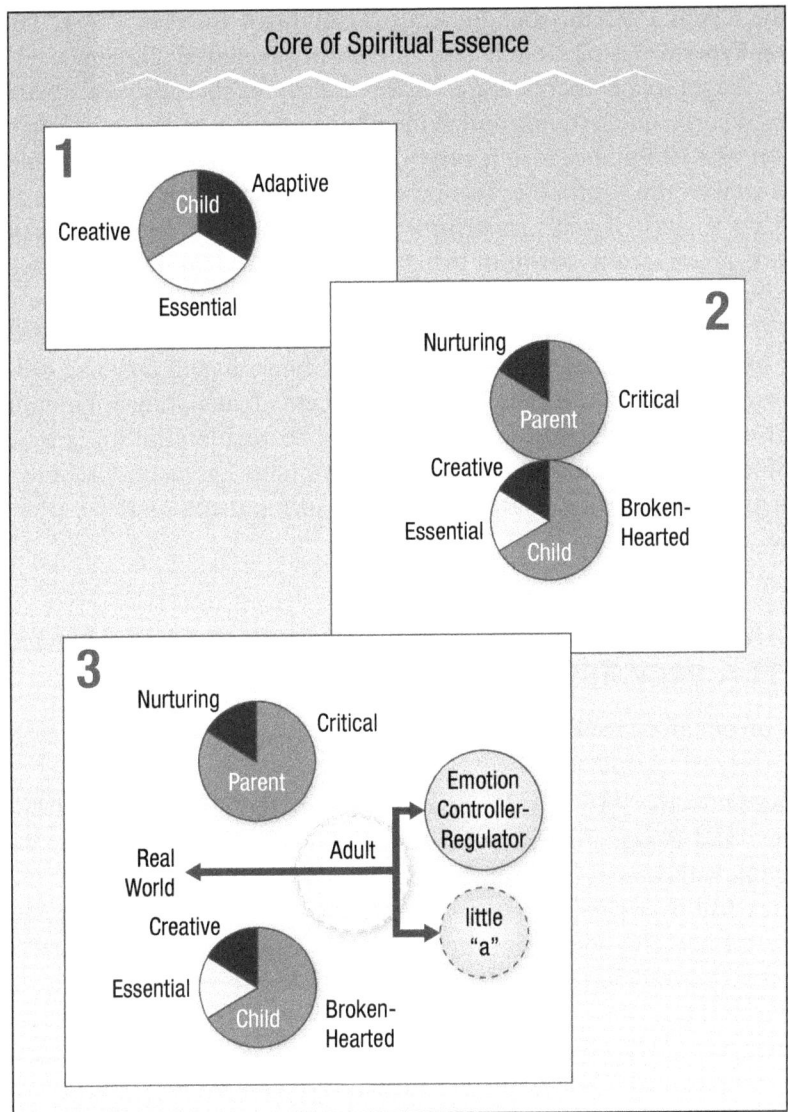

FIGURE 7.3 P-A-C diagrams: Invalidating childhood environment.
Source: Adapted from Berne, E. (1964). *Games people play: The basic handbook of transactional analysis*. Random House; Bradshaw, J. (1990). *Homecoming: Reclaiming and healing your inner child*. Bantam Publishing; and Potter, A. E. (1994). *Inside out: Rebuilding self and personality through inner child therapy* (therapist manual and client workbook). Taylor and Francis Group.

2. Discuss What Aspects of Discussion Apply and/or Don't Apply to the Client

The therapist offers clients an opportunity to pause and ask questions as well as reflect on ways cognitive materials can be applied to their lives. Clients at this point are usually able to relate information to their own experiences and may have emotional reactions about viewing their childhood experiences within the context of an "invalidating" environment.

3. Have the Client Describe and Illustrate Their Own Internal P-A-C Diagram by Drawing on Paper or Using a Sand Tray or Another Preferred Therapy

The *P-A-C diagrams* protocols are completed early in therapy. We want clients to be able to absorb, understand, and remember as much of the psychoeducational information as possible because it provides the foundation for the whole AFTT-A process as well as the protocols. To that end, it's essential for therapists to provide clients with a variety of ways to express their emotions in regulated ways so they can process information without being flooded with emotions. Sometimes, it's helpful for clients to create a visual representation of how they picture their own P-A-C diagram. Expressive therapies are utilized to describe clients' perception of their own internal P-A-C diagrams. Drawing or using a sand tray can aid clients in making abstract ideas more tangible and concrete. Translating their inner system into visual images also facilitates clients' ability to regulate on an emotional level by providing them a means to project their thoughts, perceptions, and emotions outside of themselves; thus, making intense emotional topics more objective and observable.

P-A-C DIAGRAMS PROTOCOL #3: STEPS FOR EXPLANATION OF THE AFTT-A PROCESS

For more information, see Protocol Script 3 at the end of the chapter.

1. Describe How the AFTT-A Process Heals and Reconstructs the Client's Inner Attachments and Personality Structure and Enhances Their Capability for Healthy and Satisfying Attachment Relationships in Their Adult Life

Clients often feel overwhelmed or pessimistic about their ability to change. Since in their minds the negative cognitions they learned in childhood are still very much true, they tend not to have much confidence in their ability to repair and heal. Therapists have an essential task at this early point in therapy—to demonstrate their unshakable belief in the fact that clients have everything they need to heal and that they, as therapists, are partners in the healing process. It's important to emphasize that clients won't return to a pre-trauma state as if nothing bad had ever happened to them but, as with the objects that go through the Kintsugi transformation process, their scars are viewed as precious, are accented and even celebrated, and show the clients' strength and resilience. Therapists use the comparison between clients' own P-A-C diagram, Figure 7.2 *P-A-C Diagrams: Validating Childhood Environment*, and Figure 7.3 *P-A-C Diagrams: Invalidating Childhood Environment* to illustrate how the AFTT-A process corrects and heals the impacts of attachment trauma while also presenting a mini-overview of the steps of the AFTT-A process.

2. Have the Client Describe and Illustrate Their Internal P-A-C Diagram as They Would Like It to Be by Drawing on Paper, Using a Sand Tray, or Through Another Preferred Therapy

Again, an expressive therapy such as drawing or using a sand tray assists clients to externalize their thoughts, perceptions, and emotions. The second drawing or sand tray design is meant to reflect what clients would like their inner systems to look like and how they imagine their parts will relate to each other and function together when they have completed the AFTT-A process. With this step, clients are basically describing their goals and making them real and more defined.

POINTS TO REMEMBER

- Normalize process and elements of development and clients' reactions to discussion of parts.
- Emphasize the impact of external messages from real-life attachment figures on development and the disconnection from Spiritual Essence.
- Remind clients that when they were children, their brains did what they were supposed to do, which was to internalize the messages from attachment figures in their lives.
- Explain how an invalidating environment affects the maturing of the Competent Adult part of Self or "Adult Brain."
- Show the link between optimal pathways/validating environments and positive adulthood behaviors and relationships and the link between nonoptimal pathways/invalidating environments and challenges with adulthood behaviors and relationships.

TROUBLESHOOTING

- Clients sometimes get defensive when discussing parents or other caregivers, reacting to the assumption that therapists are being judgmental about their parents or telling them they had "bad" parents. AFTT-A emphasizes that most childhoods are not perfect; even optimal environments aren't perfect. Parents are imperfect, make mistakes, are hurtful or neglectful, and act out of their own parts of Self and attachment patterns that developed in their invalidating or nonoptimal childhood environments. It's important to let clients know that they didn't deserve to be abused or neglected. It's challenging for therapists to avoid negative labels for parents especially when clients' abuse and/or neglect was severe.
- Use examples from other clients if the client has difficulty identifying how their internal personality parts were impacted by their childhood environment. Listen for an overprotective Critical Parent or Emotion Controller-Regulator that might be discouraging the client from sharing insights.

PAUSE AND REFLECT FOR THE THERAPIST

At this point, take some time to think about a challenging client with whom you work; perhaps someone who has difficulty following through with assignments, someone who is stuck and doesn't seem to be able to move forward, someone who seems to need more than you feel you can offer, or someone who is critical of you as a therapist. Instead of focusing on the client, consider your own feelings and thoughts about and reactions to the client. What do those self-observations tell you about your own internal P-A-C diagram? Jot down/draw what you imagine your own parts look like, their relationship with you as an adult and therapist, and with each other as well as in relationship to your challenging client. Then draw a second picture of what changes you would like to see in your parts, their relationships with each other, and how you would like your system to function as a whole. How would these changes affect how you interact with your challenging client?

USEFUL TERMS AND DEFINITIONS

"Adult Brain": The parts of the brain that house EMDR's adaptive information processing (AIP) system and include higher cognitive processes such as learning, problem-solving, decision-making, language, understanding of emotions, and narrative memory.

AFTT-A: Attachment-Focused Trauma Therapy for Adults

AIP: adaptive information processing

EMDR: Eye Movement Desensitization and Reprocessing

"Kid Brain": The neural network clusters in the emotional/social part of the brain that store unprocessed memories of adverse events and are disconnected from a sense of time and from the parts of the brain capable of processing memories and transferring them into narrative memory. AFTT-A views the neural networks as encapsulating more than memories of adverse events and includes the experiences, cognitive development, learning during a particular client age.

P-A-C diagrams: Parent-Adult-Child diagrams

PROTOCOL SCRIPT 1. PARENT-ADULT-CHILD (P-A-C) DIAGRAMS PROTOCOL #1: VALIDATING CHILDHOOD ENVIRONMENT

Adapted from Berne, E. (1964). *Games people play: The basic handbook of transactional analysis*. Random House; Bradshaw, J. (1990). *Homecoming: Reclaiming and healing your inner child*. Bantam Publishing; and Potter, A. E. (1994). *Inside out: Rebuilding self and personality through inner child therapy* (therapist manual and client workbook). Taylor and Francis Group.

Say... "Before we start, I want to make sure you understand that I want you to ask questions, stop me if you don't understand something, ask me to slow down (or tell me to hurry up because I'm getting repetitious and boring! Ha!). We're going to be doing a lot of what we call psychoeducation in this session and maybe even our next session depending on how much we talk about today. I'll be giving you some basic information that we'll be using and building on throughout the therapy we've started." *Ask...* "Any questions or concerns before we start?"

1. Introduce Concepts of Personality Parts and Aspects of Self. *Say...* "We all have different aspects or parts of ourselves and having parts is normal. We show different qualities or characteristics or wear different 'hats,' so to speak, depending on who we're with and what the situation is." *Use an example from your own life here.* ("For example, when I see clients, I tap into parts of myself that help me be attuned to how clients are feeling and what clients need, but when I'm in a business meeting about how we run the practice, I use parts of myself that are very factual, detail-oriented, and have problem-solving skills.") *Say...* "Many times when I first talk about parts to clients, they think it's weird or it means something is wrong with them. I want to reassure you that nothing is wrong with you. It's about what happened to you as you were growing up, not about you. And what happened to you was not your fault. You were a child and couldn't have known how to handle what was happening to you and around you any other way than the way you did." *Ask...* "Making sense? Any questions?"

Say... "The Parent-Adult-Child diagrams, or P-A-C diagrams, are examples of how our personality is put together as a structure, how it develops while we are growing up, and how it works when we are adults. As with all people, we're individuals and we have tendencies toward different kinds of personalities depending on what we genetically inherit from our families. However, how our personality develops depends quite a bit on the kind of environment we grow up in, especially the relationships we have with people who raise us like parents or other caregivers that we call attachment relationships. We also are affected by the messages that those important people give us about ourselves, other people, and the world in general; so, messages about our worth, whether others are trustworthy, and in general, if our world is a safe place. We'll go over both the P-A-C diagrams in more detail as we go along." *Ask...* "Any questions?"

2. Explain the Concept of Spiritual Essence and Its Relationship to Personality Development and Integration. *Say...* "First of all, one of the core assumptions of the AFTT-A model is that all of us are born with a Spiritual Essence, a core of goodness that is open to be loved and capable of loving others with a sense of optimism, joy, wonder, and hope for life. We all are born with this spiritual center that enlivens and energizes all parts of us. Our Spiritual Essence helps us feel connected at a very deep and basic level to all living things—other people, nature, to our world as a whole, and to a sense that we are part of a larger spirituality, as the 12-step programs say, 'a power greater than ourselves.' Depending on the person, the idea of a Spiritual Essence may or may not be related to religious beliefs."

3. Describe the Process of Development. Use P-A-C Diagrams: Validating Childhood Environment. *Say...* "Now let's look at the P-A-C diagrams that show us what happens to the Spiritual Essence and personality when children are raised in an optimal or validating environment." *Show P-A-C Diagrams: Validating Childhood Environment to the client. Point to each part of diagram being described. Say...* "In all situations, we start out as babies who have that spiritual core we just talked about. We start as basically a Child/Adolescent part (or what we might also call 'Kid Brain') infused with that Spiritual Essence. In a validating environment, the spiritual energy is nurtured and allowed to grow. Even as very young children, we have aspects of ourselves that we need to grow up. The Creative part of our inner Child is curious, awe-filled, and wants to learn and explore. It's the part that we might imagine holds our innate wisdom and intuition. The Essential Child/Adolescent part is full of emotions, wants, and impulses; the part 'wants what it wants when it wants it.'"

Say... "In an optimal situation, we interact with parents or other attachment figures (those people with whom we develop attachment relationships) who are loving and protective. They believe we are remarkable and amazing. They love us unconditionally, meaning that we don't have to earn their love by having to do certain things or act in certain ways. Parents in validating environments are also protective. They are in charge as adults and that gives us as children a sense of safety, consistency, and dependability. They establish rules that keep us and others from harm such as 'Look both ways before you cross the street' or 'Treat other people the way you want to be treated.' We listen to and absorb the real-life messages we are told as children such as 'You are worthwhile,' 'You are lovable,' and 'You deserve good things to happen in your life' as well as 'It's okay for you to trust others' and 'Your world is safe.' We do what children are meant to do with those messages of nurturing and safety: We internalize the messages and then make them our own messages by creating an internal nurturing and protective parent part of ourselves. We give our own voice to those real-life messages from others and they are transformed into 'I am worthwhile,' 'I am lovable,' and 'I deserve good things to happen in my life,' as well as 'It's okay for me to trust others' and 'My world is safe.'" *Ask...* "Making sense so far? Anything you need me to clarify or explain?"

Continue to describe each part of the P-A-C Diagrams: Validating Childhood Environment. Say... "On this diagram, you can see how the nurturing and protective internalized Parent part communicates and interacts with the aspects of the inner Child/Adolescent part of us. We have a part of that internal child called the Adaptive Child whose job it is to respond and adapt to real-life parental messages and then, over time, to the internalized messages we give ourselves from our own Nurturing and Protective Parent part of Self. Needless to say, the Essential Child, full of impulses, wants, and emotions, doesn't always get to do what it wants when it wants. Instead, the Adaptive Child takes in and learns the rules and guidelines real-life parents teach us as children and modifies the behavior of all the parts of the inner Child so as to adhere to those parental instructions. So, if your ball rolls out into the street, it wouldn't be okay to run after it without looking both ways to make sure there aren't any cars close by.

"The Adaptive Child also helps us learn how to manage and regulate feelings based on what we're taught about feelings and what we see modeled by others in terms of how they manage and express their feelings."

Say... "As we grow into adolescence and adulthood, areas of our brains develop that are capable of understanding emotions and regulating our emotions, thoughts, and behaviors. These parts of our brains make it possible to reason, consider alternatives, set goals, make and follow through with plans, and solve problems. We call these developing parts of our brain, our Competent Adult part, the 'Thinking Brain,' or 'Adult Brain.' As you can see in this part of the diagram, the Adult part of our personality is inserted in between the Parent and Child/Adolescent parts so it can mediate and coordinate the internal Parent and Child/Adolescent parts of our personality and be in charge of making decisions about how we express ourselves as well interact and communicate with others in real-life."

Say... "As you can see on the last part of the P-A-C diagram, each of our personality parts is equally well-developed and relates to each other in ways that are most helpful to us. As I said before, the Competent Adult part of us or our 'Adult Brain' is in charge and the Parent and Child/Adolescent parts no longer communicate with each other but communicate directly with the Adult part whose job it is to decide what's needed both internally in order for us to feel competent and confident within ourselves and in our real-life in order to respond to situations or circumstances in ways that are also competent and helpful.

"So, let's say you had a disagreement with a coworker. The Adult part of you gets input from the Parent and Child/Adolescent parts such as 'Hey, don't trust them,' 'You should tell your boss,' or 'You should just tell them off. They deserve it!' The Adult part also takes in information from the environment; for example, it's the first disagreement you had with your coworker, the company policies about handling such disagreements, and any safety issues in the situation. The Adult part might tap into the related protective Parent part having stronger boundaries if the coworker isn't trustworthy or there are safety issues. The Adult part might also help manage any feelings of anger or anxiety from the Child/Adolescent part while still connecting to some of the energy from those feelings from the Child/Adolescent part in order to set and follow through with appropriate boundaries." *Ask...* "Making sense? Any questions?"

4. Discuss What Aspects of Discussion Apply and/or Don't Apply to the Client. *Ask...* "Help me understand what parts of what we've talked about so far about optimal or validating environments fit or don't fit with how you were raised? What do you notice about how you react as an adult? What does that tell you about how your personality has developed?"

_____

_____

PROTOCOL SCRIPT 2. PARENT-ADULT-CHILD (P-A-C) DIAGRAMS PROTOCOL #2: INVALIDATING CHILDHOOD ENVIRONMENT

Adapted from Berne, E. (1964). *Games people play: The basic handbook of transactional analysis.* Random House; Bradshaw, J. (1990). *Homecoming: Reclaiming and healing your inner child.* Bantam Publishing; and Potter, A. E. (1994). *Inside out: Rebuilding self and personality through inner child therapy* (therapist manual and client workbook). Taylor and Francis Group.

1. Describe How the Process of Personality Development Is Altered by Attachment Trauma. *Use Figure 7.3 P-A-C Diagrams: Invalidating Childhood Environment.* *Say...* "As I said before, I want you to remember that it's not your fault that you have parts that are under- or overdeveloped and that don't work well together. It's not about you. It's about what happened to you and how what happened to you affected the way you grew up.

"So, with that reminder, let's go back to the P-A-C diagrams to see how personality development is impacted by a nonoptimal or invalidating environment." *Show P-A-C*

Diagrams: Invalidating Childhood Environment. Point to each part of diagram being described. Say... "As you can see on the top part of the diagram, even in an invalidating environment, we start with the inner Child/Adolescent part of Self that has the Essential, Creative, and Adaptive aspects to it and that is connected to a Spiritual Essence or a core of goodness."

Show P-A-C Invalidating Childhood Environment. Point to each part of diagram being described. Say... "What is different in this situation are the messages that real-life parents or other primary attachment figures give to their children either indirectly through behaviors, body language, or facial expressions, or directly through what they say and how they act. Typically, if you were raised in an invalidating environment, you would get very few nurturing messages and those you did get usually came with conditions or obligations. You can see in the next part of the diagram that the nurturing aspect of the Parent part is very small and underdeveloped. Instead of a strong inner Nurturing Parent part of Self that cares for us as well as care for others, we may end up with a very small Nurturing Parent.

"The Protective Parent part whose messages were intended to keep us safe from harm overdevelops into a distorted version called the Critical Parent whose derogatory and disapproving messages instead *cause* harm by cutting us off from our spiritual core and preventing that essence from growing and helping us experience ourselves as good and lovable. Parental abuse and neglect give us, either directly or indirectly, messages like 'You're bad,' 'You will never be good enough,' 'You don't deserve respect or happiness,' 'Other people will hurt you,' and 'The world is a dangerous place.' Additionally, those messages might also be spoken out loud. The Critical Parent really did not want to harm us as we were growing up and even now as we are adults. Believe it or not, its function was still protection. What caused this part to become harmful were the messages from real-life attachment figures. We, like children are supposed to, internalized the external negative and hurtful messages. So, the problem wasn't with the Protective Parent part but rather with the effect the external negative messages had on the part. The original Protective Parent was prevented from being protective in healthy and helpful ways because the messages that were provided sabotaged the part's ability to be protective in effective ways. So you can see, the Protective Parent didn't have the tools it needed to do its job in a helpful way. Instead, the Critical Parent overdevelops and controls what we believe about ourselves and other people.

"In this part of the diagram, the internalized Parent is comprised mostly of the Critical part. Again, we do what our 'Kid Brains' are supposed to do and internalize those external messages from real-life adults, making them a part of ourselves: 'I'm bad,' 'I'll never be good enough,' 'I don't deserve respect or happiness,' 'People will hurt me,' and 'My world is a dangerous place.' In invalidating environments, the messages damage how we feel about ourselves and form the foundation of negative cognitions or beliefs that haunt us even into our adult lives. You can see in the diagram that the Creative and the Essential aspects of the Child/Adolescent part of Self shrink and weaken. Unfortunately, those two parts of our inner Child/Adolescent aren't nurtured and encouraged to grow so we're don't experience some of the curiosity, the desire to learn and have fun, or spontaneous and playful feelings, and, as a result, can't bring those positive qualities with us into adulthood.

"The Adaptive Child is in a no-win situation. How can it possibly adapt to such demeaning and frightening messages? In its efforts to respond to the critical and harsh messages, the adaptive part of our inner Child overdevelops and becomes the Broken-Hearted Child. The very people who should be taking care of and protecting us are hurting us instead. Of course, our hearts are broken!" ***Give a few examples of how clients try to compensate for the negative cognitions or beliefs.*** ("As a therapist, I see people who try again and again to achieve and win and somehow convince themselves and others that they *are* good enough. Or other people who just give up trying to fight those negative messages and act out in ways that end up proving how true those critical messages are. The Critical Parent part then gets to say, 'I told you so. You really *are* bad.'")

"In the diagram, it looks like one Child/Adolescent part of Self, but it can actually be more than one Child/Adolescent part; maybe an infant, a toddler, a little elementary school-age part of Self, or an adolescent part. Yet, as adults, we carry the experiences, thoughts, and feelings from those younger ages.

"Broken-Hearted Child/Adolescent parts of Self may be cut off from the rest of your internal personality and need to be encouraged to come closer and share more about their held feelings, thoughts, and experiences. Broken-Hearted Child/Adolescent parts might instead be blended or enmeshed with other parts, especially the Adult and/or Critical Parent, so we call them the "Velcro Kids." They need to be a little more separate from other parts and to learn that their only job is to be a Child/Adolescent part; they no longer have to be in charge and run the show." ***Ask…*** "Making sense so far? Anything you need me to clarify or explain?"

Say… "As with any children, our brains develop as we move into adolescence and adulthood. If you were raised in an invalidating environment, your Competent Adult part of Self or 'Adult Brain' didn't get the encouragement and the age-appropriate learning experiences needed to learn to understand and regulate how you feel, think, and act. Instead, the parts of our brains we need to be able to reason, consider options, set goals, make and follow through with plans, and solve problems, tend to either overdevelop or underdevelop.

"Let's use the example of a disagreement with a coworker again. In this scenario, the Competent Adult part of you is either underdeveloped and is not strong enough to mediate among your inner parts or overdeveloped so you need to control feelings and behaviors. Either way, the Critical Parent and Broken-Hearted Child/Adolescent parts are still in direct communication. The Critical Parent may tell you use some choice words for your coworker about how you are right and they aren't; maybe even to the point of being sarcastic or bullying. The little "a" Adult part might not be strong enough to moderate the feelings from your Child/Adolescent part and you might act out by yelling or throwing something. The Emotion Controller-Regulator might have you swallow your feelings and walk away without saying anything but then add that disagreement to your pile of resentments toward the coworker and start looking for an opportunity to make them look bad."

Continue to point to each part of diagram being described. Say… "If our 'Adult Brain' is underdeveloped, we have a part called the 'little a,' a very childish, impulsive, and self-centered part that doesn't consider the effects of its behavior on others or the consequences of its actions. Someone who functions out of little 'a' often has addictions, has difficulty in relationships and jobs, and might even have legal problems. Little 'a' isn't strong enough to mediate between the Critical Parent and Broken-Hearted Child/Adolescent parts. Weak boundaries separate those parts and the Broken-Hearted Child/Adolescent part is left defenseless against the Critical Parent part's harsh, judgmental messages; thus, setting up a vicious cycle of negative messages and acting-out behavior. Little 'a' also isn't able to make healthy decisions in adult life.

"If parts of our 'Adult Brain' overdevelop, we end up with a distorted inner part called the Emotion Controller-Regulator. This part of 'Adult Brain' is basically stuck in one function: to avoid and control emotions. The Emotion Controller-Regulator is formed when children have to learn to cope with intense emotions, chaotic situations, and unfathomable harm without support or guidance from an adult. Their nervous systems are forced to cycle between being hypervigilant and braced for danger or overwhelmed, frozen, and numb. As a result, the Emotion Controller-Regulator becomes very protective and defensive by shutting down feelings that made us feel vulnerable or by pushing people away.

"Again, you can see how the problem wasn't with your part but the events and circumstances which your part was forced to survive and try to cope with in some way. As with the Critical Parent part, the Emotion Controller-Regulator always had your best interests at heart but was thwarted in doing its intended jobs of mediating and balancing internal parts as well as responding in competent and authentic ways to situations and relationships in adult life. Unfortunately, with its overprotectiveness, the Emotion Controller-Regulator often prevents you from having close connections, being able to feel your feelings, or even asking for help from me as you work through your memories."

2. Discuss What Aspects of Discussion Apply and/or Don't Apply to the Client. *Ask...* "Help me understand what parts of what we've talked about so far related to an invalidating childhood environment fit or don't fit with how you were raised? What do you notice about how you react as an adult? What does that tell you about how your personality has developed?"

_____

_____

3. Have the Client Describe and Illustrate Their Own Internal P-A-C Diagram by Drawing on Paper, Using a Sand Tray, or Another Preferred Therapy. *Say...* "Now that we've talked about how the environment we're raised in can affect us as adults and you've told me a bit about how the information relates to you, I'd like us to get a picture of what your own inner P-A-C diagram looks like. So that you and I both can see how the inside of you looks and feels to you related to what we've talked about. I'd like to invite you to (*describe whatever therapy modality you'll be using*) how you see and feel your own Self, Spiritual Essence, and inner parts, what they look like, what size they are, how close or far away they are from each other. Where you sense the Adult part of you, if you sense more than one Child/Adolescent part, and anything else you think would be helpful for us to know." **Wait until client is finished with**

project. Say... "I'd like to understand what your *(whatever is created by the therapy modality, e.g., drawing, sand tray design)* tells us about you. What would you like me to know about your *(whatever is created by the therapy modality, e.g., drawing, sand tray design)*?"

PROTOCOL SCRIPT 3. PARENT-ADULT-CHILD (P-A-C) DIAGRAMS PROTOCOL #3: EXPLANATION OF PROCESS FOR ATTACHMENT-FOCUSED TRAUMA THERAPY FOR ADULTS

Adapted from Berne, E. (1964). *Games people play: The basic handbook of transactional analysis*. Random House; Bradshaw, J. (1990). *Homecoming: Reclaiming and healing your inner child*. Bantam Publishing; and Potter, A. E. (1994). *Inside out: Rebuilding self and personality through inner child therapy* (therapist manual and client workbook). Taylor and Francis Group.

1. Describe How the Attachment-Focused Trauma Therapy for Adults (AFTT-A) Process Heals and Reconstructs the Client's Inner Attachments and Personality Structure and Enhances Their Capability for Healthy and Satisfying Attachment Relationships in Their Adult Life. *Use P-A-C Diagrams: Validating Childhood Environment and client's drawing or sand tray design, etc. Say...* "I know changing how you are inside and how you feel inside might seem pretty overwhelming. The good news is that we have a step-by-step process designed to help you start here *(point to client's drawing or design)* and heal, rebuild, and transform to here *(point to P-A-C Diagrams: Validating Childhood Environment)*. It won't be like you are going back to your original personality structure as if nothing bad ever happened, but it'll be more like moving forward to develop inside of you an Authentic Self with parts that are healthy and secure as well as able to function together as a whole. *(Use Kintsugi pottery as analogy for therapy process.)* We will talk about these topics and steps many, many times, so I don't want you to think you have to remember all of this information from today but, to begin with, I'd like you to have at least have an overall idea of the therapy process."

Point to each part of the diagram being described. Say... "First, we work on strengthening the Competent Adult part of you by filling in any gaps in skills to help you learn more flexible and balanced ways to think and feel about yourself as well as act in relationships. You'll create a place of respite for yourself as an adult and will gather a team of inner strengths and resources to help you feel inner support and encouragement.

"Next, we want to help any Broken-Hearted Child/Adolescent or Kid parts to get settled into a sense of being nurtured and protected. It's the way you and all of your parts will be able to start telling the difference between 'back then' where the danger was real and 'now' when the danger has passed. The Critical Parent and the Emotion Controller-Regulator/little 'a' parts will be offered the opportunity to change, become nurturing and protective in more helpful ways, and become members of your Inner Resource Team. Ultimately, you will develop a sense of a healthy Competent Adult part of Self that can stay in the driver's seat; solve problems and run your life from your 'Adult Brain' while still being able to access and experience feelings in a regulated way. You will be able to tap into and express the playfulness, spontaneity, and curiosity from your Child/Adolescent part through your Competent Adult part in safe situations with safe people. And lastly, you can reconnect to that sense of your innate goodness, your Spiritual Essence, that sense of being a part of something greater than yourself. You can be immersed in its positive energy and light throughout your whole Self, what we call your Authentic Self. It will be from this place of inner strength and support you have created that you then move into the next phase of therapy in which you resolve traumatic memories."

2. Have the Client Describe and Illustrate Their Internal P-A-C Diagram *as They Would Like It to Be* **by Drawing on Paper, Using a Sand Tray, or Through Another Preferred Therapy. Say…**"Now I would like you to (*describe whatever therapy modality you'll be using*) how you imagine the inside of you looks and feels *when it is exactly how you would like or want it to be*. When you resolved whatever you needed to resolve, healed whatever needed to be healed, and overcame whatever challenges you needed to get through. And anything else you think would be helpful for us to know." **Wait until client is finished with project. Say…**"I'd like to understand what your (*whatever is created by the therapy modality, e.g., drawing, sand tray design*) tells us about you. What would you like me to know about your (*whatever is created by the therapy modality, e.g., drawing, sand tray design*)?"

REFERENCES

Anonymous. (2001). *Alcoholics anonymous* (4th ed.). Alcoholics Anonymous World Services, Inc.
Berne, E. (1964). *Games people play: The basic handbook of transactional analysis*. Random House.
Black, C. (1982). *It will never happen to me*. Central Recovery Press.
Boon, S., Steele, K., & van der Hart, O. (2011). *Coping with trauma-related dissociation*. W. W. Norton & Company.
Bradshaw, J. (1990). *Homecoming: Reclaiming and healing your inner child*. Bantam Publishing.
Brill, A. A. (Trans., Ed.) (1995). *The basic writings of Sigmund Freud*. The Modern Library.
Bryant, D., Kessler, J., & Shirar, L. (1992). *The family inside: Working with the multiple*. W. W. Norton & Company.
Carvalho, E. R. (2012). *Healing the folks who live inside: How EMDR can heal our inner gallery of roles*. Self-Published.
Fisher, J. (2017). *Healing the fragmented selves of trauma survivors: Overcoming internal self-alienation*. Routledge.
Forgash, C., & Copeley, M. (Eds.) (2008). *Healing the heart of trauma and dissociation with EMDR and ego state therapy*. Springer Publishing Company.
Fraser, G. A. (1991). The Dissociative Table Technique: A strategy for working with ego states and dissociative disorders and ego-state therapy. *Dissociation: Progress in the Dissociative Disorders*, 4(4), 205–213.

Fraser, G. A. (2003). Fraser's "Dissociative Table Technique" revisited, revised: A strategy for working with ego states in dissociative disorders and ego-state therapy. *Journal of Trauma and Dissociation*, 4(4), 5–28. https://doi.org/10.1300/J229v04n04_02

Gonzales, A., & Mosquera, D. (2012). *EMDR and dissociation: A progressive approach* (1st ed., revised). Self-Published.

Harris, T. (1969). *I'm O.K., You're O.K.* Harper & Row Publishers.

Holmes, T., & Holmes, L. (2007). *Parts work: An illustrated guide to your inner life.* Winged Heart Press.

Knipe, J. (2015). *EMDR toolbox: Theory and treatment of complex PTSD and dissociation.* Springer Publishing Company.

Lanius, U., & Paulsen, S. (2014). *Neurobiology and treatment of traumatic dissociation: Towards an embodied self.* Springer Publishing Company.

Linehan, M. (1993). *Cognitive-behavioral treatment of borderline personality disorder.* Guilford Press.

Manfield, P. (2010). *Dyadic resourcing: Creating a foundation for processing trauma.* CreateSpace Independent Publishing.

Martin, K. M. (2012). How to use Fraser's Dissociative Table Technique to access and work with emotional parts of the personality. *Journal of EMDR Practice and Research*, 6(4), 179–186. https://doi.org/10.1891/1933-3196.6.4.179

Parnell, L. (1999). *EMDR in the treatment of adults abused as children.* W. W. Norton & Company.

Paulsen, S. (2009). *Looking through the eyes of trauma and dissociation.* The Bainbridge Institute for Integrative Psychology.

Potter, A. E. (1994a). *Inside out: Rebuilding self and personality through inner child therapy* (therapist manual). Accelerated Development, Inc.

Potter, A. E. (1994b). *Inside out: Rebuilding self and personality through inner child therapy* (client workbook). Accelerated Development, Inc.

Satir, V. (1972). *Peoplemaking.* Science and Behavior Books, Inc.

Schmidt, S. L. (2009). *The developmental needs meeting strategy (DNMS): An ego state therapy for healing adults with childhood trauma and attachment wounds.* DNMS Institute LLC.

Schmidt, S. L. (2020). *Ego state therapy interventions to prepare attachment-wounded adults for EMDR.* DNMS Institute LLC.

Schwartz, R. C. (1995). *Internal family systems therapy.* The Guilford Press.

Shapiro, R. (2016). *Easy ego state intervention: Strategies for working with parts.* W. W. Norton & Company.

Van der Hart, O., & Nijenhuis, E. (2006). *The haunted self: Structural dissociation and the treatment of chronic traumatization.* W. W. Norton & Company.

Walker, P. (2013). *Complex PTSD: From surviving to thriving.* CreateSpace Independent Publishing: Azure Coyote Book.

Watkins, J. G., & Watkins, H. H. (1997). *Ego states: Theory and therapy.* W. W. Norton & Company.

Whitfield, C. (1987). *Healing the child within: Discovery and recovery for adult children of dysfunctional families.* Health Communications, Inc.

Wildwind, L. (1992). *Treating chronic depression.* Presentation, EMDRIA Conference, Sunnydale, California.

Woititz, J. (1983). *Adult children of alcoholics.* Health Communications, Inc.

CHAPTER 8

Safe Place and Higher Power for Adult Part of Self in Attachment-Focused Trauma Therapy for Adults

INTRODUCTION

Everyone naturally has needs throughout their lifetime for nurturing, connection, protection, and safety; the need to belong and be accepted, to be in relationship with others, and to feel a sense of security and stability. Throughout childhood, clients have needs for safety and nurturing; knowing that they are "good enough," that they are lovable and worthwhile, and that they deserve good things to happen in their lives. Children are dependent on the adults in their lives to meet such needs and to give them messages of love and protection, first with attachment figures such as parents or other primary caregivers and then, as they mature, with extended family, teachers, religious leaders, and other authority figures. As a part of normal development, children integrate others' external messages to form the foundation or the core of their beliefs about themselves, others, and the world.

Adults raised in relatively validating or optimal environments have well-developed parts of Self that assist them in coping with varying circumstances in their lives. Additionally, inner parts form attachments or relationships among themselves to establish the cooperation and coordination needed to respond effectively to the complex aspects of the familial, cultural, and social aspects of their adult lives.

Parts of Self perform a range of roles depending on what is required in certain situations so clients successfully manage their adult lives and navigate healthy adult relationships. For example, the Child/Adolescent part of Self provides emotions, playfulness, fun, humor, the ability to be absorbed in the present moment, passion for ideals, intuition or innate wisdom, and the ability to respond to situations in adaptive ways. The parts of Self formed by internalizing messages from real-life adults during childhood and adolescence become the True Parent part of Self, that is, the nurturing and protective aspects of Self that contribute needed encouragement and reassurance; reminders of morals, principles, and conscience; and alerts to the need for self-protection. The Competent Adult part of Self regulates affect and emotions, acts as mediator among the other internal parts, and assesses and coordinates clients' reactions to and behaviors in real-life situations and relationships.

Often in invalidating environments, the encouraging and supportive messages from primary attachment figures are absent, inconsistent, or conditional. Instead, negative messages hurt, belittle, and damage children's ability to grow into competent and confident adults. Children begin to believe that they are not good enough, they must earn love and affection, and they are undeserving or unworthy of getting their needs met.

Adults with a history of attachment trauma have a poorly-developed sense of Self and either under- or overdeveloped internal aspects of themselves with overly close (blended/enmeshed) or overly distant (detached or dissociated) internal relationships. As a result, internal attachment patterns are reflected in external relationships in their adult lives. Clients may come to therapy with Child parts "in charge" of their lives and relationships. They present as overly emotional and impulsive and engage in intense and sometimes volatile relationships. In such an instance, the Child part overdevelops, and the Parent and Adult parts of Self are underdeveloped. The Child part tends to be blended or enmeshed with the Adult aspect of Self and detached from the Parent part. As a result, the Child part does the Adult part's job of directing clients' behaviors and reactions with only the child-like cognitive resources and without the ability to reason or problem-solve or the benefit of parental guidance or wisdom. Meanwhile, the Adult and Parent parts of Self abdicate their roles of either moral compass and protector or of regulator, mediator, and orchestrator.

Conversely, clients may also present in an opposite manner: They overcontrol emotions and behavior, lack spontaneity, come across as controlling and/or critical, and keep others at a distance. In this case, the Adult and Parent parts of Self are overdeveloped and closely connected while the Child part remains underdeveloped and cut off from the other parts. Such clients tend to be rigid about following rules, hypervigilant to avoid emotional vulnerability, overfocused on achievement, and controlling in relationships.

The Attachment-Focused Trauma Therapy for Adults (AFTT-A) model enhances Eye Movement Desensitization and Reprocessing (EMDR) therapy's preparation phase (phase 2) and aims to address internal and external barriers to clients' ability to reprocess memories of adverse events. One of the EMDR preparation phase standard protocols, *Safe/Calm Place,* focuses on developing an internal sense of safety and emotion regulation so clients can tolerate the intense affect involved in phases 3 to 8 (Shapiro, 2018). The first protocol in the AFTT-A model, *Safe Place and Higher Power for the Adult Part of Self,* augments the standard Safe/Calm Place protocol by placing the client within the context of a corrective attachment relationship in their Safe Place and, as a result, strengthens clients' sense of safety and adds qualities of nurturing and acceptance to their experience.

SAFE/CALM PLACE OR STATE AND EMDR THERAPY

The concept of a "Safe/Calm Place," most recently re-designated as a "Safe/Calm State," is taught to clients in the preparation phase of EMDR therapy as a method for emotional stabilization at the end of therapy sessions when EMDR reprocessing is incomplete, and when emotional disturbance is experienced in between sessions. The eight-part Safe/Calm State protocol in EMDR therapy assists clients in making associations to a positive feeling state while also learning to accommodate bilateral stimulation (BLS), through slow tapping, eye movement, or audible tones or music, into the therapy process prior to the desensitization and reprocessing of traumatic material. The newly linked positive affect can then be accessed to reassure clients of their capability for managing challenging negative affect as well as regaining a balance with positive affect (Shapiro, 2018, pp. 117–119, 246–248; 2021, pp. 36–39).

Leeds (2016) dropped the word "Safe" from the protocol with the reworked title of "Calm Place." In addition to the previously mentioned purposes, Leeds also utilized the protocol in the EMDR therapy preparation phase as an assessment of clients' readiness to move to the subsequent phases of desensitization and reprocessing. Clients who can access and maintain connection to positive affect as well as successfully apply the protocol in and outside of sessions are deemed to have the necessary affect regulation skills to begin processing traumatic material (Leeds, 2016, pp. 123–125).

Parnell (2007) expanded Shapiro's Safe/Calm Place protocol to include a Meeting Place for clients and their inner resources such as spirituality and strength and allies such as wise, protective, and/or nurturing figures (pp. 69–82). Reddeman developed an imagery script called "Inner Safe Place," one of the stabilization techniques within Psychodynamic Imaginative Trauma Therapy (PITT) used in general to prepare clients for trauma therapy and in particular as a resource in EMDR therapy. Reddeman's script allows clients to choose whether an "inner helper" is present in the Inner Safe Place and gives clients opportunities throughout the script to make changes until all aspects of the place meet clients' needs and purposes for protection and a sense of "wellness" (Reddeman, 2009, pp. 71–72).

SAFE PLACE AND HIGHER POWER IN THE AFTT-A MODEL

Decades of clinical experience show us that adults who experienced childhood attachment trauma require more time in the preparation phase with enhancement of standard protocols as well as additional protocols. One of the underlying assumptions of the AFTT-A model is that adverse childhood experiences encompass more than discrete events of abuse and neglect. Because those traumatic events occur within attachment relationships, self-worth is damaged, trust and boundaries are violated, unhealthy relationship patterns are modeled and learned, and skills needed for healthy adult functioning are not taught. Therefore, prior to reprocessing traumatic incidents, clients need to heal and reconstruct the inner structure of their Authentic Self and begin to repair the effects of ruptured attachments.

Experiences of abuse and/or neglect by attachment figures during childhood and adolescence negatively impact clients in many areas of their lives. Clients enter adulthood with strong negative self-beliefs. They repeat patterns in relationships that helped them survive the pain and shame involved in traumatic events. They try to get unmet childhood needs met in their current relationships but find that their attempts interfere with closeness in their adult relationships.

In the AFTT-A model, the enhanced *Safe Place and Higher Power for the Adult Part of Self* protocol helps clients with a history of attachment trauma create an internal way of meeting their needs for safety and love despite negative self-beliefs or cognitions they developed in childhood. Connecting to and strengthening an inner sense of safety and nurturing provide the Adult part of Self with an inner place of respite or a place of "being" independent from stressors and negative aspects of their current circumstances.

The AFTT-A process incorporates the steps of differentiation, protection, nurturing and strengthening, reconnection, and integration in the Kintsugi pottery restoration into a framework to address the issues of under- and overdeveloped parts of Self and enmeshed or dissociated types of attachments among internal parts. The *Safe Place and Higher Power for the Adult Part of Self* protocol fosters healthy differentiation between the Adult and Child/Adolescent parts of Self; building firm and flexible inner boundaries among parts of Self and as a result, strengthens and empowers the Competent Adult part of Self to take charge of clients' present-day lives. Healthy internal boundaries also serve as the foundation of time orientation for clients. Clients can discern the difference between "back then" when there was danger, negative cognitions were believed to be true, and old coping strategies were used for survival, and "now" when they have a strong belief of their own inherent goodness, all their needs are met within their newly developing Authentic Self, and they are certain that the danger from the past is over.

Additionally, the protocol aims to reconnect clients' parts of Self with their core of spiritual goodness through positive representatives of attachment figures or Higher Powers that have an unshakable belief in their worthiness and can meet needs for safety and unconditional love. The process of internalizing strong and supportive attachment relationships among parts of Self starts to correct clients' past experiences with real-life attachment figures and expands clients' capacity for forming healthy relationships in their present-day lives.

STEPS FOR ADULT SAFE PLACE AND HIGHER POWER PROTOCOL

The *Safe Place and Higher Power for the Adult Part of Self* protocol is the first step in the AFTT-A process of tapping into and strengthening clients' Competent Adult part of Self (see Protocol Script 4 at the end of the chapter). The protocol reconnects clients to their own goodness, instills a positive self-image, and encourages the development of healthy internal and external attachments.

Clients often initially react to the protocol with fear and/or shame. They don't think they have a very good "imagination." They're afraid they will make mistakes, won't get it "right," or the process won't work for them. They may even be anxious about being vulnerable or looking silly or foolish. They sometimes think that what's involved in the protocol is imaginary and therefore not "real," and might even be critical or dismissive of the process. Sometimes clients fear that they won't be able to find any positive aspects to themselves or will be overwhelmed by negative feelings and thoughts. Luckily, clients' fear- and shame-based responses to the initial protocol offer therapists a wonderful opportunity to intervene with a balance between acknowledgment of how understandable clients' reactions are and a demonstration of their unshakable belief that clients already have what they need to be able to embrace the process and make the changes to which they aspire. Clients are also taught that their images are not "etched in stone"; they can be changed at any time as needed.

1. Discuss Concept of and Purposes for *Safe Place and Higher Power for the Adult Part of Self* Protocol

Psycho-education introduces the AFTT-A model to clients, including an explanation about the idea and purposes of creating a Safe Place for themselves with a Higher Power figure. Clients can go to their Safe Place with their Higher Power in their minds to get grounded and centered and to be free of real-world stresses, problems, and conflicts. The Safe Place is a place of "respite" and a place of "being." Clients use their Safe Place to get reconnected to and strengthen a sense of nurturing and safety. The positive affect linked to their Safe Place and Higher Power helps them regulate emotions during therapy sessions when needed and to regulate and recharge in between sessions.

Client Safe Places contain a figure, being, or entity called a "Higher Power" that represents a link to their Spiritual Essence, their core of inherent goodness. The term "Higher Power" is derived from the 12-step approach to addiction recovery and is viewed as "… a Power greater than ourselves" (Alcoholics Anonymous, 2001, p. 59); someone or something that incorporates the concepts of a helper, guide, protector, and/or advisor, but yet is more than just those concepts combined. Client Higher Powers are meant to be stronger and more powerful as well as more loving, understanding, and compassionate than clients themselves and anyone in clients' past and present life. AFTT-A's introduction of a Higher Power figure in the enhanced version of EMDR's Safe/Calm Place protocol extends the sense of caring and safety connected to the place itself to include a corrective attachment experience with a consistent, loving, protective, and attuned Higher Power within which clients' needs are met.

2. Identify Needs of the Adult Part of Self for Nurturing and Protection

Clients with a history of attachment trauma often have been taught during childhood that they should not have needs, they were bad if they had needs, and if they had needs, they shouldn't expect to have those needs met. They may even have learned that it was their responsibility to take care of others' needs while ignoring their own. As a result, clients tend to have either a difficult time identifying their needs and be somewhat disdainful of the idea they have needs (dismissive attachment pattern) or are overly dependent on others to meet their needs (preoccupied attachment pattern). The first type of client often comes across in relationships as aloof, cold, or distant while the second type might be labeled as "needy" and "high-maintenance."

The therapist normalizes clients' lifelong needs for nurturing and protection. Clients start the *Safe Place and Higher Power for the Adult Part of Self* protocol by identifying a few unmet needs in their present-day lives. Sometimes, clients need help identifying their unmet needs and therapists might offer examples of the two main types of needs to be met in their Safe Place with their Higher Power:

- Nurturing—Love, acceptance, respect, compassion, understanding, encouragement
- Safety—Protection, security, control, limits, boundaries, reassurance, respite

3. Brainstorm Ideas for a Safe Place for the Adult Part of Self

Once clients identify a few unmet adulthood needs, the therapist helps them brainstorm ideas for a place where they can feel safe, calm, grounded, and/or centered; a place to which they can attach the most unambiguous positive feelings possible. They might suggest thinking about a place they have seen in a movie or online, read about in a book, visited on vacation (in the mountains or on a beach), or have always wanted to visit (the Grand Tetons or the over-the-water huts on stilts in Bora Bora), as long as the place brings to mind a sense of peace, safety, and relaxation. We want clients to begin to experience the affect linked to strong positive cognitions or beliefs such as "I'm okay no matter what," "I am enough," and "I am lovable and worthwhile."

Prior to installation, clients test the place they have chosen to make certain that it includes both nurturing and protective properties. Clients might create a place that is very comfortable and relaxing, (e.g., a cabin on the top of a mountain that has soft furniture and relaxing music) but is vulnerable to negative people or messages. Safety measures are brainstormed and added to reinforce a sense of security. Conversely, clients may design a safe place that is very protective, (e.g., a castle with an alligator-invested moat and a knight that guards the drawbridge) but is also dark, cold, and dank so, nurturing, warm, and welcoming characteristics are brainstormed and included to balance the well-developed sense of protection.

4. Install the Safe Place

Once clients have chosen a Safe Place, the protocol guides them into the installation by asking them to decide how they want to arrive in their place and focus their sensory experiences. What do they see? What sounds are heard? What scents and textures are noticed? After the clients report positive affect related to their new Safe Place (e.g., easing or relaxing; a sense of calm, being grounded or centered; or feeling safe or secure), BLS is started through the use of hand-held tappers or clients doing butterfly taps (arms crossed with tapping back and forth on their upper arms) or alternate tapping on the tops of their thighs. Since clients are connecting to and strengthening positive affect, the sets of BLS are very short and very slow; perhaps only three or four round trips. Positive affect is strengthened, deepened, and expanded through short sets of slow BLS.

5. Containment/Mindfulness

Clients are often able to focus on and reinforce positive affect during installation of the Safe Place and Higher Power for their Adult part of Self without therapist intervention. Sometimes, clients find focusing on positive affect challenging, distracted by distressing cognitions, emotions, body sensations, or memories. AFTT-A views such experiences as time disorientation, when clients are confused between "now" in the present moment and "back then" from stored traumatic material that intrudes during the protocol. If clients have a difficult time getting or staying connected to positive affect during installation, therapists can intervene containment and mindfulness approaches aimed at time orientation (Martin, 2018). The AFTT-A model looks at clients' experience of negative affect or difficulty staying with positive affect as a perfect opportunity to teach containment and mindfulness skills. One of the benefits of the practice of containing and setting aside negative affect during the protocol aimed at connecting to and strengthening positive aspects is that clients learn elemental ways to be mindful in the present moment, a skill that is applicable in EMDR therapy trauma reprocessing and many areas of their lives. Being able to notice negative affect and treat it as a distraction rather than as evidence of something wrong becomes a foundational piece of clients' affect or emotion regulation and provides valuable information to therapists about client readiness for subsequent phases of EMDR therapy (Murray, 2011).

Therapists normalize how negative thoughts or affect might interrupt their positive focus. Clients are encouraged to notice the negative affect (thoughts, feelings, and body sensations) without judging it as "bad." Therapists then remind clients that the purpose of the protocol is to tap into and strengthen a positive state of mind. Clients are reassured that all of their feelings are important and they are not being told *not* to feel their feelings, but rather that negative affect is just not the focus of this particular protocol. Clients are guided to separate out their negative affect to "set aside" and refocus on positive impressions. Sometimes, clients can mentally separate and separate negative affect from the protocol focus without further therapist intervention. However, if not, they can create an imaginary container that is outside of the boundaries of their Safe Place and is strong enough to hold the negative affect at least until they have completed the protocol. They utilize the container as needed if subsequent distressing thoughts, emotions, or memories intrude while they are completing the protocol. If they wish, they can always pick up or take back what they have put in the container on their way out of their Safe Place.

Often clients with a history of attachment trauma experience triggered affect and memories outside therapy sessions. The image and practice of a container can be helpful to clients in separating negative affect and traumatic materials brought up and examined in therapy sessions from their lives outside the therapy office. Clients can imagine using a container such as a safe, a lidded bin, or a burn barrel in their adult lives where they can set aside distressing material until they take it out and bring it back to their next therapy session. Clients can also imagine a container in the therapy office where they can leave behind negative affect and memories when they leave sessions. I (A.P.) have clients who have left distressing material in my file cabinet, under the couch, on top of the bookshelf, or in an invisible recycling bin in the waiting room.

6. Brainstorm Ideas for a Higher Power for the Adult Part of Self

The next step in the Adult Safe Place and Higher Power protocol focuses on talking about the concept and the purposes of a Higher Power. Some clients may have a problem with the idea because they immediately think of a religious figure or the 12-step programs, but one of the main purposes of having a Higher Power is to introduce the concept and the experience of a healthy attachment relationship into their Safe Place. In addition to the sense of "I'm okay no matter what," a relationship with a Higher Power figure helps clients start to develop a sense of being supported and encouraged with positive beliefs such as "I am loved unconditionally."

As with clients' Safe Places, Higher Powers also encompass both qualities of nurturance and safety. Additionally, the Higher Power figure or entity represents someone or something with whom clients can experience a corrective attachment relationship. Higher Power figures can be anyone or anything if the being, creature, animal, person, or force of nature is protective and accepting. Clients can use religious figures, such as dieties, prophets, leaders, holy or enlightened beings, saints, or angels, or entities from indigenous spiritual, religious, and cultural traditions. Higher Powers don't have to have religious foundations. Agnostic and atheist clients generate nonreligious characters. Higher Powers can also be family members, famous people or leaders clients admire, characters from books or video games, or superheroes from comics or movies.

If a client chooses a family member who is living, the therapist needs to make sure that the person is given special characteristics, qualities, or powers that the real-life person doesn't have so the client can differentiate between the actual person and the person representing their Higher Power. If the client selects someone from their childhood, they face a hard truth—that no matter how much the person from their past loved them or tried to protect them, bad things still happened. So, a childhood figure as a Higher Power needs to be stronger and more powerful as well as more loving and nurturing than anyone in the clients' past or present life. For example, a client who wanted her grandfather as her Higher Power transformed him into a grandfather figure who had a laser finger that could disintegrate any danger that got close to their Safe Place.

If a client chooses a family member or other person who has died, that person also needs to be given a special quality or power to help them separate the real-life person from the client's Higher Power. One client's grandmother became "Angel Grandma" who sat with them on a swing and wrapped her wings around them in their Safe Place. Depending on their belief system, clients also imagine the person who died as their "most-evolved" self in the afterlife as their Higher Power.

Additionally, the therapist wants to ensure that the client has unambiguous positive feelings toward any person from their past or present life as their Higher Power. Clients don't have to eliminate someone as their Higher Power just because they are still angry at that person, still hope for a relationship, miss the person, or feel grief about the person's death. If clients can utilize their container to set aside their feelings of sadness, anger, longing, or grief and refocus on their positive feelings, the person can still represent their Higher Power in their Safe Place. If the client is not able to set aside the negative affect associated with their potential Higher Power, then brainstorming another Higher Power is necessary.

The final step prior to installing the client's Higher Power in their Safe Place is discussing ways the Higher Power figure might be tested to refine it as needed. For example, clients might create a Higher Power who is extremely protective and able to guarantee safety, but warmth and connection are lacking so those characteristics are added before installation.

BOX 8.1 CLIENT EXAMPLE: CLIENT BRAINSTORMING A SAFE PLACE AND HIGHER POWER FOR ADULT PART OF SELF

Therapist: Okay, like we talked about last time, the Safe Place for the Adult part of you can be a real place or an imaginary place. A place you've been or maybe a place you've always wanted to visit, as long as when you think about it, you get a sense of "now there's a place I could go and leave everything else behind. Like worries or concerns. Troubling situations ...."

Client: Well, I was thinking of using Mr. Mendez from The Butterfly Circus as my Higher Power because he's so accepting and wise but doesn't let any circus members get hurt, so what do you think about me using the Butterfly Circus for my Safe Place?

Therapist: Help me understand how that would work for you.

Client: Well, it wouldn't be when everyone is in the sideshow, but while they're sitting around in their camp with the caravans circled. Everyone's there with me, and I can just be myself.

Therapist: Sounds very caring and nurturing. How about safe?

Client: Well, it feels like when they are circled together, there's something there that keeps anyone that shouldn't be there from coming into the circle.

7. Install the Higher Power in the Safe Place

First, the therapist guides the client back into their Safe Place to get reconnected to feeling calm, safe, grounded, centered, or whatever words they use to describe the positive affect associated with their Safe Place. A couple of short sets of BLS reinforces their positive affect. The therapist elicits a description of the client's Higher Power and lets the client choose how the Higher Power is going to be added to the Safe Place. Sometimes clients want their Higher Power to be waiting for them or join them, or for them to go to the Safe Place together. The therapist asks about and obtains positive feelings, thoughts, and body sensations about being connected to their Higher Power in their Safe Place. Again, the positive affect is strengthened and reinforced with short sets of slow BLS. If negative affect comes up, the therapist prompts the client to use their container to set aside negative affect and refocus on the positive emotions, thoughts, and sensations being generated.

8. Add a Boundary Around the Safe Place With the Higher Power

Inner boundaries represent both protection and differentiation. In the AFTT-A model, clients create a Safe Place in which they feel safe and nurtured regardless of what is happening in their adult lives. The AFTT-A *Safe Place and Higher Power for the Adult Part of Self* protocol provides a boundary to protect clients' positive internal experiences related to their Safe Place and Higher Power from any stressful or negative circumstance in their present-day lives. Once clients have connected to and reinforced the positive affect related to their Safe and Higher Power, therapists assist them in surrounding their Safe Place with a protective boundary so the internalized sense of being loved, accepted, safe, calm, grounded, and/or centered can be experienced consistently, regardless of present circumstances or situations.

Clients use many substances or objects for boundaries, for example, a force field, deflector shield, wall, cloak of invisibility, or snow globe. They may use people to guard the perimeter of the Safe Place such as Secret Service agents, Jedi warriors, ninjas, knights, Scottish Highlanders, or figures with magical, protective powers or objects like wands, lightning, or light sabers.

Clients install the boundary around their Safe Place and focus on positive thoughts, emotions, and sensations associated with the addition of the boundary. The therapist encourages clients to experience the steadfastness of their positive beliefs and affect while imagining whatever events might take place or what people might do or say outside the boundary, watching how the boundary deflects, averts, or prevents any potential threats to the clients' positive affect from gaining access to their Safe Place. Positive thoughts, emotions, and body sensations linked to the boundary are strengthened and reinforced with short sets of slow BLS.

9. Anchor and Word

EMDR therapy utilizes both a word or phrase and a place on clients' bodies as ways to reconnect them to the positive affect gained in the Safe Place protocol. The AFTT-A model also employs the same techniques so clients can readily apply what they experienced in therapy sessions to their lives between sessions.

First, therapists brainstorm with clients a place on their body (or a piece of jewelry they always wear). Clients often choose one of their fingers, a place on their hand or arm, their ear, on their chest over their heart, a ring, an object on a necklace, or even a motion like running their hand through their hair or a body posture like straightening their shoulders or backs. Once clients anchor their positive affect, short sets of slow BLS strengthen and reinforce the affect.

Therapists explore with their clients a word or a phrase that exemplifies the affirming beliefs and emotions they want to take from their Safe Place and Higher Power into their present-day life. Clients may pick one of the aspects of themselves they realized during the *Safe Place and Higher Power for the Adult Part of Self* protocol such as "proud," "strong," "safe," "calm," "serene," or "grounded." They may opt for a positive cognition or belief that came up during the protocol such as "I'm okay no matter what," "I'm capable," "I'm lovable," or "I deserve respect." Once clients link the word or phrase to positive affect, short sets of slow BLS strengthen and reinforce the link to their affirmation.

Clients are encouraged to practice stepping into their Safe Place and visiting their Higher Power at least daily. They can take a few moments while they're getting ready for the day and use their word, phrase, or body anchor to remind themselves of their connection to their sense of being calm and capable. Practice! Practice! Practice!

10. Test the Effectiveness of the Installations With a Challenging Situation From Present-Day Life

The final test for the client's newly installed Safe Place and Higher Power is whether the client finds using it helpful in between therapy sessions. The therapist sets up a mini-Future Rehearsal by asking the client to think of a potentially challenging situation that might occur before they meet again. The therapist guides the client to imagine briefly visiting their Safe Place with their Higher Power surrounded by the boundary prior to going into the difficult situation, reinforcing positive affect with short sets of slow BLS. The therapist then encourages the client to step into the setting and use their anchor and/or word to access how it feels to be in the situation connected to their positive characteristics, emotions, and beliefs and protected by their Higher Power and Safe Place boundary.

11. Refine and Install the Revised Safe Place and Higher Power as Needed

Sometimes, clients return to therapy after having practiced using their Safe Place and Higher Power between therapy sessions and report that some aspect didn't seem right or didn't work, or they had difficulty connecting to the images and affect. The therapist normalizes the client's experience since they are new to the process and to the *Safe Place and Higher Power for the Adult Part of Self* protocol. Together, they troubleshoot the client's barriers to accessing or applying their new Safe Place with their Higher Power and modify either or both as needed. The therapist guides the client in installing the revised Safe Place and Higher Power using the steps of the *Safe Place and Higher Power for the Adult Part of Self* protocol.

POINTS TO REMEMBER

- Images are not "etched in stone." They can be seen as a starting point and can be changed at any point if needed.

- The purposes of the Safe Place are to provide a place of respite, of being calm and grounded, while helping clients connect to and strengthen an unshakable belief in "I'm okay no matter what."
- Both the Safe Place and the Higher Power figure contain aspects of nurturing and protection.
- The Adult Safe Place cannot be the same as the Safe Place(s) for the Child part(s) of Self.
- Higher Powers can be shared between the Adult and Child/Adolescent parts of Self.
- Higher Powers based on real-life people need to be given special powers or characteristics.
- Use short sets of slow BLS using tappers or butterfly tapping.
- Link the positive affect associated with the Safe Place and Higher Power with a word or phrase and/or a body anchor.
- Consider the client's social, religious/nonreligious, and cultural identity and influences when brainstorming Safe Places and Higher Powers.

TROUBLESHOOTING

- Clients who have difficulty creating a sense of inner safety and protection often have a Child part involved that is disoriented to time and truly can't conceive of a place of safety and protection. Therapists take the opportunity to help them separate their Adult part from Child/Adolescent parts of Self, thus freeing them to imagine a sense of safety despite adverse childhood experiences.
- Phrases to use when clients have difficulty coming up with ideas: "There's no right or wrong way to do this." "Give it a try. If it works, great! If it doesn't work, we'll figure out how to make it work." "Nothing's etched in stone. We can always change it to be more helpful."
- If clients protest that they can't complete the protocol because they don't have a good imagination, therapists can give examples of ideas other clients have used.
- If clients fear they won't do it right or perfectly, therapists can identify negative cognitions or beliefs that can actually help them create a place that addresses and modifies those beliefs.
- If clients emphasize either the nurturing or protective aspect of the Safe Place or Higher Power, acknowledge the quality they described and remind them to generate ideas for the other characteristic.
- If clients have problems with the concept of a Higher Power, remind them that their "Higher Power" can be represented by any real or imagined being, animal, or part of nature that is more powerful and more loving than the client and anyone in their actual lives. Clients can even use a spiritual aspect of themselves connected to a sense of their own goodness and innate wisdom; for example, Highest Self, Best Self, or Inner Wisdom.

PAUSE AND REFLECT FOR THE THERAPIST

At this point, take some time to think about a challenging client with whom you work; perhaps someone who has difficulty following through with assignments, someone who is stuck and doesn't seem to be able to move forward, someone who seems to need more than you can offer, or someone who is critical of you as a therapist. Instead of focusing on the client, consider your own feelings and thoughts about and reactions to the client. What do you notice when you're in session with them? Anxiety? Frustration? Self-blame for the client not making progress? Do you notice a sense of worry or dread when you see that client's name on your schedule? Do any negative cognitions or self-beliefs come up as you think about being in session with the client? Jot down what you might need to be able to feel confident and competent, in order to bring your Authentic Self into future sessions with the client.

Next, create for yourself a Safe Place and a Higher Power that will help you connect to what you need. Somewhere you can go to get centered, to recharge and regroup, to quiet any doubts, and to connect to a Higher Power who believes in you, your worth, and your capabilities. Include accepting, nurturing, and encouraging aspects as well as a sense of safety and security to both the Safe Place and the Higher Power. Imagine yourself there and, if you like, when you notice positive feelings, sensations, body posture, and thoughts, you can do some slow BLS by tapping back and forth on the tops of your thighs or use butterfly taps on your upper arms. Jot down a word or phrase that will help you tap into the confidence and competence you gained and remind you of the sense of protection and acceptance you felt. Anchor the positive affect with a gesture or a part of your body you can connect to like your hand over your heart and again reinforce with slow tapping.

Now, imagine taking a moment before you meet with the client again to call to mind whatever you need from your Safe Place and Higher Power to be able to go into the session with your Competent Adult part of Self, your most Authentic Self. Picture yourself having at your fingertips the helpful and encouraging thoughts and the positive feelings any time you might need them during the next session with the client. Again, if you like, you can strengthen and reinforce positive feelings, sensations, thoughts by doing more slow tapping back and forth.

USEFUL TERMS AND DEFINITIONS

AA: Alcoholics Anonymous

AFTT-A: Attachment-Focused Trauma Therapy for Adults

BLS: bilateral stimulation

EMDR: Eye Movement Desensitization and Reprocessing

PROTOCOL SCRIPT 4. SAFE PLACE AND HIGHER POWER FOR THE ADULT PART OF SELF

Adapted from Leeds, A. (2016). *A guide to the standard EMDR protocols for clinicians, supervisors, and consultants* (2nd ed.). Springer Publishing Company; Parnell, L. (2007). *A therapist's guide to*

EMDR: Tools and techniques for successful treatment. W. W. Norton & Company; Reddemann, L. (2009). The inner safe place. In M. Luber (Ed.), *EMDR scripted protocols: Basics and special situations* (pp. 71–72). Springer Publishing Company; Shapiro, F. (2021). *Weekend 1 training manual of the two-part EMDR therapy basic training* (revised). EMDR Institute, Inc; and Shapiro, F. (2018). *Eye movement desensitization and reprocessing (EMDR) therapy: Basic principles, protocols, and procedures* (2nd ed.). Guilford Press.

1. Discuss Concept of and Purpose for Safe Place and Higher Power for the Adult Part of Self. *Say…* "What we want to create for you and give to you is a place of respite, a place you can go to just be, a place where you can get away from any stress or worries or conflicts, a place where you will have a sense of safety and acceptance, where all of your needs are met in the present moment. We want you to develop an unshakable belief in your own inherent goodness; that you are okay, you are enough, you are lovable. We do that with both a place and what we call a Higher Power or a caregiver. We want you to have a place that only belongs to you where you can feel secure and loved no matter what within a caring and protective attachment relationship with that Higher Power. Your Safe Place and Higher Power are also another way you can tell the difference between 'now' and 'back then,' reminding you that the danger is past and, in this present moment in your Safe Place, all of your needs are being met."

2. Identify Needs of the Adult Part of Self for Nurturing and Protection. *Say…* "We've talked about the needs for nurturing and protection throughout our lives. Even as adults, we need affection and a sense of safety." *Ask…* "What do you think your needs are?"

_____

_____

3. Brainstorm Ideas for the Safe Place for the Adult Part of Self. *Say…* "Your Safe Place can be anywhere … real or imagined, someplace you may already have been or someplace you'd like to go to. What kind of Safe Place do you think you need so you can feel safe and protected, loved and nurtured?"

_____

If the client describes only one aspect of the Safe Place, either nurturing or protective, brainstorm ideas about the other side. Make changes as needed.

_____

_____

4. Install the Safe Place. *Say…* "Imagine everything about your Safe Place … use all of your senses … what you see, hear, any scents, any textures, what time of day, what season of the year, the temperature of the air." *Access and reinforce positive affect with short sets of slow BLS with tappers or butterfly taps. Practice using the container for setting aside negative affect if needed.*

5. Containment/Mindfulness. (Use if client reports negative affect.) *Say...* "Sometimes, people have challenges with staying focused on positive feelings and thoughts and might get distracted by more distressing feelings, thoughts, or experiences. I invite you just to notice whatever is coming up for you without judging it as bad or as evidence you're doing something wrong but rather as a distraction from what we're doing today with this exercise. I don't want you to think that I'm saying you shouldn't have your feelings or your feelings aren't important—they're just not what we're focusing on right now in this visualization." *Ask...* "What are you noticing?"

_____

_____

Say... "Let's set that aside for now. Imagine putting it in some kind of a container outside your Safe Place. Wherever you think you can leave it for now while you return your attention to what you experience as you imagine being in your Safe Place." *Ask...* "What do you notice?"

_____

_____

6. Brainstorm Ideas for the Higher Power for the Adult Part of Self. *Say...* "As we talked about earlier, we want you to experience a healthy attachment relationship within your Safe Place. With someone or something that will be both more powerful and more nurturing than anyone in your real life, past or present. Your Higher Power can be anyone ... someone real or imagined, somebody you knew in the past or know now or someone you've never met. A hero or heroine, a famous person, someone you admired or admire. Your Higher Power can even be an animal or part of nature. It's whatever you think that you need as an adult to feel safe and nurturing in the present moment."

_____

_____

If the client describes only one aspect of the Safe Place, either nurturing or protective, brainstorm ideas about the other side. Make changes as needed.

_____

_____

Access and reinforce the positive affect with short sets of slow BLS.

7. Install the Higher Power in the Safe Place. *Say...* "Let's talk about how you and your Higher Power will be in your Safe Place. For example, some people like to already be in their Safe Place and their Higher Power joins them, or their Higher Power is already in their Safe Place and welcomes them as they come in, or they and their Higher Power may go to their Safe Place together." *Ask...* "How do you want to be in your Safe Place with your Higher Power? How do you feel being in your Safe Place with your Higher Power?" *Access and reinforce the positive affect with short sets of slow BLS.*

8. Add a Boundary Around the Safe Place With the Higher Power. *Say…* "Now I invite you to imagine a boundary that surrounds you and your Higher Power in your Safe Place. A boundary that protects you and the beliefs and feelings of (*repeat the client's description of positive beliefs and affect here*) from your Safe Place so that you can feel it … any time, no matter what is happening outside of you. No matter what anyone says or does or no matter what happens, you can still feel it … and believe…. The boundary needs to be strong and flexible. It can be made of any material you can imagine if it keeps anything that might lead you to doubt those beliefs of … , or those feelings of…. What do you imagine that boundary would be made of?"

_____

_____

"Now imagine how the boundary will work to help you sustain those beliefs and feelings. Notice that whatever it is outside of the boundary that might weaken your beliefs and feelings maybe just slides off or bounces off the outside of the boundary all while you are able to experience the feelings and beliefs in your Safe Place. How do you see that boundary working for you?"

_____

_____

Access and reinforce the positive affect with short sets of slow BLS. Ask… "What needs to be said or done to complete this scene?" *Access and reinforce the positive affect with short sets of slow BLS.*

9. Anchor and Word. *Say…* "In order to be able to bring from your Safe Place and Higher Power your sense of (*repeat client's words*), your feelings of (*repeat client's words*), and your beliefs of (*repeat client's words*) into your everyday life, we want you to anchor it in your body so that when you touch your hand or chest or wherever you choose, you bring that sense into the present moment, the present situation, or relationship. And we want you to be able to do the same with a word or phrase: When you see it or say it, you bring those feelings and beliefs from your Safe Place and Higher Power into your present-day life. Let's start with the anchor. I want you to choose a place on or connected to your body—it could be your hand, a piece of jewelry, your hand over your heart, anywhere you want so that when you touch it, you can connect to your experience of your Safe Place and Higher Power." *Ask…* "Where do you think you would like to anchor those feelings and those unshakable beliefs of (*repeat client's beliefs*) from your Safe Place?"

_____

_____

Say… "Put your hand (*repeat location of client's anchor*) and bring up all that you noticed in your Safe Place with your Higher Power." *Access and reinforce the positive affect with short sets of slow BLS.*

Say... "Now let's think of a word or phrase that, when you see it or you say it, you bring from your Safe Place and Higher Power those feelings and beliefs into your present-day life."

_____

_____

Say... "Hold in mind (*repeat client's word or phrase*) while you bring up the feelings and beliefs from your Safe Place and Higher Power." *Ask...* "What do you notice? Where do you notice it in your body?" *Access and reinforce the positive affect with short sets of slow BLS.*

10. Test the Effectiveness of Installations With a Challenging Situation From Present-Day Life. *Say...* "Let's practice how you can use your anchor and word to connect the feelings and beliefs from your Safe Place and Higher Power to a challenging situation this week. What might be a good example of when you would want to deal with something or someone from your most Competent Adult part of Self?"

_____

_____

Say... "Imagine using your anchor of (*use client's words*) and the word or phrase of (*use client's words*) to connect those feelings and beliefs of (use client's words) from your Safe Place and Higher Power to that situation." *Ask...* "What do you notice? Where do you feel that in your body?" *Access and reinforce the positive affect with short sets of slow BLS.*

11. Refine and Install the Revised Safe Place and Higher Power as Needed. *Review nurturing and protective aspects of both the Safe Place and Higher Power. Revise as needed. Strengthen and reinforce positive affect connected to revised images with BLS.*

REFERENCES

Anonymous. (2001). *Alcoholics anonymous* (4th ed.). Alcoholics Anonymous World Services, Inc.

Leeds, A. (2016). *A guide to the standard EMDR protocols for clinicians, supervisors, and consultants* (2nd ed.). Springer Publishing Company.

Martin, K. M. (2012). How to use Fraser's Dissociative Table Technique to access and work with emotional parts of the personality. *Journal of EMDR Practice and Research, 6*(4), 179–186. https://doi.org/10.1891/1933-3196.6.4.179

Martin, K. (2018, April). *Mastering the treatment of complex trauma: Transforming theory into practice.* Presentation, Omaha, Nebraska.

Murray, K. (2011). Container. *Journal of EMDR Practice and Research, 5*(1), 29–32. https://doi.org/10.1891/1933-3196.5.1.29

Parnell, L. (2007). *A therapist's guide to EMDR: Tools and techniques for successful treatment.* W. W. Norton & Company.

Shapiro, F. (2021). *Weekend 1 training manual of the two-part EMDR therapy basic training* (revised). EMDR Institute, Inc.

Shapiro, F. (2018). *Eye movement desensitization and reprocessing (EMDR) therapy: Basic principles, protocols, and procedures* (2nd ed.). Guilford Press.

CHAPTER 9

Safe Place and Higher Power for Child/Adolescent Part(s) of Self in Attachment-Focused Trauma Therapy for Adults

INTRODUCTION

Everyone naturally has needs throughout their lifetime for nurturing, acceptance, protection, and safety; the need to belong and be accepted, to be in relationships with others, and to feel a sense of security and stability. Chapter 8 showed how the creation of the enhanced Safe Place and Higher Power for the Adult part of Self helps meet those needs in present-day life. Connecting to a sense of safety and nurturing provides the Adult part of Self with a place of respite, a place of "being" regardless of what is going on in day-to-day life. The Adult Safe Place and Higher Power protocol also begins the process of healthy differentiation between the Adult and Child/Adolescent parts of Self, building firm and flexible inner boundaries among parts of Self, and strengthening the Competent Adult part of Self.

Children also have needs for safety and nurturing: knowing that they are "good enough," that they are lovable and worthwhile, and that they deserve good things to happen in their lives. As illustrated in Attachment-Focused Trauma Therapy for Adults (AFTT-A) Parent-Adult-Child (P-A-C) diagrams, children are dependent on the adults in their lives to meet those needs and to give them messages of love and protection; first with attachment figures such as parents or other primary caregivers, and as they mature, with extended family, teachers, religious leaders, other authority figures, and social-cultural groups.

Often in invalidating childhood environments, those encouraging and supportive messages are absent, inconsistent, or conditional and, instead, messages are given that are hurtful, belittling, and damaging to children's growth into competent and confident adults. Children begin to believe that they are not good enough, they must earn love and affection, and they are undeserving or unworthy of getting their needs met.

Cultural and Social Considerations

Chang (2017) advises therapists working with transgender or gender nonconforming clients to discuss the gender of Child/Adolescent parts and pronouns to be used in referring to each part prior to imagining the Child/Adolescent parts. Otherwise, clients can be confused about whether they are visualizing their younger parts as their gender assigned at birth or as the gender with which they identify. Having an open conversation with transgender or gender nonconforming clients will build a comfort level and may prevent memories of childhood confusion being triggered.

A SAFE PLACE AND HIGHER POWER FOR CHILD/ADOLESCENT PARTS

The AFTT-A process reconstructs clients' inner system and its component parts. Up to this point, AFTT-A, which enhances and extends Eye Movement Desensitization and Reprocessing (EMDR) therapy's preparation phase, provides clients with psychosocial education about personality development, parts of Self, and how personality development and attachment relationships are adversely impacted in an invalidating childhood environment (see Chapters 3 to 5 and 7). The first AFTT-A protocol focused on strengthening the client Competent Adult part of Self by creating an inner sense of safety and acceptance through installation of a Safe Place and Higher Power (see Chapter 8).

The next step in assisting clients to integrate an inner sense of safety and acceptance is to develop Safe Places and Higher Powers for Child/Adolescent parts of Self. The ideas of Safe Place and Higher Power for Child/Adolescent parts of Self are similar in many ways to those provided for the Adult part of Self. The experience of safety/protection and nurturing/acceptance are provided to Child/Adolescent parts through the *Safe Place and Higher Power for Child/Adolescent Parts of Self* protocol. Time orientation is reinforced when younger parts experience protection and nurturing in their Safe Places within the context of a corrective attachment relationship with their Higher Power figures, thus discerning the difference between "now" in the present moment when danger is past and all their needs are met and "back then" when danger was real and childhood needs were unmet.

Strong and flexible boundaries form around and between client Child/Adolescent and Adult parts. The Competent Adult part of Self continues to be differentiated from other inner personality parts and is empowered to provide leadership to clients' internal systems. Although the preparation phase of EMDR therapy does not include this step, it is essential in the AFTT-A process to rebuild personality parts, reconstruct internal attachments, and begin to form positive attachment relationships with others prior to desensitizing and reprocessing traumatic events.

STEPS FOR A SAFE PLACE AND HIGHER POWER FOR CHILD/ADOLESCENT PARTS

The *Safe Place and Higher Power for Child/Adolescent Parts of Self* protocol is the second step in AFTT-A's process of tapping into and strengthening clients' Authentic Self. (Use Protocol Script 5 at the end of this chapter throughout the following explanation of protocol steps.) As Child/Adolescent parts are separated out from the Competent Adult part of Self and provided with a sense of caring and protection in the present moment, a client's Competent Adult part is freed to focus on and manage real-life relationships and situations.

1. Identify Child/Adolescent Parts From Patterns in Adult Life

Therapists might begin discovering the presence of Child/Adolescent parts through answers to questions during an initial assessment or at the beginning of therapy sessions when discussing issues, patterns, behaviors, or even memories. The "How did it go since the last time you were here?" is sometimes seen as a time-waster at the beginning of a therapy session but can be an invaluable tool to an attuned therapist in gaining insight into how Child/Adolescent parts are or have been present in clients' adult lives and relationships.

Typically, a Child/Adolescent part is involved in present-day relationships or interactions when clients describe one or more of the following situations related to their emotions: (a) an intense emotional reaction that seems out of proportion for a situation, (b) similar emotional reactions across different situations, and/or (c) getting "stuck" in and not being able to move through an emotion even though the situation has ended. In therapy sessions, Child/Adolescent parts might be identified by a change in tone or pitch of voice, body posture or use of gestures, eye contact, way of relating to the therapist, or emotions being expressed.

EMDR therapy uses the term "touchstone event" to refer to a past traumatic event unprocessed through the adaptive information processing (AIP) system that underlies clients' negative cognitions or core beliefs (Shapiro, 2018, 2021). In AFTT-A, "touchstone" also refers to a specific client age or a client's Child/Adolescent part of Self. When clients report a maladaptive pattern of behavior or relationship conflict, therapists ask, "How old did you feel when that happened?"

When therapists observe the possible blending of Child/Adolescent parts with the Adult part of Self in session, they inquire, "How old do you feel as you say that?" or "How old do you feel while you talk about that?" That question begins to connect or link a pattern, issue, or emotion in clients' adult lives to a Child/Adolescent part of Self that has unmet needs and is attempting to get those unmet childhood needs met in adult life. As an example, someone who tends to come across in their present-day relationships in a very distant or dismissive way might find a younger Child/Adolescent part that was abandoned or rejected and is pretending not to care, thus acting out in a dismissive way to prevent further hurt or loss in adult relationships.

2. Brainstorm Unmet Needs of Child/Adolescent Parts

Once therapists have helped clients identify a Child/Adolescent part and the part's approximate age, the next step in creating a Safe Place and Higher Power is to brainstorm clients' unmet needs for nurturing and protection at the age of that Child/Adolescent part. Unmet needs could include affection, safety, firm but flexible rules and boundaries, independence and autonomy, identifying and expressing emotions in healthy ways, and skills for self-care and relationships. Unmet childhood needs tend to be age-dependent, so the needs of Child/Adolescent parts are unique to their age. Erickson's stages of development are helpful in understanding typical needs throughout childhood and adolescence. For example, infant parts of Self need to develop a sense of basic trust and toddler parts of Self a sense of autonomy, while the school-age child parts need to resolve issues of adequacy and industry and teen parts identify with roles related to identity (Erikson, 1993).

3. Discuss the Concept and Purposes of a Safe Place and Higher Power for Child/Adolescent Parts of Self

Safe Place and Higher Power for the Adult Part of Self is the foundational protocol in the AFTT-A model. Much of the information is the same when creating a Safe

Place and choosing a Higher Power for Child/Adolescent parts: (a) The primary characteristics are safety and nurturing; (b) the Safe Place and Higher Power can be real or imagined, known or unknown by the client; and (c) the chosen Safe Place and Higher Power are tested to ensure that both sets of characteristics are present and sufficient to meet the Child part's unmet needs.

A central purpose of Safe Places and Higher Powers for Child/Adolescent parts is to provide time orientation for Child/Adolescent parts of clients. Child/Adolescent parts represent the parts of clients that are confused about time or the difference between the past and the present, then and now. The Child/Adolescent parts' reality is contained in the neural networks that are disconnected from the AIP system and so the events, beliefs, and emotions are not connected to time; their negative cognitions are true, memories and flashbacks feel real in the present moment, and the danger is not past. Creating a Safe Place and a Higher Power where unmet childhood needs are fulfilled demonstrates for clients the real differences between the past, when needs remained unmet, and the present moment, in which all those same needs are realized.

4. Brainstorm Ideas for a Safe Place for Child/Adolescent Parts of Self

One of the main differences between Safe Places for the Adult and Child/Adolescent parts of Self is that they need to be age-appropriate for younger parts; for example, a nursery for an infant, a playroom for a toddler, a playground for a school-age child, a sleepover with safe friends in a teen's bedroom for an adolescent. Other examples of Safe Places for Child/Adolescent parts are a swing set, a rocking chair, a castle, a farm with animals and a vegetable garden, a library, or a swimming pool. Depending on the age of the Child/Adolescent part, clients might choose settings from children's books, television shows, or movies like *Mr. Roger's Neighborhood*, *Sesame Street*, the Harry Potter series, *The Hobbit*, the *Star Trek* series, or *Avatar*. Safe Places for older adolescents might also include scenes or places from video games, movies, books, or television shows.

5. Install a Safe Place

Once clients choose a Safe Place for their Child/Adolescent part, the protocol guides them into the installation by asking them to decide how the Child/Adolescent part will be introduced to their Safe Place. Is the younger part already in their Safe Place? What do they need to hear? Does the Adult part of Self need to find them and take them to their Safe Place? Again, a sensory description of the Safe Place helps to make it more real and immediate. What do they see? What sounds are heard? What scents and textures are noticed? Clients are then asked to notice how their Child/Adolescent part seems to feel about being in the Safe Place.

As with the *Safe Place and Higher Power for the Adult Part of Self* protocol, Child/Adolescent parts may also have ambivalent or negative feelings about being separated from the Adult part of Self and installed in their Safe Place. Feelings of fear, anxiety, anger, reluctance, or abandonment are normalized and can be set aside in some kind of imagined container at the edge or outside of the Child/Adolescent's Safe Place, given to the Adult part of Self to place in their container, or eventually entrusted to their new Higher Power (Murray, 2011).

Child/Adolescent parts sometimes have a hard time giving up the magical thinking of "what ifs." They cling to the belief and hope that if they just get the adult in their present-day life to do something more, ask for less, change something, or act in a different way, those childhood needs will finally be met. Letting go of magical thinking lays bare the grief of all that was lost and cannot be regained. Therapists can say, "Well, there's good news and bad news. The bad news is that no matter how hard you try, you cannot get those unmet childhood needs met in your adult life. It doesn't work. The good news is that you cannot get your unmet childhood needs met in your adult life. You can get your *adulthood* needs met and your Child/Adolescent part can get *their* needs met all of the time now in their Safe Place with their Higher Power. Nothing can make up for what you didn't get or what happened to you as a child, but I will be here for you while you grieve those losses."

After clients report that their Child/Adolescent part is connected to a positive affect related to their new Safe Place, therapists then refocus on the Adult part of Self, the client sitting in their office, by asking how *they* feel as they watch their Child/Adolescent part in their Safe Place, knowing that they are providing the gift of safety and acceptance to the younger part of themselves. Clients often experience relief or happiness, sometimes even pride. They may describe feeling more ease and relaxation or a lessening of tension, a sense of calm, or being grounded and centered. Bilateral stimulation (BLS) is used to strengthen positive affect *from the client as an adult* and started through the use of hand-held tappers or clients doing butterfly taps (arms crossed with tapping back and forth on their upper arms) or tapping on the tops of their thighs. Since clients are connecting to and strengthening positive affect, the sets of BLS are very short and very slow, perhaps only three or four sets.

6. Brainstorm Ideas for a Higher Power for the Child/Adolescent Parts of Self

Higher Powers for Child/Adolescent parts also need to demonstrate attributes of acceptance and safety. The main goal for creating a Higher Power for Child/Adolescent parts is to provide clients with an initial experience of an internal, corrective attachment relationship so the confidence and competence clients develop as a result of those restructured inner bonds can then be carried into real-life relationships.

Higher Powers also need to be age-appropriate for younger parts and can be modeled after someone from their past or current life; real-life heroes; or imaginary beings like characters from books, comic books, movies, or television shows. Some examples might be Mary Poppins, Cinderella, fairy godmothers, video game heroes, characters from *Avatar,* or superheroes like Spiderman, Superman, Wonder Woman, and Thor. Sometimes, a Higher Power can be a figure from clients' spiritual, religious, cultural, or social groups such as a spirit, angel, diety, individual from a holy book, admired leader, or even a family member or friend who has passed and now has characteristics beyond what they possessed during their life. If clients have difficulty trusting people, Higher Powers can be animals or aspects of nature.

Higher Powers are more than a representative of an imperfect parental figure. They will always be there for Child/Adolescent parts even when clients are doing their job of running their present-day lives. So, if clients pick a person from their real life, they need to change something about or add something to that person so they become more powerful and more nurturing than anyone in their actual life; someone who will attune to the Child/Adolescent parts' needs and keep bad things from happening again.

> **BOX 9.1 CLIENT EXAMPLE: BRAINSTORMING AND INSTALLING HIGHER POWER FOR CHILD/ADOLESCENT PART OF SELF**
>
> The client discovered after installing a Safe Place for a group of Child parts of Self called the "little-littles" that the parts seemed to like their new Safe Place but balked at the idea of a Higher Power. In fact, they were afraid of anyone coming into their Safe Place. The client reported feeling stuck brainstorming a Higher Power for them.
>
> Therapist: If you think it would help, you can bring in your Resource Team.
>
> Client: Oh, yeah, my Team! I can do that.
>
> (Do slow, short BLS sets to reinforce the client's positive affect related to getting reconnected to the Safe Place, Higher Power, and Resource Team.)
>
> Therapist: How do you think your Team can help?
>
> Client: Well, I asked them about the little-littles and they think Jane Goodall, that anthropologist who studied chimpanzees, would be perfect for their Higher Power.
>
> Therapist: Tell me about that.
>
> Client: Well, when she studied chimpanzees, she observed them without trying to force herself into their lives. She let them make her a part of their world when they were ready. So, she understands that the littles are afraid and she doesn't feel like she needs to do anything. She's not going to swoop in and take over. She'll take her cues from them when they're ready to let her get closer. But she can be there quietly and make sure they're safe.
>
> Therapist: How about if you ask Jane to go into their Safe Place? How could you imagine that would happen?
>
> Client: Well, I see her sitting quietly in the room with them. Over to the side.
>
> Therapist: How does it seem that the littles feel about that?
>
> Client: You know, I think they're okay.
>
> Therapist: When you say "okay," what does that mean?
>
> Client: They noticed her but don't seem threatened. They've calmed down a little.
>
> Therapist: Wow, wonderful! How do *you* feel when you can tell they're calmer?
>
> Client: Relieved and happy.
>
> (Do slow, short BLS sets to strengthen the client's positive affect experiencing Child/Adolescent parts of Self feeling calmer.)

7. Install the Higher Power in the Safe Place

After clients select their Child/Adolescent part's Higher Power, brainstorming how the part will be introduced to them is helpful. The protocol allows clients to decide how the Child/Adolescent part is going to be introduced to their Higher Power. Sometimes, the new Higher Power is waiting for the Child/Adolescent part in the Safe Place.

Other times, they go in together or the Higher Power comes into the Safe Place after the Child/Adolescent part is already there. Again, therapists ask about what the Child/Adolescent part needs to hear or what needs to happen so they can be introduced to their Higher Power. Clients are then asked to notice how their Child/Adolescent part seems to feel about their new Higher Power. As with the Safe Place, ambivalent feelings are normalized and set aside in some kind of container at the edge or outside of the Safe Place itself.

After clients report that their Child/Adolescent part is connected to positive affect related to their new Higher Power, the therapist then refocuses on the Competent Adult part of Self as a component of the client sitting in their office. They ask their client how *they* feel about being able to give the gifts of safety, acceptance, and attuned connection to the younger part of themselves as they watch their Child/Adolescent part with their Higher Power in their Safe Place. Again, clients often experience relief or happiness, sometimes even pride. They may describe feeling more ease and relaxation or a lessening of tension, a sense of calm, or being grounded and centered. BLS is started through the use of hand-held tappers or clients doing butterfly taps (arms crossed with tapping back and forth on their upper arms) or tapping on the tops of their thighs. The positive affect of the adult aspect of the client is strengthened, deepened, and expanded through several short sets of slow BLS.

8. Test the Effectiveness of Installations With a Challenging Situation From Present-Day Life

Since therapists initially helped their clients identify Child/Adolescent parts through situations, patterns, or emotions from their present-day life, therapists can refer back to those points when testing the effectiveness of Safe Place and Higher Power in separating out their Child/Adolescent parts from real life and coping with challenging situations or emotions in their most Authentic Self. Clients are asked to imagine "tucking in" their Child/Adolescent part, talking to the Child/Adolescent part about needing to take care of "grown-up stuff," and reassuring the Child/Adolescent part that they will be safe and cared about and that nothing bad will happen to them as they are in their Safe Place with their Higher Power, even when the adult struggles in their present-day life. Remind the Child/Adolescent part that they have already survived whatever bad things happened, they can't ever happen to them again, and the danger is past. Once clients imagine their younger part in their Safe Place, they then imagine going through a particular situation or handling a certain emotion with a positive outcome. Positive affect is reinforced with short sets of slow BLS.

9. Refine and Install the Revised Safe Place and Higher Power as Needed

If, through the effectiveness tests, the new Safe Place or Higher Power has weaknesses in either the loving or protective aspects, clients can brainstorm what changes or enhancements need to be made and the positive affect related to those changes are reinforced with short sets of slow BLS.

POINTS TO REMEMBER

- Identify the Child/Adolescent parts through patterns of emotions, behaviors, and relationships in present-day life or during therapy sessions.

- Emotional reactions are clues to the presence of Child/Adolescent parts.
- Make sure that the Safe Place and Higher Power meet unmet childhood needs.
- The Safe Place and Higher Power for Child/Adolescent parts need to be age-appropriate and reflect both nurturing and protective characteristics.
- The Client's Adult part of Self helps Child/Adolescent parts with understanding and accepting the Safe Place and Higher Power.
- Use BLS to reinforce the positive affect of the client sitting in your office, *not* the Child/Adolescent part.
- A Safe Place for the Child/Adolescent parts is the foundation of time orientation.

TROUBLESHOOTING

- If the client has difficulty imagining a Safe Place, make sure the most Adult Self is in charge of doing the protocol. Say, "Let's make sure your most Adult Self is doing this visualization" or "There's no right or wrong; it's just whatever you imagine that the younger part of you needs."
- If the client feels like they need to have an answer right away, say, "Take your time," "We have plenty of time," or "Give yourself some time."
- If the client overemphasizes either the protective or nurturing aspects of either the Safe Place or the Higher Power, ask about the other aspect. For example, say, "I can see how that is nurturing; how do you imagine it can be protective?"
- If the client has problems with the concept of a Higher Power, remind them that the "Higher Power" for their Child/Adolescent parts of Self needs to be appropriate for the age of the parts and can be represented by any real or imagined being, animal, or part of nature that is more powerful and more loving than anyone in the client's childhood.
- If the client's Child/Adolescent part is reluctant to go to the Safe Place, normalize feelings. Say, "Child/Adolescent parts often have many different feelings when they first learn about their Safe Place. It's normal for Child/Adolescent parts to be unsure, afraid, or mistrustful."
- If the client feels grief or jealousy toward the Child/Adolescent part about getting their needs met when in real-life or the client's childhood needs weren't met, normalize feelings. Ask the client to set aside those feelings and focus on a positive affect related to giving the younger part of them a sense of safety and acceptance in the present moment. Use a container if needed.
- If the client blames their Child/Adolescent part or doesn't think their Child/Adolescent part deserves to feel safe and loved, remind clients of the negative messages they got during childhood and normalize believing those messages even as adults. Use a container if needed.

PAUSE AND REFLECT FOR THE THERAPIST

> **BOX 9.2 ANN'S STORY: IMPACT OF THE THERAPIST'S OWN CHILD PART OF SELF ON CLIENT PROGRESS**
>
> I worked with a challenging client who was very dependent on me to tell them what to do. When I asked them to brainstorm ideas, skills, options, and so forth, they often said, "Why don't you just tell me and I'll do it." Initially, I fell into the trap of giving them all kinds of suggestions. Even though they asked me for advice, they responded with all the reasons why my brilliant ideas (ha!) weren't going to work for them. Before and during sessions with them, I noticed tension in my body, anxiety, a sense of urgency, and the negative cognition of "I need to know the answer. If I don't have the answer, something bad will happen."
>
> I took the issues to my personal therapist and realized I had an undiscovered school-age Child part who knew that when she *didn't* know what to do, something bad *did* happen. I found her in a library frantically paging through huge reference books, trying to find the answer that would prevent scary stuff from happening in her family. She thought it was her fault that she couldn't protect her younger brother and sisters. I gave her a Safe Place of a meadow surrounded by a forest with a scientist/teacher sort of guy who takes her exploring and she gets to examine insects and plants.
>
> Once I installed my younger part in her Safe Place with her Higher Power during my own therapy, I found it helpful to check in with and make sure that the younger part of me was off exploring in the forest and my Competent Adult part of Self was in charge prior to the starting sessions with the client. My client didn't magically become more independent, but I was able to attune to them from a more competent, authentic perspective and I handled silence in sessions with them and their struggles to find their own answers with more ease.

As shown in Box 9.2, therapists with their own history of attachment trauma can be triggered and react in therapy sessions out of a part of Self other than their Competent Adult part or their most Authentic Self; for example, when a negative cognition is triggered. Think back to a session with a challenging client—perhaps someone who has difficulty following through with assignments, someone who is stuck and doesn't seem to be able to move forward, someone who seems to need more than you can offer, or someone who is critical of you as a therapist. Instead of focusing on the client, notice how you feel in your body, negative thoughts or cognitions, your emotions, any urges to react to the client in a certain way. Ask yourself how old you felt during that interaction. Ask yourself what you think that Child/Adolescent part of you needs in order to be tucked in during sessions with that client. Remind the Child/Adolescent part of you that they don't need to come to therapy sessions with you.

Write down ideas for a Safe Place and Higher Power for your Child/Adolescent Part. If you feel comfortable, imagine taking that younger part of you to their Safe Place with their Higher Power. Notice how that Child/Adolescent part of you feels to be in a place where all of their needs for acceptance and safety are being met. Notice how you feel as you think about giving this younger part of you what they need. If you like, when you notice positive feelings, sensations, body posture, and thoughts, you can do some slow BLS by tapping back and forth on the tops of your thighs or use butterfly taps on your upper arms.

If you have your own therapist, share this information in a therapy session with them.

USEFUL TERMS AND DEFINITIONS

AFTT-A: Attachment-Focused Trauma Therapy for Adults

AIP system: adaptive information processing system

BLS: bilateral stimulation

EMDR: Eye Movement Desensitization and Reprocessing

P-A-C diagrams: Parent-Adult-Child diagrams

PROTOCOL SCRIPT 5. SAFE PLACE AND HIGHER POWER FOR CHILD/ADOLESCENT PART(S) OF SELF

Adapted from Erikson, E. (1993). *Child/adolescent and society* (2nd ed.). W. W. Norton and Company; Leeds, A. (2016). *A guide to the standard EMDR protocols for clinicians, supervisors, and consultants* (2nd ed.). Springer Publishing Company; Parnell, L. (2007). *A therapist's guide to EMDR: Tools and techniques for successful treatment.* W. W. Norton & Company; Shapiro, F. (2018). *Eye movement desensitization and reprocessing (EMDR) therapy: Basic principles, protocols, and procedures* (2nd ed.). Guilford Press; and Shapiro, F. (2021). *Weekend 1 training manual of the two-part EMDR therapy basic training* (revised). EMDR Institute, Inc.

1. Identify Child/Adolescent Parts From Patterns in Adult Life. *Ask…* "How old did you feel when that was happening?" or "How old do you feel as you talk about that right now?"

_____

_____

Say… "Tell me a little bit about yourself at that age."

_____

_____

2. Brainstorm Unmet Needs of the Child/Adolescent Part. *Say…* "We've talked about children's needs for nurturing and protection as they grow up." *Ask…* "What do you think that ____-year-old part of you needed?"

_____

_____

3. Discuss the Concept and Purpose of a Safe Place and Higher Power for Child/Adolescent Parts of Self. *Say...* "What we want to create for or give to that ____-year-old part of you is a sense of safety and acceptance in the present moment, so that the younger part of you can get all their needs met now and be able to tell the difference between 'now' and 'back then.' To know that all the bad things are past, all the danger is past and in this present moment, all their needs are being met. We do that with both a place and what we call a Higher Power or a caregiver. We want that ____-year-old part of you to have a place of their own where they can feel secure and loved no matter what within a caring and protective attachment relationship with that Higher Power. You know this part of you better than anyone else, so you'll be able to give this younger part exactly what they need in this present moment."

4. Brainstorm Ideas for a Safe Place for Child/Adolescent Parts of Self. *Say...* "The Safe Place can be anywhere ... real or imagined, some place you have already been or someplace you'd like to go to. A place for a ____-year-old child/adolescent. What kind of a Safe Place do you think that ____-year-old Child/Adolescent part needs so they can feel safe and protected, loved and nurtured?"

_____

_____

If the client describes only one aspect of the Safe Place, either nurturing or protection, brainstorm ideas about other aspects. Make changes as needed.

_____

_____

5. Install a Safe Place. *Ask...* "What do you think that younger part of you needs to hear; what needs to happen so they can go to their Safe Place?"

_____

_____

With the client's Adult part of Self observing, elicit a positive affect about the Child/Adolescent part's reaction to the Safe Place. Next, focus on the positive affect the client (sitting in your office) has in observing their Child/Adolescent part, with the knowledge that they have given this place of safety and nurturance to their younger part. Access and reinforce positive affect with short sets of slow BLS with tappers or butterfly taps. Practice the container for setting aside the negative affect if needed.

6. Brainstorm Ideas for a Higher Power for the Child/Adolescent Parts of Self. *Say...* "As we talked about earlier, we want to create a corrective attachment experience for the ____-year-old part of you, someone or something that will be both more powerful or more nurturing than anyone in your real life. The Higher Power can be anyone ... someone real or imagined, somebody you knew or someone you didn't know. A Higher Power can even be an animal or part of nature. It's whatever you think that younger part of you needs to feel safe and nurtured in the present moment."

If the client describes only one aspect of the Safe Place, either nurturing or protection, brainstorm ideas about other aspects. Make changes as needed.

7. Install the Higher Power in the Safe Place. *Ask…* "What do you think that younger part of yourself needs to hear, what needs to happen so they can be with their Higher Power in their Safe Place?"

With the client's Adult part of Self observing, elicit positive affect about Child/Adolescent part's reaction to their Higher Power. Next, focus on the positive affect that the client (sitting in your office) has in observing their Child/Adolescent part, with the knowledge that they have given this special being to their younger part. Once the positive affect is accessed, do short, slow sets of BLS with tappers or butterfly taps to strengthen and reinforce the positive affect. Practice the container for setting aside the negative affect if needed.

Ask… "What needs to be said or done to complete this scene?" *Guide the client to remind their Child/Adolescent part that all their needs will be met in their Safe Place with their Higher Power, that everything bad has already happened and can't happen again, and that when they stay in their Safe Place, nothing from the client's adult life can affect them. Elicit positive affect from the client and reinforce with slow, short sets of BLS.*

8. Test the Effectiveness of Installations With a Challenging Situation From Present-Day Life. *Say…* "Let's practice how you can use the Safe Place and Higher Power to 'tuck in' your Child/Adolescent part when something challenging comes up this week. What might be a good example of when you would want to deal with something or someone from your Competent Adult part of Self?"

Say… "Imagine taking a minute to check on the Child/Adolescent part, making sure they are in their Safe Place with their Higher Power while you handle the situation in your present-day life, reminding them that they are safe and loved and really don't need to concern themselves with how you as the adult handle this situation, that you have your own Higher Power to help you now. And that no matter how you handle the situation, they will be okay." *Elicit positive affect. Strengthen and reinforce with BLS.*

___

___

9. Refine and Install the Revised Safe Place and Higher Power as Needed. *If the client has difficulty keeping the Child/Adolescent part in their Safe Place, review nurturing and protective aspects of both the Child/Adolescent part's Safe Place and Higher Power. Revise as needed. Strengthen and reinforce with BLS the positive affect connected to revised images.*

___

___

REFERENCES

Chang, S. C. (2017). EMDR therapy as affirmative care for transgender and gender nonconforming clients. In M. Nickerson (Ed.), *Cultural competence and healing culturally based trauma with EMDR therapy* (pp. 171–194). Springer Publishing Company.

Erikson, E. (1993). *Child/adolescent and society* (2nd ed.). W. W. Norton and Company.

Murray, K. (2011). Container. *Journal of EMDR Practice and Research*, 5(1), 29–32. https://doi.org/10.1891/1933-3196.5.1.29

Shapiro, F. (2018). *Eye movement desensitization and reprocessing (EMDR) therapy: Basic principles, protocols, and procedures* (2nd ed.). Guilford Press.

Shapiro, F. (2021). *Weekend 1 training manual of the two-part EMDR therapy basic training* (revised). EMDR Institute, Inc.

CHAPTER 10

Creating an Internal Resource Team in Attachment-Focused Trauma Therapy for Adults

INTRODUCTION

The preparation phase of Eye Movement Desensitization and Reprocessing (EMDR) therapy includes the identification and reinforcing of clients' inner or psychological resources as an affect regulation technique (Kiessling, 2009a, 2009b; Korn & Leeds, 2002; Laub, 2009; Leeds, 2016; Parnell, 2007; Shapiro, 2009, 2018). Resource Development and Installation (RDI) is typically used in trauma therapy with clients who have complex trauma or complex posttraumatic stress disorder (C-PTSD); who tend to have safety issues such as suicidal ideation or urges to self-harm; whose impulsive or compulsive behaviors are at risk for restarting or worsening; who demonstrate fear about or unwillingness to progress in trauma therapy; or who are at risk for affect dysregulation during trauma reprocessing (Leeds, 2016, p. 131). Standard RDI assists clients in connecting to and strengthening links between positive affect and mastery (past coping skills), relational (role models), and symbolic inner resources.

The Attachment-Focused Trauma Therapy for Adults (AFTT-A) model expands and enhances RDI by utilizing the idea of a "team" of inner resources. The client's Inner Resource Team encompasses as well as extends the concept and purposes of core resources to include figures or team members who represent clients' inner strengths needed to accomplish therapy goals. Resource Team meetings (an adaption of Fraser's Dissociative Table Technique [1991, 2003]) between clients and their Resource Team members help connect clients to their positive qualities and strengthen the inner resources needed for therapy and application to real-life situations. Clients also have the chance in team meetings to identify and negotiate needed changes with old versions of Adult and Parent parts of Self so they transform into more helpful versions and play more useful roles. An equally important purpose of the Internal Resource Team is the opportunity for clients to experience corrective internal attachment relationships, thus developing the positive cognitions of "I have everything that I need" and "I am not alone."

EMDR THERAPY AND INNER RESOURCES

EMDR therapy was originally developed to assist people to resolve the experience of a single traumatic event like a death, accident, mugging, assault, or natural disaster (Shapiro, 2018). EMDR therapists began to realize that many clients who came to trauma therapy had experienced more than one traumatic event, often ongoing or chronic trauma during childhood and/or adolescence. A pilot study conducted at an agency in the Midwest serving women who had been sexually assaulted or were in domestic violence situations as adults, found that most of the participants also had experienced trauma prior to adulthood (Potter et al., 2013).

Deficits in emotion and behavior regulation are frequently noted in clients who experienced trauma prior to adulthood, especially in clients whose trauma was ongoing and within the context of their primary attachment relationships. In addition to living through what was perceived as life-threatening events and/or events that harmed clients' sense of worthiness, sense of belonging, or sense of control, clients who suffered attachment trauma often did not learn essential self-regulation skills or to integrate their own strengths and positive qualities. Clients' skills deficits not only added to the complexity of their PTSD symptomology but also significantly and negatively impacted their ability to cope with situations and relationships as adults. The expansion of the definition of traumatic stress to include (C-PTSD) or disorders of extreme stress (DES) gained recognition and credibility with clinicians in the trauma therapy field (van der Kolk et al., 2005).

EMDR therapy integrated RDI as an affect regulation technique (Kiessling, 2009a, 2009b; Korn & Leeds, 2002; Leeds, 2016; Shapiro, 2018). RDI uses the same framework as the Safe/Calm Place/State protocol to tap into and strengthen clients' positive affect and the adaptive behaviors they want to have or perhaps already demonstrate in some situations (Shapiro, 2018, pp. 248–250). Laub (2009) created a protocol that includes client statements of traumatic events followed by a positive memory and its associated affect and uses the cue word associated with the positive affect to decrease emotional disturbance during trauma reprocessing. Shapiro (2016) utilizes a "Resource Map" to encompass all aspects of and links to each installed resource (p. 101).

Leeds identified seven steps for RDI (2016, p. 133):

1. Identify the target situation from adult life (which client wants to handle more skillfully).

2. Select mastery (memory of positive coping), relational (role models and support figures), and symbolic (representative images) internal resources that are linked to positive affect and needed in order to improve the client's response to the target situation.

3. Access resources through guided imagery and enhance as many aspects of resources as needed.

4. Strengthen and reinforce positive affect with short sets of slow bilateral stimulation (BLS).

5. Repeat steps 2 to 4 with as many memories and images as needed.

6. Practice Future Rehearsal protocol for the target situation.

7. Verify stability of resources in the target situation through the client's feedback and tracking log.

Potter (1994a, 1994b) introduced the idea of the need to repair and reconstruct relationships (what we now know as attachments) among internal parts of Self and a process to rebuild the inner relationships. Manfield (2010), Parnell (1999), and Schmidt (2009) integrated the element of attachment into RDI by evaluating, repairing, and strengthening the relationship between the inner Adult and Child parts of Self. Parnell's approach helps clients resolve inner conflict by identifying resources that will aid in repairing and improving the dyadic relationship and utilizing a variety of inner resources such as an inner advisor; nurturing figures; protectors; animals; a spiritual resource; inner strengths; wise beings; figures from books, stories, movies, or cartoons; historical figures; positive memories; music; movement; and parts of nature types (Parnell, 2007, pp. 75–84). The AFTT-A model also adds positive representatives for social or cultural identities and social or cultural groups to the options for potential inner resources.

AFTT-A AND THE INNER RESOURCE TEAM

AFTT-A incorporates the overall RDI steps into the framework of both internal and real-life attachments. At the same time therapists demonstrate their unshakable belief that clients have everything that they need to do their emotional work in therapy, they also normalize the fact that most clients do not have similar positive perceptions of themselves. The negative messages they got from real-life attachment figures often led them to believe that they either didn't have positive qualities or resources at all or the inner resources they did have weren't accessible to them based on negative cognitions such as "I don't deserve to feel good about myself" or "Being proud of myself is ... sinful, selfish, vain, arrogant, self-centered, cocky." The AFTT-A model transforms negative self-beliefs into positive cognitions in the context of a supportive and encouraging team of resources.

As with any of the AFTT-A protocols, clients may find focusing on positive images and affect challenging and may get distracted by distressing cognitions, emotions, body sensations, or memories. AFTT-A views such experiences as time disorientation, when clients are confused between "now" in the present moment, and "back then" from stored traumatic material that intrudes during the protocol. If clients have a difficult time getting or staying connected to positive affect during installation, therapists can intervene with containment and mindfulness approaches aimed at time orientation (Martin, 2018). The AFTT-A model looks at clients' experience of negative affect or difficulty staying with positive affect as a perfect opportunity to teach containment and mindfulness skills. One of the benefits of the practice of containing and setting aside negative affect during the protocol aimed at connecting to and strengthening positive aspects is that clients learn elemental ways to be mindful in the present moment, skills that are applicable in both EMDR therapy trauma reprocessing and many areas of their lives. The ability to notice negative affect and treat it as a distraction rather than as evidence of something wrong becomes a foundational part of client affect or emotion regulation skills and provides valuable information to therapists about client readiness for subsequent phases of EMDR therapy (Murray, 2011).

STEPS FOR BRAINSTORMING RESOURCE TEAM MEMBERS

For more information, see Protocol Script 6 at the end of this chapter.

1. Explain the Concept and Purposes of a Resource Team

Clients build on the foundation of new beliefs about worthiness, lovability, safety, and protection gained from their Safe Place and Higher Power. Just as the Safe Place serves as a place of respite and "being," the Meeting Place with the Resource Team functions as a place of action, a place of "doing."

In the *Brainstorming Internal Resource Team Members* protocol, clients set goals, identify needed strengths, and select representatives of their strengths to form an Inner Resource Team with whom they connect to their own positive qualities. The Resource Team concretizes and internalizes the client's own strengths so the negative affect surrounding the possibility of having positive attributes is less likely to trigger a cascade of negative thoughts and emotions. At the same time, clients begin to experience corrective attachment relationships with Resource Team members that begin to offset and replace prior negative cognitions. Clients' Resource Team members are accepting, protective, and have an unwavering commitment to be helpful.

Clients and their team initially meet to brainstorm ways team members will help them to achieve their goals for therapy. Additionally, Resource Team meetings can be used at any time or at any step in the therapy process to help clients feel less alone and find solutions to barriers and stuck points in therapy sessions as well as real-life situations.

2. Identify Client Goals for the Attachment-Focused Trauma Therapy for Adults Process

When clients first begin to work with an Inner Resource Team, therapists want them to identify overall or general goals for therapy. The therapist and client then rework the goals to make them concrete and specific so that they can evaluate together whether therapy goals have been met.

BOX 10.1 CLIENT EXAMPLE: IDENTIFYING GOALS FOR THE RESOURCE TEAM

Therapist: How did you do this week with thinking about your goals?

Client: I did okay with goals. I wasn't really sure about the rest.

Therapist: Well, let's start with the goals you thought of.

Client: Mostly, I want to get back to the person I used to be—more fun-loving, care-free, enjoying life—instead of worrying and being so serious all the time.

Therapist: And what do you think you would need to do in order to get reconnected to that part of you?

Client: Well, I would need to be okay with being uncomfortable starting to do things I used to do that I stopped doing.

Therapist: Can you give me an example of that?

Client: Well, I would go out with friends or go out to listen to music and go dancing.

Therapist: Let's say I was a fly on the wall when you were out dancing and listening to music with friends, how could I tell that you were more connected to that part of you?

(continued)

BOX 10.1 CLIENT EXAMPLE: IDENTIFYING GOALS FOR THE RESOURCE TEAM (continued)

Client: I would be laughing and talking. I wouldn't care if I looked silly.

Therapist: Anything else?

Client: You would be able to tell I was relaxed.

Therapist: How so?

Client: I would be smiling, sitting back in my chair, tapping my foot to the music. My body would be relaxed. Maybe singing along.

3. Brainstorm Strengths or Positive Characteristics Clients Need to Accomplish Their Therapy Goals

In this step, therapists review the clients' goals and explain that in order to achieve their therapy goals, they want to link the goals with positive characteristics needed to achieve those goals. Clients may or may not have difficulty identifying strengths they will need to meet their therapy goals. Sometimes, they can recognize the needed positive traits fairly easily. If not, therapists can normalize clients' challenges with seeing themselves in a positive light and reassure them that they don't already have to believe that they *have* the strength or that the quality is strong and easily accessible. Offering examples of positive qualities is often helpful:

- courage, bravery;
- self-compassion, self-acceptance, empathy;
- strength, perseverance, determination;
- clear thinking, wisdom, discernment;
- sense of humor, ability to laugh at self; and
- ease, relaxation, confidence.

BOX 10.2 CLIENT EXAMPLE: BRAINSTORMING STRENGTHS FOR RESOURCE TEAM GOALS

Therapist: Okay. Let's talk about what you might need to draw on from inside you in order to be able to be more fun loving and care free again. Characteristics or strengths that you would want to get connected to in order to be able to go out with friends and really enjoy yourself in the moment. What are you thinking?

Client: Well, I'd have to be really brave.

Therapist: So bravery or courage?

Client: Yeah, courage.

Therapist: Okay, what else?

Client: I think I would need to be nicer to myself.

Therapist: Help me understand what you mean.

(continued)

> **BOX 10.2 CLIENT EXAMPLE: BRAINSTORMING STRENGTHS FOR RESOURCE TEAM GOALS** (*continued*)
>
> **Client:** I beat myself up so much for being the way I am and that ends up being part of why I don't follow through.
>
> **Therapist:** So being nicer to yourself? Maybe kinder?
>
> **Client:** Yeah. I don't know how to do that.
>
> **Therapist:** What strength do you think you could call on to help you learn to be nicer or kinder to yourself?
>
> **Client:** Well, it would need to come from a part of me that believes I can change but isn't going to expect me to be perfect.
>
> **Therapist:** Hmmm. What strength would that be?
>
> **Client:** Maybe like self-compassion?
>
> **Therapist:** How would self-compassion help?
>
> **Client:** I could see myself as someone who has been through a lot and it's understandable that I got so serious and started worrying a lot.
>
> **Therapist:** So, having some compassion and understanding for yourself as you are now. Sounds like those strengths will help you and even build on each other!

4. Select Resource Team Members to Represent Each Strength/Positive Quality

The AFTT-A model does not include Child parts of Self on the Resource Team nor invites younger parts to participate in Team meetings. Therapists help clients understand that Resource Team meetings involve "grown-up" work. Younger parts stay in their Safe Places with their Higher Powers so they can just be the ages they are and maintain a sense of safety and nurturance. A Resource Team member is assigned as a representative of Child parts in case any of them has information important to the team. The therapist clarifies which Resource Team member communicates back and forth with Child parts, passing on information from Child parts to the Resource Team.

One of the most important points to make with clients when they're brainstorming team members that represent each needed strength is that there is no right or wrong answer and that nothing is etched in stone. Clients sometimes feel pressure to come up with the "perfect" answer immediately. Therapists can encourage clients to slow down, take their time, and remind them that any ideas they generate can always be changed if needed. Again, examples of Resource Team members as representatives of strengths or positive qualities are helpful if clients have difficulty coming up with ideas on their own:

- someone they know and admire;
- public figure, cultural or social group leader, author, athlete, musician, or artist;
- religious deity, prophet, saint, angel, or holy/enlightened being;
- fictional characters from books, cartoons, or movies;

- animals; or
- aspects of nature.

> **BOX 10.3 CLIENT EXAMPLE: SELECTING RESOURCE TEAM MEMBERS TO REPRESENT POSITIVE QUALITIES**
>
> **Therapist:** The last step is to brainstorm members of your Resource Team. People or beings who will represent your inner strengths of courage and self-compassion. And, like we talked about last week, you can also have team members who are your cheerleaders or mentors.
>
> **Client:** I thought of a couple of people already. I had a third grade teacher, Mrs. T., who took time to really help me with math. I was really bad at math! But her attitude was always like, "I know you can do this."
>
> **Therapist:** How would it be helpful for Mrs. T. to be a part of your team?
>
> **Client:** She could be one of my cheerleaders but also someone who taught me not to be so hard on myself.
>
> **Therapist:** She sounds great! What about the other people you mentioned?
>
> **Client:** My Aunt D. needs to be on my team. She's been through a lot and somehow has managed to stay the person she's always been—caring, outgoing. But she's also different too. In a good way. Like she doesn't let people take advantage of her like she used to. She's not mean or anything, just knows how to say "no" more and stick to it.
>
> **Therapist:** How would she add to the team?
>
> **Client:** Well, she could be a mentor and my representative for courage.

5. Add Cheerleader and/or Mentors as Members to the Resource Team

Clients often need Resource Team members that do not necessarily represent a specific strength but offer unconditional acceptance and encouragement or are a role model for how to grow and learn from difficult experiences. If clients have not already identified Resource Team members who are either a mentor (someone who has been through a difficult time and made it through to the other side in a positive way) or a cheerleader (someone who believes in the client no matter what, will have their back, and encourages them to grow and improve), therapists can suggest that clients add team members with those roles to their Resource Team.

6. Review Client's Therapy Goals, Necessary Strengths, and Resource Team Members and Make Changes if Needed

As a means of closure to the brainstorming aspect of developing an inner team of strengths and resources, clients find it helpful to review their goals, strengths, and their representative Resource Team members. They have the opportunity to re-examine; assess the accuracy, relevance, and importance of; and revise any of their choices.

STEPS FOR INSTALLING THE INTERNAL RESOURCE TEAM

For more information, see Protocol Script 7 at the end of this chapter.

1. Introduce the Idea of a Meeting Place for the Client and Their Resource Team Members

Now that clients have brainstormed goals, strengths or positive inner resources, and representatives for those inner resources on their Resource Team, they are ready to create a place or a space where they can meet with their team. Therapists want to emphasize the following aspects of a Meeting Place:

- It is separate from the client's Safe Place. It can be connected to their Safe Place, but it can't be the exact same place since their Safe Place is a place of respite or "being" and their Meeting Place is a place for action or "doing."
- It needs to have aspects of both nurturing and safety.
- It assists clients with time orientation. Clients with a Resource Team in their Meeting Place develop a sense of "I have everything I need" and "I am not alone." These new beliefs help clients tell the difference between "back then" when the danger was real and they felt isolated, scared, and unprotected, and "now" when the danger is past, their needs are being met, and they feel accepted, safe, and supported.

2. Brainstorm a Meeting Place for the Client and Their Resource Team Members Including Protective and Nurturing Attributes and Placement of Transitional Object From the Client's Adult Safe Place With Their Higher Power

The Meeting Place can be anywhere real or imagined. Just as with the Safe Place, therapists encourage clients to find a place that is connected to unambiguous positive feelings, thoughts, and sensations. If negative affect comes up, clients can still use their choice for the Meeting Place as long as they are able to set aside or contain any negative affect associated with the place and can refocus on and reinforce the links between the place and positive affect.

3. Transition the Client From the Adult Safe Place With Higher Power With Transitional Object to the Meeting Place With Resource Team Members

When starting to install the client's Resource Team in their Meeting Place, the therapist invites the client to revisit their Safe Place with their Higher Power and reconnect with the sense of being loved, accepted, safe, calm, centered, quiet, grounded, and so forth. Clients select a "transitional object" to take with them from their Safe Place into the Meeting Place; something that will bring to mind the experience of nurturing and protection and the beliefs such as "I am okay," "I am enough," "I am loved no matter what," and/or "I am worthwhile and deserve respect." As a result, the positive affect and beliefs from the client's Safe Place are linked to the new Meeting Place and become the foundation for the positive cognitions of "No matter what, I have what I need" and "I am not alone anymore" that clients develop with their Resource Team. Since the Resource Team installation builds and reinforces links between inner resources and positive affect, do short sets of slow BLS with tappers or butterfly taps.

4. Install the Resource Team and Meeting Place
In the AFTT-A model, therapists ask open-ended questions and offer a nondirective approach to creating the Meeting Place. Offering clients choices and encouraging them to draw ideas from their own internal and real-life experiences also enhance their sense of competence and confidence. For example, therapists ask clients to decide how they want to gather their team into the Meeting Place, what they want to do with the object they brought from their Safe Place, and what they want to add to the Meeting Place that will boost their sense of confidence and competence. Positive affect is again elicited and reinforced with short sets of slow BLS.

5. Discuss Ways in Which Resource Team Members Will Assist Clients in Meeting Goals for Therapy
Clients have an initial discussion with their Resource Team members about the general ways the team will be helpful to them in meeting their goals for therapy. The initial meeting allows the client to see how they and their Resource Team are going to work together to brainstorm ideas, offer support and encouragement, and make and follow through with decisions. Equally important in how the Resource Team will function is how the team offers clients the experience of a corrective attachment relationship; for example, their teams' unwavering support and willingness to help and their commitment to and their unshakable positive beliefs about the clients.

6. Anchor and Cue Word
Now clients are ready to find ways to activate the positive affect associated with their Resource Team. Typically, a body anchor and a cue word are used to activate the positive affect linked to the Resource Team and the Meeting Place. Once the body anchor and the cue words are selected, clients practice using them to begin to create an automatic response that then can be utilized when needed. Positive affect is again elicited and reinforced with short sets of slow BLS.

7. Test the Effectiveness of the Installation With a Challenging Present-Day Situation
The last major step in the *Installing the Internal Resource Team* protocol is to link the positive affect from clients' Meeting Place with their Resource Team with challenging situations from their adult lives. Basically, the therapist does a mini-Future Rehearsal with their client. The client has the opportunity to experience a difficult situation with the support and guidance from their team. One of the twelve promises in the Alcoholics Anonymous *Big Book* states, "We will instinctively know how to handle situations that used to baffle us" (2001, p. 84).

Clients no longer have to figure out what to do or how to respond by themselves. They are part of a team that has their backs. Clients now view circumstances or people through the filter of their new positive cognitions and increased sense of competence and self-confidence.

> **BOX 10.4 CLIENT EXAMPLE: USE OF RESOURCE TEAM IN FUTURE REHEARSAL**
>
> **Therapist:** So let's take your Resource Team and your sense of happiness and being loved and supported into this next week. How do you think they might help you this week?
>
> **Client:** Well, I can imagine them with me while I go through my week reminding me that I can follow through with my goals so I can get better. I can feel them with me so I don't feel like I have to do this all by myself.
>
> **Therapist:** When you think about them connected to you, supporting you, what do you notice?
>
> **Client:** I feel more confident like "I can do this!"
>
> **Therapist:** I was just going to ask if there is a positive cognition that goes with your experience with your team and the sense of them being with you through the week. Does "I can do this" feel right to you?
>
> **Client:** Well, my thought is that I can do this because I have the help I need. I can ask for the help I need from my team any time I need it.
>
> **Therapist:** What positive cognition fits for that?
>
> **Client:** How about "I have the help I need this week?"
>
> **Therapist:** Okay, hold in mind your Resource Team going through your week with you, feeling happy, confident, loved, and supported, while you say to yourself, "I have the help I need this week."
>
> (Slow, short BLS sets reinforced the client's positive affect as they imagined using their Resource Team throughout the upcoming week.)

8. Refine and Install the Revised Resource Team and Meeting Place as Needed

The good news is that if something about a client's Resource Team or Meeting Place doesn't seem to fit or isn't helpful, any aspect can be modified to become more effective. Positive affect linked to the revised team or place is elicited and reinforced with BLS. Clients are encouraged to practice connecting to their Resource Team in the Meeting Place with the use of their anchor and cue word in between sessions and report back to the therapist so they can reinforce what was helpful and revise and reinforce any needed improvements.

POINTS TO REMEMBER

Brainstorming Resource Team Members

- Initially, client goals for the Resource Team are more general; for example, what the client wants to accomplish in therapy. As clients transition from preparation phase to phases 3 to 8 of EMDR therapy, client goals are generated for specific ways the Resource Team can be helpful in subsequent phases.

- The therapist demonstrates an unshakable belief that clients have the inner strengths and support they need in order to meet their trauma therapy goals.
- In addition to Resource Team members who represent the clients' strengths or positive characteristics, clients may have team members who are cheerleaders and mentors.
- Clients don't have to have Resource Team members who are perfect. They can have faults or unlikable qualities; their only job is to embody the needed strength in team meetings.

Installing the Resource Team

- The Resource Team builds on the foundational beliefs of "I am okay" and "I am lovable" initiated in the client Adult Safe Place and Higher Power by tapping into and strengthening two main positive cognitions: "No matter what, I have what I need" and "I am not alone anymore."
- Like the Safe Places and Higher Powers for the Adult and Child parts of Self, the Meeting Place includes both nurturing and protective characteristics.
- Clients carry transitional objects from the Adult Safe Place to integrate sense of being calm, grounded, centered, and so forth into their Meeting Place.
- Clients can add objects, music, wall hangings, photos, and so on to their Meeting Place as long as they enhance the positive affect already linked the Meeting Place.
- Child parts do not directly attend or participate in Resource Team meetings. It's "grown-up stuff." Clients can figure out methods for Child parts' feelings, doubts, fears, and so forth to be communicated to and taken into consideration by the team without Child parts needing to leave their Safe Places and Higher Powers.

TROUBLESHOOTING

- If clients have difficulty identifying positive characteristics, remind them that they don't have to already possess the positive qualities or the qualities do not already have to be strong. Give examples from other clients to normalize client perception.
- Explore pros and cons of using real-life persons from clients' lives, especially if a potential Resource Team member has died. Ensure that the client is able to focus on the positive aspects of their choice for a team member as well as positive affect about the team member. Use the container to contain or set aside any negative affect.
- Remember that nothing is etched in stone. Consider changing an aspect of the Meeting Place or a Resource Team member if clients have difficulty staying focused on or strengthening positive affect. Consider the presence of a Critical Parent, Emotion Controller-Regulator, little "a," or Child part of Self. Work with the whole team to generate ideas about how to deal with parts of Self not yet members of the Resource Team or, as with Child parts, not intended to be a part

of the team. Use the container if needed for setting aside distressing material or affect.

PAUSE AND REFLECT FOR THE THERAPIST

Brainstorming a Resource Team Member

At this point, take some time to think about a challenging client with whom you work; perhaps someone who has difficulty following through with assignments, is stuck and doesn't seem to be able to move forward, has frequent crises, often late-cancels or no-shows for appointments, seems to need more than you can offer, or is critical of you as a therapist. Instead of focusing on the client, consider your own feelings and thoughts about and reactions to the client. Is there something you're doing or not doing with the client that could be enabling the client to continue behaviors that get in the way of the them making progress? Are you not saying something because you feel anxious or somewhat intimidated? Are you focusing too much on problem-solving and not enough on being attuned to their emotional state? Do you view the client as too fragile or feel over-responsible for their reactions or feelings? Write down a goal you could set for yourself that would address what would be in your client's best interest for you to change. Then identify a positive quality you would need to tap into and/or strengthen in order to accomplish that goal. Brainstorm ideas for a team member that would represent that positive characteristic on your Resource Team.

Installing the Resource Team

Brainstorm a Meeting Place where you'll talk with the Resource Team member you identified to represent the inner strength needed to achieve the goal you have for yourself in working with your challenging client. Take a few moments to imagine tucking in any younger parts who might have snuck out of their Safe Place.

Next, imagine being in your Safe Place with your Higher Power so you can reconnect to a sense of being okay, grounded, calm, and so forth. If you like, do a couple of short sets of slow BLS to help you reconnect to that positive affect. Select an object in your Safe Place that you will take with you to your Meeting Place to remind you of the affirming aspects of your Safe Place and Higher Power.

Make your way to your Meeting Place and use all of your senses to take in the sights, sounds, scents, and textures involved in the space. Absorb the accepting, nurturing, and encouraging aspects as well as a sense of safety and security of your Meeting Place. If you like, when you notice positive feelings, sensations, body posture, and thoughts, you can do some slow BLS by tapping back and forth on the tops of your thighs or use butterfly taps on your upper arms. Decide how you want to bring your Resource Team member into the Meeting Place and imagine that figure coming into the space with you. Notice how it feels to have a team member who is committed to helping you reach your goal with your challenging client. Again, if you like, when you notice positive feelings, sensations, body posture, and thoughts, you can do some slow BLS by tapping back and forth on the tops of your thighs or use butterfly taps on your upper arms.

Jot down a word or phrase that will help reconnect you to the confidence and competence you have gained and remind you of the sense of protection and acceptance you are feeling. Anchor the positive affect with a gesture or a part of your body you can connect to like your hand over your heart and again reinforce with slow tapping.

Now, imagine taking a moment before you meet with the client again to call to mind whatever you need from your Resource Team member in your Meeting Place to take into the session as your Competent Adult part of Self, being connecting to everything you need to approach your client in this more effective way. Picture yourself calling on your Resource Team member to remind you that you have at your fingertips whatever helpful and encouraging thoughts and the positive feelings any time you need them during the next session with the client. Again, if you like, you can strengthen and reinforce positive feelings, sensations, thoughts by doing short sets of slow BLS.

USEFUL TERMS AND DEFINITIONS

AFTT-A: Attachment-Focused Trauma Therapy for Adults

BLS: bilateral stimulation

DES: disorders of extreme stress

EMDR: Eye Movement Desensitization and Reprocessing

PTSD: posttraumatic stress disorder

RDI: Resource Development and Installation

PROTOCOL SCRIPT 6. BRAINSTORMING INTERNAL RESOURCE TEAM MEMBERS

Adapted from Fraser, G. A. (2003). Fraser's "Dissociative Table Technique" revisited, revised: A strategy for working with ego states in dissociative disorders and ego-state therapy. *Journal of Trauma and Dissociation*, 4(4), 5–28. https://doi.org/10.1300/J229v04n04_02; Leeds, A. (2016). *A guide to the standard EMDR protocols for clinicians, supervisors, and consultants* (2nd ed.). Springer Publishing Company; Korn, D., & Leeds, A. (2002). Preliminary evidence of efficacy for EMDR resource development and installation in the stabilization phase of treatment of complex posttraumatic stress disorder. *Journal of Clinical Psychology*, 58(12), 1465–1487. https://doi.org/10.1002/jclp.10099; Manfield, P. (2010). *Dyadic resourcing: Creating a foundation for processing trauma*. CreateSpace Independent Publishing; Schmidt, S. L. (2020). *Ego state therapy interventions to prepare attachment-wounded adults or EMDR*. DNMS Institute LLC; Shapiro, F. (2018). *Eye movement desensitization and reprocessing (EMDR) therapy: Basic principles, protocols, and procedures* (2nd ed.). Guilford Press; and Shapiro, R. (2016). *Easy ego state intervention: Strategies for working with parts*. W. W. Norton & Company.

1. **Explain the Concept and Purposes of the Resource Team.** *Say...* "So far, you have created for yourself a place of respite and safety or what we call a place of 'being' for that Adult part of you; that place (***describe the client's Safe Place for Adult part of Self here***) where you can go to get grounded, calm, and centered, and where you can connect with your Higher Power (***describe client's Higher Power here***). The place

where you know you are okay, you're lovable, and you deserve good things in your life. The next step is to help you tap into and strengthen positive parts or characteristics of yourself that will help you accomplish your goals in therapy and be where you want to be by the time you finish therapy. Sometimes, especially early in therapy, people don't believe they have strengths, or if they do, they think those characteristics are not very strong or they think they don't deserve to feel good about themselves or to recognize something positive about themselves.

"The good news is that I have an 'unshakable belief' that you have everything you need inside to do this work and reach goals for therapy. You may have been led to believe that you don't by the way you were raised, the messages you got, and the hurt you experienced as you grew up, but it isn't true. It may *feel* true, but it isn't. What we're going to do in this part of therapy is to identify your goals for therapy and help you tap into and reinforce the positive qualities you will use to accomplish what you want in therapy.

"Then we're going to create a team inside you that will be made up of team members that represent your strengths. It's sometimes hard to get connected to positive qualities because they can be abstract, so we make them real and more approachable by having a person, being, creature, animal, whatever you want, to stand in for each strength that you identified. We want all your strengths and resources at your fingertips whenever they're needed. No matter what the situation or circumstances, your Inner Resource Team will help you develop your own unshakable belief that you have what you need inside of you.

"One of the most important purposes of the Resource Team is to offer another opportunity for you to experience corrective attachment relationships within yourself. You'll build on the foundation of the relationship you started with your Higher Power; a relationship that contains aspects of both acceptance and safety. The relationships among Resource Team members who work together to help you and the relationship between you and your Resource Team also include those same characteristics of nurturing and protection. We want you to know that you are not doing this work alone. You will have all the help you need. Your Resource Team has your back. You're not alone anymore." *Ask…* "Make sense so far? Any questions?"

2. Identify the Client's Goals for the Attachment-Focused Trauma Therapy Process. *Say…* "So, the first step is to identify your goals; where you want to be when you finish therapy, how you want to feel about yourself, what you want your life to look like. There's no right or wrong answer, it's whatever you think. We might need to tweak them a little bit here and there to make them as useful to you as possible, but I want them to be *your* goals." *Ask…* "What would you like to get out of therapy?"

_____

_____

3. Brainstorm Strengths or Positive Characteristics Clients Need to Accomplish Their Goals. *Say…* "What I'd like you to do next is brainstorm ideas about the strengths or positive qualities you will need to tap into and/or strengthen so that you can reach the goals of (*repeat client's goals here*)."

4. Select Resource Team Members to Represent Each Strength/Positive Characteristic. *Say...* "The last step is to create a team inside of you made up of the qualities, strengths, and resources of (***repeat client's identified strengths/resources here***); to bring together an inner group that will help you know what strengths you need and will work together to help you tap into and use those positive characteristics when needed. As we talked about a little while ago, this group is your 'Resource Team'; a team that will be there for you no matter what, so you know you're not alone anymore and that you have everything you need.

"Much as you did in choosing a Higher Power, you will pick someone or something to represent each of the strengths you identified. Let's use the example I gave earlier about having a goal to be more direct in getting my needs met. Since that goal might include me learning to be more assertive, I decided that a positive quality I might need to be more assertive is courage or bravery. Some examples of Resource Team members that represent courage or bravery might be a lion, a Scottish Highlander, a ninja, or even someone you admire who is able to be direct in a healthy way despite its difficulty or if they're afraid. Team members can be someone you know or someone you don't know but admire—a public figure, author, or leader in your social or cultural groups. Team members could be fictional characters from a movie, book, or cartoons. They can even be an animal or a part of nature. They just need to embody the quality that you want them to bring to the team. They don't need to be perfect or have a lot of positive qualities, they just need to represent the one quality you assign to them." *Ask...* "Any questions? Let's go down your list of strengths and brainstorm some ideas of Resource Team members."

5. Add Cheerleader and/or Mentor Members to the Resource Team. *Say...* "If you'd like, we can add two other kinds of Resource Team members even though their purpose is not to represent a specific strength. One is a cheerleader-type member and the other is a mentor. The cheerleader is someone who believes in you, wants what's best for you, is in your corner, and has your back. The mentor is someone who has been through a difficult situation or time and has made it through to the other side, having learned from and having been made better by the experience. Again, cheerleaders and mentors can be people you know or someone you don't know but you admire—public figures, authors, or leaders. Cheerleaders and mentors could be fictional characters from a movie, book, or cartoons. They can even be an animal or a part of nature." *Ask...* "Would you like to add a cheerleader or mentor to your Resource Team?" ***Brainstorm ideas for cheerleader and/or mentor members to add to the team.***

6. Review the Client's Therapy Goals, Strengths, and Resource Team Members and Make Changes if Needed.

___

___

PROTOCOL SCRIPT 7. INSTALLING THE INTERNAL RESOURCE TEAM

Adapted from Fraser, G. A. (2003). Fraser's "Dissociative Table Technique" revisited, revised: A strategy for working with ego states in dissociative disorders and ego-state therapy. *Journal of Trauma and Dissociation, 4*(4), 5–28. https://doi.org/10.1300/J229v04n04_02; Leeds, A. (2016). *A guide to the standard EMDR protocols for clinicians, supervisors, and consultants* (2nd ed.). Springer Publishing Company; Korn, D., & Leeds, A. (2002). Preliminary evidence of efficacy for EMDR resource development and installation in the stabilization phase of treatment of Complex Posttraumatic Stress Disorder. *Journal of Clinical Psychology, 58,* 1465–1487. https://doi.org/10.1002/jclp.10099; Manfield, P. (2010). *Dyadic resourcing: Creating a foundation for processing trauma.* CreateSpace Independent Publishing; Schmidt, S. L. (2020). *Ego state therapy interventions to prepare attachment-wounded adults or EMDR.* DNMS Institute LLC; Shapiro, F. (2018). *Eye movement desensitization and reprocessing (EMDR) therapy: Basic principles, protocols, and procedures* (2nd ed.). Guilford Press; and Shapiro, R. (2016). *Easy ego state intervention: Strategies for working with parts.* W. W. Norton & Company.

1. Introduce the Idea of a Meeting Place for the Client and Their Resource Team. *Say…* "Now that you have your goals, strengths, and Resource Team members identified, we want to create a place for you to meet with your team—a Meeting Place or Gathering Space; somewhere separate from your Safe Place where you and your team can meet. The place where you meet with your team can be connected to your Safe Place but it can't be the exact same place. Remember that your Safe Place is a place of 'being' where you can go to be calm, grounded, and free from whatever is going on in your adult life. The Meeting Place or Gathering Space is a place of 'doing'; a space where you and your team meet to discuss, look at options, make decisions, and solve problems." ***Give an example here.*** (For example, someone's Safe Place might be by a stream in the mountains and the Meeting Place is in a nearby cabin. There's a path with a gate separating the two places.) *Ask…* "Make sense? Any questions?" *Say…* "Your Resource Team and the Meeting Place are also another way you can tell the difference between 'now' and 'back then.' Your team and the Meeting Place remind you that the danger is past and, in this present moment, all of your needs are being met. You have everything you need and you are not alone anymore." *Ask…* "Any questions?"

2. Brainstorm Meeting Place/Gathering Space for the Client and Their Resource Team Members Including Safety and Nurturing Attributes and Placement of Transitional Object From the Client's Adult Safe Place With Their Higher Power. *Say…* "Just like with your Safe Place, Your Meeting Place also needs to be both nurturing and protective." ***Give an example here.*** (For example, someone might choose a large, flat rock extending out from a forest in the mountains. The area was quiet, peaceful, and lush with the sound of a breeze in the trees and a nearby stream. There's only one path through the trees to get to the Meeting Place and a Secret Service Agent is posted at the top of the path so no one can get to the Meeting Place without clearance.) *Say...* "Your Meeting Place can be anywhere ... real or imagined, someplace you may already have been or someplace you'd like to go to." *Ask...* "What kind of Meeting Place do you think you need so you can feel accepted and safe while you and your team meet?"

If the client describes only one aspect of the Meeting Place, either nurturing or protection, brainstorm ideas about the other side. Make changes as needed.

Access and reinforce positive affect with short sets of slow BLS. Practice use of a container to set aside negative affect if needed.

3. Transition the Client From the Adult Safe Place With the Higher Power With Transitional Object Into the Meeting Place With Resource Team Members. *Say...* "I invite you to go back to your Safe Place with your Higher Power and get reconnected to all the sights, sounds, and scents; all of your positive thoughts, feelings, and sensations." *Access and reinforce positive affect with short sets of slow BLS. Say...* "Now I'd like you to choose something to take from your Safe Place to your Meeting Place; something that will remind you of (*repeat positive affect client expressed*). Something you can have with your team in your Meeting Place so all you need to do is look at it or touch it or hear it and be able to bring up (*repeat positive affect client expressed*)."

Reinforce the positive affect with short set of slow BLS.

4. Install the Resource Team and Meeting Place. *Ask...* "How would you like you and your team to meet in your Gathering Space?"

"How do you feel now that you are with your team? How does it seem that your team feels about meeting?"

Access and reinforce the positive affect.

Add the object from the Safe Place to the Meeting Place. Ask… "What would you like to do with (***name object***) that you brought from your Safe Place?"

_____

_____

Ask… "How do you feel now that you've put (***name object***) in your Meeting Place?"

_____

_____

Access and reinforce the positive affect with short, slow sets of BLS. Ask… "Is there anything else you would like to add to the Meeting Place that would help you feel accepted, protected, competent, and confident?"

_____

_____

Access and reinforce the positive affect.

5. Discuss Ways in Which Resource Team Members Will Assist Clients in Meeting Goals for Therapy. *Say…* "Let's have a short meeting with your team now. I want you to get a sense of their commitment to you and their willingness to help you with your therapy process." *Ask…* "What would you like to ask of or to say to your team about what you will need from them going forward?"

_____

_____

Ask… "How does your team respond to that?"

_____

_____

Access and reinforce the positive affect.

Ask… "What needs to be said or done to complete the scene?"

_____

_____

Access and reinforce positive affect with short sets of BLS.

6. Anchor and Cue Word. *Say…* "I'd like you to anchor that sense of (***repeat client's words***), your feelings of (***repeat client's words***), and your beliefs of (***repeat client's words***) in your body so that when you touch your hand or chest or wherever you choose, you can bring it into the present moment. I want you to be able to do the same with a word or phrase: When you see it or say it, you bring those feelings and beliefs from your team into your present-day life. Let's start with the anchor. I want you to choose a place on or connected to your body—it could be your hand,

10. CREATING AN INTERNAL RESOURCE TEAM   139

a piece of jewelry, your hand over your heart, anywhere you want so that when you touch it, you can connect to your experience of your Resource Team in the Meeting Place." *Ask...* "Where do you think you would like to anchor those feelings and those unshakable beliefs of (*repeat client's beliefs*) from your Resource Team?"

_____

_____

Access and reinforce the positive affect. Say... "Now let's think of a word or phrase that when you see it, hear it, or say it, you will reconnect to those feelings and beliefs from your Resource Team into your present-day life."

_____

_____

Say... "Hold in mind (*repeat client's word or phrase*) while you bring up the feelings and beliefs from your team in the Meeting Place." *Access and reinforce the positive affect with short sets of slow BLS.*

7. Test the Effectiveness of the Installation With a Challenging Situation From Present-Day Life. *Say...* "Let's practice how you can use your anchor and word to connect the feelings and beliefs from your Resource Team in the Meeting Place to a challenging situation that might come up between therapy sessions. What might be a good example of a situation when you would want to deal with this from your Competent Adult part of Self?"

_____

_____

Say... "Imagine using your anchor of (*repeat client's words*) and the word or phrase of (*repeat client's words*) to connect those feelings and beliefs of (*repeat client's words*) from your Resource Team in the Meeting Place to handle that situation easily and successfully." *Access and reinforce the positive affect.*

_____

_____

8. Refine and Install the Revised Resource Team and Meeting Place as Needed. *Review nurturing and protective aspects of both the Resource Team and Meeting Place. Revise as needed. Strengthen and reinforce positive affect connected to revised images with BLS.*

_____

_____

REFERENCES

Anonymous. (2001). *Alcoholics anonymous* (4th ed.). Alcoholics Anonymous World Services, Inc.

Fraser, G. A. (1991). The Dissociative Table Technique: A strategy for working with ego states and dissociative disorders and ego-state therapy. *Dissociation: Progress in the Dissociative Disorders*, 4(4), 205–213.

Fraser, G. A. (2003). Fraser's "Dissociative Table Technique" revisited, revised: A strategy for working with ego states in dissociative disorders and ego-state therapy. *Journal of Trauma and Dissociation*, 4(4), 5–28. https://doi.org/10.1300/J229v04n04_02

Kiessling, R. (2009a). Resource strengthening. In M. Luber (Ed.). *EMDR scripted protocols: Basics and special situations* (pp. 85–86). Springer Publishing Company.

Kiessling, R. (2009b). Extending resources. In M. Luber (Ed.). *EMDR scripted protocols: Basics and special situations* (pp. 87–89). Springer Publishing Company.

Korn, D., & Leeds, A. (2002). Preliminary evidence of efficacy for EMDR resource development and installation in the stabilization phase of treatment of complex posttraumatic stress disorder. *Journal of Clinical Psychology*, 58(12), 1465–1487. https://doi.org/10.1002/jclp.10099

Laub, B. (2009). Resource connection envelope (RCE) in EMDR standard protocol. In M. Luber (Ed.), *EMDR scripted protocols: Basics and special situations* (pp. 93–99). Springer Publishing Company.

Leeds, A. (2016). *A guide to the standard EMDR protocols for clinicians, supervisors, and consultants* (2nd ed.). Springer Publishing Company.

Manfield, P. (2010). *Dyadic resourcing: Creating a foundation for processing trauma*. CreateSpace Independent Publishing.

Martin, K. (2018, April). *Mastering the treatment of complex trauma: Transforming theory into practice*. Presentation, Omaha, Nebraska.

Murray, K. (2011). Container. *Journal of EMDR Practice and Research*, 1(5), 29–32. https://doi.org/10.1891/1933-3196.5.1.29

Parnell, L. (1999). *EMDR in the treatment of adults abused as children*. W. W. Norton & Company.

Parnell, L. (2007). *A therapist's guide to EMDR: Tools and techniques for successful treatment*. W. W. Norton & Company.

Potter, A. E. (1994a). *Inside out: Rebuilding self and personality through inner child therapy* (therapist manual). Taylor and Francis Group.

Potter, A. E. (1994b). *Inside out: Rebuilding self and personality through inner child therapy* (client workbook). Taylor and Francis Group.

Potter, A., Davidson, M., & Wesselmann, D. (2013). Utilizing EMDR as phase-based trauma treatment: A case study series. In L. C. Stewart (Ed.), *Eye Movement: Developmental perspectives, dysfunctions, and disorders in humans* (pp. 49–72). Nova Publishers.

Schmidt, S. L. (2009). *The Developmental Needs Meeting Strategy (DNMS): An ego state therapy for healing adults with childhood trauma and attachment wounds*. DNMS Institute LLC.

Shapiro, E. (2009). The resource map. In M. Luber (Ed.), *EMDR scripted protocols: Basics and special situations* (pp. 101–104). Springer Publishing Company.

Shapiro, F. (2018). *Eye movement desensitization and reprocessing (EMDR) therapy: Basic principles, protocols, and procedures* (2nd ed.). Guilford Press.

Shapiro, R. (2016). *Easy ego state intervention: Strategies for working with parts*. W. W. Norton & Company.

van der Kolk, B. A., Roth, S., Pelcovitz, D., Sunday, S., & Spinazzola, J. (2005). Disorders of extreme stress: The empirical foundation of a complex adaptation to trauma. *Journal of Traumatic Stress*, 18(5), 389–399. https://doi.org/10.1002/jts.20047

CHAPTER 11

Strengthening the Competent Adult Part of Self in Attachment-Focused Trauma Therapy for Adults

INTRODUCTION

Self-efficacy, as described in the seminal work by Bandura (1977), is confidence in one's own capacity to master challenges and accomplish goals. High self-efficacy is linked with positive well-being and acceptance of life's challenges, while low self-efficacy is associated with avoidance of tasks and more mental health symptoms. In a longitudinal study of 143 assault victims, high self-efficacy appeared helpful in reducing traumatic stress symptoms over time, but self-efficacy was also shown to be negatively impacted by trauma (Nygaard et al., 2017).

The adaptive information processing (AIP) model (Shapiro, 2018) explains that clients who experience symptoms related to early attachment trauma have unprocessed disturbing memories that are stored in an unprocessed form along with the affect and beliefs present at the time of the trauma. Attachment-Focused Trauma Therapy for Adults (AFTT-A) conceptualizes activation of childhood negative memory networks holding distressing emotions, sensations, and perceptions that were experienced over an extended period of time as a Child/Adolescent part of Self that is hypervigilant and easily activated by relationships in present-day adult life. The younger part of Self is commonly activated while the Adult part of Self is simultaneously attempting interpersonal relationships and other adulthood tasks. This results in a "blend" of "Adult Brain" and "Kid Brain," leading to overall decreased self-efficacy, negatively impacting capacity to communicate, problem-solve, and self-regulate.

Enmeshed "Velcro Kid" Child Parts

When the Child and Adult parts of Self are blended on a regular basis, it is as if the parts are attached with "Velcro." One client stated that it felt more like "Super Glue." When the "Velcro Kid" feelings and thoughts are frequently interwoven with feelings and thoughts belonging to the Adult part, the client may have difficulty holding onto the differentiated adult state. Clients are usually initially unaware of the hypervigilant Child/Adolescent parts of Self, but when the AFTT-A therapist asks about a recent situation they had difficulty managing and asks, "Hold old did you feel that day?" the client usually responds with an immediate, gut-level answer related to a much younger age.

Some clients have a Child/Adolescent part of Self who operated as a pseudo-adult when they were very young due to neglect in the family and a need to take on adult caregiving roles. They may confuse the pseudo-adult part as an Adult part of Self. The therapist can clarify whether or not the client is operating from a "pseudo-adult" young part by asking, "When you bring up that recent situation in your mind, does it make you feel genuinely competent and truly adult? Or do you feel like you are 'faking it' or feeling 'little' while 'acting big'?"

COMPETENT ADULT PART: CONDUCTOR OF THE ORCHESTRA

The AFTT-A model overall provides sets of protocols that utilize slow bilateral stimulation (BLS), as part of the preparation phase of Eye Movement Desensitization and Reprocessing (EMDR) therapy to create a healthy internal system through appropriate internal boundaries and increased connection to internal resources. Over time, the protocols lead to healthy functioning from the Authentic Self, incorporating strengthened competent and nurturing adult qualities.

The protocol for differentiating and strengthening of the Competent Adult part of Self specifically helps ensure a boundary with the Child/Adolescent part of Self and empowers the Competent Adult part of Self to operate with greater self-efficacy and with access to adulthood resources and skills. The strengthened Adult part is able to notice the internal shift when the younger part of Self is activated. The awareness allows the Adult part to take action to move the Child/Adolescent part of Self back to an internal place of safety and protection. The differentiated and empowered Competent Adult part of Self has greater capacity to grow in the skills of adulthood (e.g., communication, self-regulation, problem-solving) and make healthy choices in adult life. The strengthened Competent Adult part of Self is able to reflect upon their internal state and consider their own emotions and needs as well as the emotions and needs of significant others and their children. The empowered, Competent Adult part of Self can facilitate change in the internal system like a conductor leading an orchestra—providing Child/Adolescent parts of Self with safety and care, negotiating and dialoguing with younger parts of Self, and increasing compassion and empathy for younger parts.

Strengthening Through Resourcing

EMDR Resource Development and Installation (RDI) was developed by Korn and Leeds (2002) as a way to increase adaptive resources during the preparation phase of EMDR therapy using mastery experiences, positive relationships, or symbols to access inner resources and slow BLS to deepen the positive affect. Shapiro (2018) implements slow BLS to deepen a sense of safety associated with a "Safe/Calm Place." The Strengthening of the Competent Adult part of Self procedure accesses a memory in which the client felt both competent and adult for the resource activity.

The first step in the *Strengthening the Competent Adult Part of Self* protocol begins with a therapist and client collaboration to identify a memory that is associated with a felt state of adult competency. If the client struggles, the AFTT-A therapist provides some general suggestions such as a past accomplishment, a time they overcame a fear, a time they were with someone who made them feel good about themselves, or a time they felt included in a cultural or social group.

Once a memory is identified, the therapist uses the two-step guided imagery method inspired by the positive state protocol by Popky (2005). The client is instructed to first view the memory on a screen. Viewing the memory from a distance is useful because it allows the client to observe body position, facial expression, and voice tone. Slow BLS is added once they achieve the visual picture to deepen any positive shift. As a second step, the therapist instructs the client to "step into the movie," noticing their emotions and sensations as they think about their body, facial expression, and voice tone in the memory. Again, slow BLS is implemented to deepen any positive affect or sensations. The therapist also asks clients to find an associated cue word or phrase, as suggested in the original protocol (Korn & Leeds, 2002). The cue word or phrase is paired with the memory along with slow BLS.

Finally, the therapist asks the client to experiment with the combination of competency memory, cue word, and body position/facial expression/voice tone to find the combination that is most helpful for accessing the Competent Adult part of Self. Most importantly, the therapist encourages clients to use the combination that works best to access the Competent Adult part of Self on a daily basis outside of therapy. The client is instructed in the use of the butterfly tap to apply at home as a slow, short set of alternate taps by crossing their arms and tapping on upper arms, shoulders, or collarbone. The protocol is repeated in subsequent therapy sessions, as well, for further deepening and strengthening as needed.

While this chapter focuses on the development of the Competent Adult part of Self, the *Corrective Attachment Experiences Between the Child/Adolescent and True Parent Parts of Self* protocol in Chapter 12 enhances the True Parent aspect of Self. The True Parent and the Competent Adult part of Self are important aspects for moving toward and reclaiming the Authentic Self.

Moving Toward the Reprocessing Phases of EMDR Therapy

During the reprocessing phases of EMDR therapy, the empowered Competent Adult part has a stronger capacity to hold onto the present-day, adult perspective while accessing memory networks holding unprocessed childhood trauma. Metaphorically speaking, this allows the client to keep one foot in the past and one foot in the present for effective EMDR reprocessing. When both perspectives are activated along with BLS, EMDR reprocessing can proceed unhindered by dissociation, avoidance, or an overactive "Kid Brain."

As you read the following overview of steps for the *Strengthening the Competent Adult Part of Self* protocol, you may wish to refer to Protocol Script 8 at the end of the chapter.

OVERVIEW OF STEPS FOR STRENGTHENING THE COMPETENT ADULT PART OF SELF PROTOCOL

1. Explanation
Explain that the activity will increase the client's feelings of confidence and help differentiate the Adult part from the Child/Adolescent parts of themselves.

2. Create a Drawing That Illustrates the Current Strength of the Competent Adult Part of Self in Relationship to Child/Adolescent Part(s) of Self (Optional)

Suggest the client draws a picture using circles (or any other shape or visual the client wishes to use) to illustrate their felt sense regarding the Competent Adult part of Self in relationship to any identified Child/Adolescent parts of Self. Explain that the size of the Competent Adult circle in relationship to the Child/Adolescent circle(s) illustrates the felt strength of the Competent Adult part. Close placement of the circles can illustrate a "Velcro Kid" or enmeshed Child/Adolescent part. Greater distance between the circles might illustrate a dismissive or rejecting attitude on the part of the Adult part toward a Child part of Self. Remind the client that for the purposes of the protocol, the drawing is based only upon their intuition. They needn't worry about getting it "exactly right."

3. Brainstorm Memories of Operating From the Competent Adult Part of Self
Ask the client to think back to a memory or memories involving a situation in which they felt a sense of functioning from a competent adult state. If the client has difficulty, brainstorm together and assist the client by providing examples such as a first job, a job success, holding their child for the first time, solving a problem, overcoming a fear, building something, or fixing something. Another option is a memory of being with someone who demonstrates belief in their potential or their talents or a memory of feeling included or respected by their identified cultural or social group. (Note that the protocol can be repeated with more than one memory of adult competency for further strengthening of the Competent Adult part of Self.)

4. Note the Details
Ask the client to describe what they remember in detail. Write down what they say.

5. Direct the Client to Watch the Memory on a Movie Screen as You Provide Guided Imagery and Slow BLS
The client's eyes may be open or closed for the visualization. Use your notes to guide the client's imagination. Add a slow, short set of BLS (for resourcing, clients often prefer tactile BLS) as you provide the imagery. Check to make sure the memory did not have any negative associations. If so, ask the client to "put parentheses" around the positive part of the memory or choose an alternate memory.

6. Call the Client's Attention to What They Observe on the Screen Regarding Their Body Posture, Facial Expression, and Voice, and Deepen With Slow BLS
The client's observations about their body posture, facial expression, and voice tone provide the client with options for accessing the Competent Adult part of Self quickly when needed. Changing one's body posture, facial expression, or voice tone like an actor in a movie is something that can easily be managed and allows the body to send messages to the brain regarding affect state. Observing their body and voice on the screen allows them to gain insight into the body changes. A slow, short set of BLS deepens their awareness.

7. Direct the Client to "Step Into" the Movie and Deepen Positive Affect With Slow BLS
Ask the client to keep in mind the associated body position as well as any associated facial expression or voice tone. Ask the client to "step into" the movie and notice their

affect and the feeling in their body in the here and now. Add a slow, short set of BLS to deepen the positive experience.

8. Pair the Memory With a Cue Word Using Slow BLS
Ask the client to think of a word or phrase and bring up the memory. Direct the client to adjust their body position to match the adult state while thinking of the cue word. Repeat the slow, short set of BLS.

9. Help the Client Identify Their Preferred Method(s) for Accessing the Competent Adult Part of Self
Ask the client to experiment with picturing the memory, changing body posture and facial expressions, and bringing up their cue word. Ask them to find the most helpful method or combination of methods for accessing the Competent Adult part of Self.

BOX 11.1 CLIENT EXAMPLE: OBSERVING BODY POSTURE, FACIAL EXPRESSION, AND VOICE TONE TO ASSIST WITH ACCESSING THE COMPETENT ADULT PART OF SELF

Client has chosen a "Competent Adult" memory about working as a volunteer for a local politician.

Therapist: (Running tappers slowly) See yourself there on the screen, in the big basement room full of activity, people on the phones, people putting together mailers and signs… you with the other volunteer, putting mailers together and deeply engrossed in conversation. Notice how you look as you are sitting there, especially how you are holding your body. Notice your face, your expression, and notice anything at all about your voice (stopping BLS). What did you notice?

Client: I could see that I was completely comfortable, with no self-consciousness.

Therapist: What did you notice about your body?

Client: My body was relaxed, I was sitting fairly straight, though, not all hunched over like I do sometimes. I was looking up from my work, making eye contact.

Therapist: What did you notice about your face?

Client: My face was relaxed, an open expression. When I smiled, I smiled with my eyes.

Therapist: What about your voice?

Client: It had a relaxed sound, not strained.

Therapist: That's wonderful. Let's do it again, but this time I would like you to step right into the movie. As I start the tappers again now (adding slow BLS) imagine yourself there, engrossed in conversation, activity all around you. Notice how your face feels, with muscles loose, not tense, your forehead relaxed, smiling, your voice relaxed. Let me check in now (stopping BLS). What are you noticing?

(continued)

> **BOX 11.1 CLIENT EXAMPLE: OBSERVING BODY POSTURE, FACIAL EXPRESSION, AND VOICE TONE TO ASSIST WITH ACCESSING THE COMPETENT ADULT PART OF SELF** (*continued*)
>
> **Client:** Comfortable in my own skin. Even just sitting here, I notice my spine is nice and straight, my shoulders feel relaxed and more drooping, not pulled up, and my body feels kind of open. My face feels natural, relaxed. My kid self must be all tucked in right now, because I really do feel fully adult right now.
>
> **Therapist:** That's great. Is there a word or phrase we could pair with this memory to help you find this adult self when you need to?
>
> **Client:** I like the phrase "comfortable in my skin."
>
> **Therapist:** Okay. I'm just going to run the tappers a little bit while you remember the feeling in your body and you hold in mind the phrase "comfortable in my skin." (Resumes tappers for a few seconds and then stops.) How did that go?
>
> **Client:** Really well. I wish I could hold onto this feeling.
>
> **Therapist:** Well, let's see if we can help you learn to recapture this adult state whenever you need to or want to. You have three ways to do that now. One is through the memory itself. The second way is by putting your body in the relaxed but confident position, with your face relaxed and open. And the third is through the cue word. Take a moment to experiment and see what works best for you. You might like using one way, two ways, or all three of the ways to step into your Competent Adult part of Self. You can even apply a very short and slow set of self-tapping with the butterfly hug. (Therapist demonstrates crossing the arms and tapping bilaterally on shoulders.) At home, I'd like you to practice accessing your Competent Adult part of Self each day.

FURTHER STEPS TO HELP BRING THE COMPETENT ADULT PART OF SELF TO FUTURE CHALLENGES

To assist the client with bringing the Competent Adult part of Self to their present and future adult life and build overall feelings of confidence, conduct a Future Rehearsal as a final step of this adaptation of the RDI procedure.

10. Find a Present-Day Challenging Situation

Ask the client to think of a challenging situation that happens often. Find a situation that is challenging without being overwhelming.

11. Invite the Client to Access the Competent Adult Part of Self

Ask the client to utilize the method or combination of methods that seem most effective for "stepping into" the state of adult competency. Ask the client to let you know when they have accessed the Competent Adult part of Self.

12. Direct the Client to View a Future Rehearsal on a Screen
Once the client has accessed the Competent Adult part of Self, ask the client to consider how they would hope to handle the present-day challenge. Discuss and problem-solve with the client as needed. Suggest the client visualize the Competent Adult part of Self handling the situation on a movie screen.

13. Check in and Deepen the Experience With Slow BLS
Ask the client how they saw themselves handling the situation from their Competent Adult part of Self in the future. Ask the client to describe their feelings in the present. If the response is positive, deepen the client's felt sense with a slow short set of BLS.

14. Encourage the Client to "Step Into" the Future Rehearsal if the Client Feels Ready and Then Deepen With Slow BLS
Ask the client if they are ready to "step into" the movie of the Future Rehearsal on the screen and experiment with how it feels in their body to respond to the challenging situation with their Competent Adult part of Self. Invite them to bring along a Resource Team member to help if needed. Deepen positive affect with a slow, short set of BLS.

15. Encourage the Client to Practice Accessing the Competent Adult Part of Self at Home
Suggest the client use their favorite method for accessing the Competent Adult part of Self at home. Show the client how to use a slow, short set of butterfly taps (crossing their arms and alternating slow taps on their upper arms or shoulders) to reinforce the Competent Adult part of Self, especially at the start of each day.

POINTS TO REMEMBER

- Clients with a history of attachment trauma may struggle with confidence in their own capacity to master life's challenges due to stored, unprocessed memories associated with negative feelings and beliefs related to a loss of self-efficacy.
- The Child/Adolescent part of Self may be enmeshed with the Adult part of Self. This "Velcro Kid" prevents the Adult part from thinking, interacting, and problem-solving as a mature, wise, and differentiated Adult.
- The Child/Adolescent part of Self may act as a "pseudo-adult," especially if during childhood, the client had to take care of adults or siblings.
- The differentiated and empowered Competent Adult part of Self can make healthy choices in adult life and facilitate healthy changes in the internal system.
- The strengthened Competent Adult part of Self can stay present while accessing memory networks for EMDR reprocessing.
- Viewing a memory or situation associated with adult competence first on a screen encourages awareness of changes in the body, the facial expression, and the voice tone. This awareness later helps the client access and hold onto the Competent Adult part of Self.
- The exercise provides three possible "doors" to shifting the affect state: the memory itself, the body, and cue word(s).

- Bringing the Competent Adult part of Self into EMDR Future Rehearsal helps bring the Competent Adult into adult life.

TROUBLESHOOTING

If the client has difficulty remembering an experience related to feeling competent and adult, follow these steps to help them access a Competent Adult state:

- Ground the client by asking them to describe their surroundings, touch and notice contrasting textures of cushions and clothing items, and notice the feeling of the soles of their feet solidly making contact with the floor. Additionally, suggest taking some slow, deep breaths along with you, followed by a slow exhale. Reinforce their sense of being grounded with a slow, short set of BLS.
- Time-orient the client by directing them to observe their hands, their rings, and the size of their shoes. Direct the client to stand and notice their height and how high they can reach. Reinforce the present-day Adult state with a slow, short set of BLS.
- Suggest the client shift their body into a tall, straight posture with shoulders down. Model the position for the client. Explain that the body position sends signals of confidence to their nervous system and deepen this state with a slow, short set of BLS.

PAUSE AND REFLECT FOR THE THERAPIST

Think of some examples of times when you have felt strongly connected to your most Competent Adult part of Self. You may have someone in your life with whom you feel connected who reflects back a positive view of yourself. Or you may have an activity in which you participate that increases your sense of confidence and competence. You may have conducted sessions as a therapist in which you felt in touch with your inner wisdom and purpose. Choose an experience and practice looking at yourself in the situation from a distance, observing your body posture, facial expression, and voice. Step into the felt sense of the experience, and do a short, slow set of butterfly taps to deepen this competent, adult state. Identify a cue word to represent this positive state and bring up the felt sense of the experience along with the cue word. Deepen with a slow, short set of BLS. Practice bringing this Competent Adult part of you, with your competent body posture and cue word, into a future situation with a client that you have found challenging in the past. Imagine how you will respond to the situation as your most Competent Adult part of Self. If you feel good about it, deepen the positive felt sense with some short, slow taps. Practice this activity frequently to build a stronger capacity to step into the Competent Adult part of you.

USEFUL TERMS AND DEFINITIONS

AFTT-A: Attachment-Focused Trauma Therapy for Adults

AIP: adaptive information processing

BLS: bilateral stimulation

EMDR: Eye Movement Desensitization and Reprocessing

RDI: Resource Development and Installation

PROTOCOL SCRIPT 8. STRENGTHENING THE COMPETENT ADULT PART OF SELF

Adapted from Korn, D., & Leeds, A. (2002). Preliminary evidence of efficacy for EMDR resource development and installation in the stabilization phase of treatment of complex posttraumatic stress disorder. *Journal of Clinical Psychology*, 58(12), 1465–1487. https://doi.org/10.1002/jclp.10099; and Popky, A. J. (2005). DeTUR, an urge reduction protocol for addictions and dysfunctional behaviors. In R. Shapiro (Ed.), *EMDR solutions: Pathways to healing* (pp. 167–188). W. W. Norton & Company.

1. Explanation. *Say...* "We all function most effectively and feel confident when we're able to access our most Competent Adult part of Self. Everything we're doing is designed to help you move in this healthy direction. Even if the Competent Adult state feels unfamiliar to you due to very active 'kid parts,' we can help you get more familiar with it by accessing and strengthening this part of you. Over time, your capacity to access and hold onto the Competent Adult state will become more natural. From this state, you'll be able to notice changes that signal activated Child/Adolescent parts—and you'll have more capacity for settling them back into their Safe Places."

2. Create a Drawing That Illustrates the Current Strength of the Competent Adult Part of Self in Relationship to Child/Adolescent Part(s) of Self. *Say...* "On this piece of paper, I'd like you to use circles of various sizes to show the current strength of your most Competent Adult part of Self in relationship to the felt strength of the Child/Adolescent parts of Self on the inside. You can also show which Child/Adolescent parts of Self are most blended with the Competent Adult part by drawing them close to or partially on top of the Adult part. Some you may feel are separate but still large on the page. Perhaps there is a strong felt sense of the Child/Adolescent parts, even though they are successfully pushed away. Or perhaps they take over and take control, pushing the Adult part away. Don't overthink this. The drawing is just to get a general idea, an estimate, through a visual picture. We can look back at this later and see what's changed."

3. Brainstorm Memories of Operating From the Competent Adult Part of Self. *Say...* "Think back to a situation, whether recent or a while ago, in which you felt you were operating from your most competent adult state. You may have one memory or more than one memory come to mind. Take your time, and then let me know what comes to you. If nothing comes to you, let me know, and I can give you some possible ideas."

If the client struggles with finding a memory, *say...* "I can give you some possible ideas. It might be getting hired for your first job, a job success, holding your child for the first time, solving a problem of some kind, overcoming a fear, building something, or fixing something. Another option is a memory of being with someone who is supportive to you, or a time when you felt included or respected by _____ (a cultural or social group to which the client belongs)."

If the client recalls multiple memories, *say...* "Which memory seems the most powerful or most positive to start with? After that, we may choose a couple more and repeat the protocol with those memories."

_____

_____

4. Note the Details. *Say...* "Tell me about the memory in detail. I'm going to take notes."

_____

_____

5. Direct the Client to Watch the Memory on a Movie Screen as You Provide Guided Imagery and Slow BLS. *Say...* "I'm going to help you bring up this memory in your mind with a little guided imagery. What I'd like you to do is picture the memory on a movie screen in your mind. You can close your eyes or leave your eyes open. Notice what all happens in the movie, who's there, and so forth. Take your time. I'll add a little slow BLS to help with deepening the experience." (*Read the details of the memory from your notes while adding a short set of slow BLS through tactile pulsars. Alternatively, show the client how to add the BLS with the butterfly tap.*) "I'd like to check in. Did this go okay?" _____ (*If there are unexpected negative associations, suggest putting parentheses around the positive part of the memory or suggest choosing an alternate memory.*)

6. Call the Client's Attention to What They Observe on the Screen Regarding Their Body Posture, Facial Expression, and Voice, and Deepen With Slow BLS. *Say...* "Now, this part is really important. I'd like you to observe anything about your body posture in the memory, notice your facial expression, and listen to your voice tone. Take your time. When you're ready, tell me what you noticed." (***Deepen positive affect with a short set of slow BLS.***)

_____

_____

Say... "Stay with that and let's add a little slow tapping to deepen that." (***Add a slow, short set of BLS.***)

7. Direct the Client to "Step Into" the Memory and Deepen Positive Affect With Slow BLS. *Say...* "I'd like you to 'step into' the memory now. Notice what you can see in this memory, what you can hear, touch, or smell. Remember your body posture, facial expression, voice tone. Notice how it feels in your body right now as you remember this moment. If it's okay, I'd like to add a slow, short set of tapping to help deepen the sense of it." (*Add a slow, short set of BLS.*)

8. Pair the Memory With a Cue Word Using Slow BLS. *Say...* "What word or phrase could represent this memory?"

"I'd like you to bring up the memory, adjust your body position, and hold in mind the cue word(s) while I add some slow bilateral stimulation to deepen the connection."

9. Help the Client Identify Their Preferred Method(s) for Accessing the Competent Adult Part of Self. *Say...* "This is the Competent Adult part of you. What do you think might be the easiest way for you to access the Competent Adult part of Self when you want to? Some people use the memory, and some people can take a short-cut by adjusting their body position or thinking of the cue word. Some people like using more than one method. Take your time to experiment and see what works best for you."

---

10. Find a Present-Day Challenging Situation. *Say...* "I'd like you to tell me about a present-day challenge that commonly presents itself. Pick something that's somewhat challenging without being overwhelming."

---

11. Invite the Client to Access the Competent Adult Part of Self. *Say...* "Use the memory, your body posture, or your cue word, in whatever combination works best, to find that Competent Adult part of you. Take your time. Let me know when you have it."

---

12. Direct the Client to View a Future Rehearsal on a Screen. *Say...* "Now picture yourself on a screen, handling this situation from the Competent Adult part of you at some point in the future. Remember that you don't actually have to change anything about what you're doing right now.

"This is just an experiment to imagine what the Competent Adult part of you *might* want to do at some point when it feels more natural. Let me know when you're finished."

13. Check in and Deepen the Experience With Slow BLS. *Say…*"How did you see yourself handling the situation from your Competent Adult part of Self at some point in the future?"

_____
_____

Say…"What do you notice about how you're feeling right now?"

_____
_____

If the response is positive, say…"Just notice that." (*Add a slow, short set of BLS.*)

14. Encourage the Client to "Step Into" the Future Rehearsal if the Client Feels Ready and Then Deepen With Slow BLS. *Say…*"Do you feel ready to step into the screen as an experiment?" _____ *If yes, say…*"Go ahead, then, and step into the screen. Imagine your future self, whenever it is that you're ready to handle this situation from your most Competent Adult state. Feel free to bring along any Resource Team member you feel will be supportive to you with this effort. Let me know when you're finished." (*Add a slow, short set of BLS.*) *Say…*"What are you noticing?" _____ (*If the response is positive, say…*"Let's deepen that a little more." (*Add another slow, short set of BLS.*)

15. Encourage the Client to Practice Accessing the Competent Adult Part of Self at Home. *Say…*"At home, I'd like you to practice bringing up the most Competent Adult part of you. A good time might be at the beginning of the day, even before you get out of bed. It would be helpful to repeat it whenever you need a boost of confidence. If you're alone, you can use the butterfly tap, just a slow, short set, to reinforce the positive state." (***Demonstrate the butterfly tap for the client by crossing your arms and tapping alternate taps on your shoulders or arms.***) "If you're at work or in public, you can always tap your feet, one and then the other, or even just tap your toes back-and-forth inside your shoes."

REFERENCES

Bandura, A. (1977). Self-efficacy: Toward a unifying theory of behavioral change. *Psychological Review*, 84(2), 191–215. https://doi.org/10.10370033-295s.34.2.191

Korn, D. L., & Leeds, A. M. (2002). Preliminary evidence of efficacy for EMDR resource development and installation in the stabilization phase of treatment of complex posttraumatic stress disorder. *Journal of Clinical Psychology*, 58(12), 1465–1487. https://doi.org/10.1002/jclp.10099

Nygaard, E., Johansen, V. A., Siqveland, J., Hussain, A., & Heir, T. (2017, June). Longitudinal relationship between self-efficacy and posttraumatic stress symptoms 8 years after a violent assault: An autoregressive cross-lagged model. *Frontiers of Psychology*, 8, 913. https://doi.org/10.3389/fpsyg.2017.00913

Popky, A. J. (2005). DeTUR, an urge reduction protocol for addictions and dysfunctional behaviors. In R. Shapiro (Ed.), *EMDR solutions: Pathways to healing* (pp. 167–188). W. W. Norton & Company.

Shapiro, F. (2018). *Eye movement desensitization and reprocessing (EMDR) therapy: Basic principles, protocols, and procedures* (3rd ed.). Guilford Press.

CHAPTER 12

Providing Corrective Attachment Experiences Between Child/Adolescent and True Parent Parts of Self in Attachment-Focused Trauma Therapy for Adults

INTRODUCTION

All children are born with an innate sense that they need love from their attachment figures to survive. The felt sense is "I will die if I don't get the love/closeness I need." The adaptive information processing (AIP) model explains that when children don't get their needs met adequately, the many distressing experiences are stored in memory networks in unprocessed form along with the associated emotions, sensations, and beliefs. The memory networks are easily triggered by relationships later in life.

The Attachment-Focused Trauma Therapy for Adults (AFTT-A) model recognizes that activated memory networks may activate a sense of Self that was present during those childhood experiences. This Child/Adolescent part of Self may carry the old wounds and defensive mechanisms that were present at the time.

If we grew up in a family that met our needs well, we may have a large store of positive attachment memories that are well integrated, and our memory networks may be a source of present-day positive expectations and secure attachment patterns for present-day relationships. Our Child/Adolescent parts of Self may be secure for the most part and function in a well-integrated way most of the time.

However, adults with a history of early attachment trauma have developed an unhealthy internal system that parallels the family system they experienced in childhood. The AFTT-A model provides protocols for restructuring the internal system as part of Eye Movement Desensitization and Reprocessing (EMDR) preparation phase work. As described in Chapters 8 through 11 of this book, the Adult part of Self is provided a Safe Place and Higher Power to access a connection to the spiritual core. Child/Adolescent parts of Self are provided a Safe Place and Higher Power/Caregiver of their own to provide internal safety and time orientation. A Resource Team enhances helpful qualities for the Adult part of Self, and the therapeutic relationship provides healthy, secure-based support. Protocol Script 9 found at the end of this chapter enhances the healthy internal system through internal corrective attachment experiences between the Child/Adolescent and True Parent parts of Self.

RATIONALE FOR CREATING CORRECTIVE ATTACHMENT EXPERIENCES BETWEEN THE CHILD/ADOLESCENT AND TRUE PARENT PARTS OF SELF

Adults who were raised with parents who had dismissive patterns and discomfort with closeness most likely learned to suppress their own feelings and needs. They may have difficulty being emotionally present with themselves and deny the vulnerable parts of themselves. Adults with a dismissive attachment pattern may have a dismissive or even derogatory stance toward the Child/Adolescent parts of Self. The Child/Adolescent parts of Self may be associated with a shut-down state and fear closeness. For adults with the dismissive attachment pattern, the creation of corrective internal attachment experiences increases self-awareness, self-compassion, and compassion for others. The emotionally corrective attachment experiences can create feelings of comfort and safety for the younger parts.

Adults with preoccupied attachment patterns may be enmeshed with younger parts of themselves, blended with the feelings and beliefs carried forward from the past, so both Adult and Child/Adolescent parts are operating in adult life at the same time. We often refer to the frequent blending of the Adult or Child parts of Self as the problem of a "Velcro Kid"—the Child/Adolescent part that seems "Velcroed" to the adult's side. Both the Adult and Child/Adolescent parts of Self may hold feelings of anxiety and unworthiness. The activated Child/Adolescent parts of Self typically attempt to get unmet childhood needs met through present-day relationships. This situation is a set up for disappointment, as the time for getting childhood needs met from others is over; adulthood relationships cannot fill the empty spot for the Child/Adolescent part of Self. Paradoxically, adulthood relationships become taxed, which further entrenches negative beliefs about Self as unlovable and unworthy.

For adults with preoccupied tendencies, the creation of corrective internal attachment experiences can further differentiate and strengthen the Adult part, strengthen healthy self-compassion, and allow the Child/Adolescent part of Self to settle. For both dismissive and preoccupied adults, working with the "Kid Brain" through the "Adult Brain" is integrative, as the child perspective is viewed through adult eyes.

Historically, therapists have utilized guided imagery or hypnotherapy methods for working with ego states and addressing the needs of younger ego states, including Bradshaw (1990), Fisher (2017), Fraser (2003), Potter (1994), Schwartz (1995), and Watkins and Watkins (1997). Many EMDR therapists have developed various methods for implementing bilateral stimulation (BLS) to enhance ego state work and address the needs of younger child states as part of EMDR preparation phase work, including Forgash (2008), Gonzales and Mosquera (2012), Knipe (2015), Paulsen (2009), Parnell (1999), Phillips (2008), Schmidt (2020), and Twombly and Schwartz (2008).

OVERVIEW OF STEPS FOR CORRECTIVE ATTACHMENT EXPERIENCES BETWEEN THE CHILD AND TRUE PARENT PARTS OF SELF

If Protocol Script 9 for *Corrective Attachment Experiences Between the Child/Adolescent and True Parent Parts of Self* is attempted when the client is operating from a Child/Adolescent part of Self or blended Child and Adult parts, the activity will be met with resistance and roadblocks. Only a differentiated Adult part of Self, resourced and grounded, can view a Child/Adolescent part with adult, present-day insight and compassion to meet their unmet needs. Thus, the protocol begins by ensuring that the client is operating from a grounded, present-oriented adult state.

The next steps of the protocol assist the differentiated Adult part with viewing the Safe Place and the Child/Adolescent part of Self from the adult perspective. From the vantage point of an adult looking in on a vulnerable child, the innocence of the younger part of Self becomes clear to the Adult part. Over time, the nurturing qualities we refer to as the True Parent part of Self become stronger, while the younger part of Self grows more content.

It's important to establish with clients a clear understanding that work with the Child/Adolescent part of Self is taking place in present day. The younger part of Self does not reside in the past; the past is over. The Adult part of Self is not time-traveling. Within the protocol, the therapist explains, "I'm going to guide you in some nurturing work with the Child/Adolescent part of Self who is a part of you now, in present-day time." If this is not made clear to the client, the Adult part may view the Child/Adolescent part of Self as still unsafe, frozen in time, waiting for bad things to happen (Martin, 2018). This confusion regarding time creates a roadblock to completion of the protocol.

The protocol includes creation of an emotional experience of connection between the True Parent part of Self and the Child/Adolescent part of Self through imaginal touch or through looking into the eyes, through words of affirmation and reassurance, and through a cord of love or light that runs heart-to-heart between Adult and Child parts and never ends. The client is encouraged to repeat small pieces of the work at home, through a small bit of imagery and internal dialogue, reinforcing positive feelings with a very short, slow "butterfly hug" (i.e., alternating self-taps by crossing the arms and tapping on the shoulders or upper arms). The therapist should not consider the internal attachment work complete after one session. If the protocol is repeated and practiced over time, the positive effects of the nurturing work are deepened.

It is contraindicated for the therapist to provide nurturing words directly to the Child/Adolescent part of Self. Although this action would likely be followed by an immediate positive response from the younger part, it would lead to a need for reassurance that the therapist will never leave and would result in increased anxiety regarding abandonment and an unhealthy dependency upon the therapist.

As you read the overview of the steps for the *Corrective Attachment Experiences Between the Child/Adolescent and True Parent Parts of Self* protocol, you may wish to refer to Protocol Script 9 at the end of this chapter.

STEPS FOR CORRECTIVE ATTACHMENT EXPERIENCES BETWEEN THE CHILD/ADOLESCENT AND TRUE PARENT PARTS OF SELF PROTOCOL

1. Introduce the Activity
The therapist explains that strong feelings stored in the "Kid Part" of the brain are easily triggered in adult life, often by adulthood relationships. The therapist goes on to explain that the client has everything they need on the inside to heal through new, corrective attachment experiences between the Adult and the Child/Adolescent parts

of Self. The work will provide feelings of contentment and worthiness to the younger parts and will also develop and strengthen the True Parent aspects of Self for self-nurturing and self-protection. Ask the client for permission to conduct guided imagery for corrective attachment experiences between the Child/Adolescent and the Adult parts and only proceed if the client is willing.

2. Time-Orient by Grounding the Client in the Present-Day Adult Part of Self
Bring the client's awareness to their feet on the floor and the appearance of their adult hands. Bring up their most Competent Adult part of Self by suggesting the client shift into the body posture associated with feelings of competence (see Protocol Script 8). Emphasize that you will not be going back in time or bringing up past memories. Reassure the client that you will be working with the Child/Adolescent parts of Self that in the here-and-now, in present time.

3. Identify the Child/Adolescent Part of Self With Which to Begin the Activity
Ask the client to identify which Child/Adolescent part/age needs the most reassurance and connection. This gives you a place to begin. Remind the client that they can tell you or signal you to stop at any point during the imagery.

4. Initiate the Guided Imagery and Dialogue
Suggest the client place a hand over their heart and think about the nurturing and protective aspects of themselves they want to bring to the internal work. Suggest the client picture the Child/Adolescent part of themselves in the Safe Place with the Higher Power/Caregiver. Invite the client to step into the Safe Place or "peek in" if they prefer. Suggest the client ask the younger part if it's okay for them to stay for a bit.

5. Encourage the Adult Part of Self to Reach Out in Some Way
Suggest the client reach out in some way that feels comfortable, perhaps by touching the younger part's hand, giving a hug, or by looking into the eyes of the younger part, if it feels okay to do so. Check in with the client. If the response is positive, strengthen the positive affect with a short set of slow BLS.

6. Get Assistance If Needed
If the Adult needs assistance with accessing the nurturing, parenting qualities of themselves, encourage the Adult part to ask for assistance from a Resource Team member (see Protocol Scripts 6 and 7) or from the Child's Higher Power/Caregiver figure (see Protocol Script 5). Following is an example of inviting the Higher Power/Caregiver figure to help a client who becomes stuck during the visualization.

> **BOX 12.1 CLIENT EXAMPLE: INVITING THE HIGHER POWER/CAREGIVER TO HELP**
>
> The client becomes stuck in the middle of the imagery work and the Higher Power/Caregiver figure is invited to help.
>
> **Therapist:** If you can, you might reach out and connect physically, perhaps with a light touch on the toddler's hand or by looking into the toddler's eyes, or with a hug if it seems okay. (*Pause*). What are you noticing?

(continued)

> **BOX 12.1 CLIENT EXAMPLE: INVITING THE HIGHER POWER/CAREGIVER TO HELP** (*continued*)
>
> **Client:** I feel frozen. I want to want to do this, but I feel like I can't.
>
> **Therapist:** You said that you can see the toddler part of you sitting on the floor with your Higher Power figure, Gandhi.
>
> **Client:** Yes, they both looked up at me and smiled when I walked in. They're playing with blocks.
>
> **Therapist:** Perhaps you could ask Gandhi for help in reaching out to the toddler part of you. Or you may wish to bring in a Resource Team member to help. Whatever you think is best. Take your time and let me know how it goes when you're ready.
>
> **Client:** (*Long pause, eyes closed. Then opens their eyes.*) That was really moving. Gandhi stood and came to me. He wrapped me in his shawl and held onto me as I picked up the toddler and held her. I don't think I could have done that without his help.
>
> **Therapist:** (*Nodding and starting the tappers at a slow speed.*) Take a moment to just notice the positive emotions and sensations you're experiencing right now.

7. Begin Providing the Nurturing Messages (With Continuous Slow BLS Throughout)
Give the client permission to change or add to anything you suggest and to dialogue aloud or silently, whichever they prefer. Remind the client to let you know or signal if they wish to check in or pause at any point during the dialogue. Begin slow BLS and continue throughout the dialogue. Suggest the Adult part reassure the Child/Adolescent part of themselves that they can stay in the Safe Place with the Higher Power/Caregiver and just be a kid without any worries or responsibilities. Suggest the Adult part reassure the younger part that they are protected and safe there and that they are part of the adult body in present day, and therefore childhood problems are in the past. Suggest they reassure the Child/Adolescent part that they are lovable and valuable just as they are and that they don't have to be perfect or do anything different to be worthy. Suggest they reassure the younger part of themselves that they belong and they are part of the Adult. Encourage the client to add anything else that comes to mind.

8. Check in Regarding the Feelings of the True Parent and Child/Adolescent Part and Reinforce a Positive Shift With Slow BLS
Ask the client how it feels to be the True Parent for the Child/Adolescent part of themselves. Ask them what they are sensing regarding the feelings of the Child/Adolescent part. If the response is positive, reinforce the positive state with a slow, short set of BLS.

9. Create the Magical Cord of Love/Light of Love (Apply Slow BLS Throughout the Dialogue)
Suggest visualizing a "beautiful light of love" or a "magical cord of love" (using the term that most resonates for the client) that runs from the heart of the True Parent part of Self to the heart of the Child/Adolescent part (Wesselmann et al., 2014).

Suggest the client reminds the Child/Adolescent part that the love is continuous and unconditional, and that as the adult participates in adult life, the loving connection remains. You may also guide the client in visualizing a magical cord of love between the Child/Adolescent part and the Higher Power/Caregiver figure as well. Deepen the sense of connection with a slow, short set of BLS.

10. Closure
Suggest the client enfold the Child/Adolescent part along with the Higher Power/Caregiver in the Safe Place inside their heart and remember the loving connection between the younger part and the True Parent aspect of themselves, even while the client is managing adult life.

11. Home Practice
Suggest the client repeat the activity, even if only briefly, providing some reassuring and loving dialogue for the Child/Adolescent parts of Self at night before falling asleep or when waking in the morning. Suggest the client add a short set of butterfly taps, just 4 or 5 times slowly back and forth, crossing their arms like a hug.

POINTS TO REMEMBER

- Adults with poor quality attachments as children frequently have Child/Adolescent parts of Self that attempt to get earlier needs for love and protection met through present-day adult relationships with partners, children, or friends, which leads to problems in those relationships.
- Adults with poor quality attachments as children frequently experience feelings of unworthiness rooted in younger parts of Self and/or feelings of disdain from the Adult part toward younger parts.
- The Corrective Attachment Experiences protocol helps create a corrective attachment relationship between the Adult part of Self and the Child/Adolescent parts of Self, developing and strengthening the nurturing and protective aspects of the Adult (the True Parent part of Self), and a healing experience of connection for the younger parts of Self.
- The client may object to the activity, insisting that the nurturing come directly from the therapist to the Child/Adolescent parts of Self. The therapist should maintain the stance that the time is past for the younger parts of Self to get needs met from outside adults. The therapist can explain that the client has everything they need inside of themselves to heal the Child/Adolescent parts of Self and give them what they need.
- Begin the activity by making sure the client is operating from their most differentiated Competent Adult part of Self, using the Competent Adult memory, body posture, or cue word established during the *Strengthening the Competent Adult Part of Self* protocol (see Protocol Script 8)
- Explain that you will not be going to the past; you'll be working with a Child/Adolescent part of Self activated in present day.

- The activity can be implemented for various ages as needed. Ask, "How old do you feel when you feel vulnerable or defensive? What age or ages on the inside were most hurt or have the most unmet needs?"
- "Enfold" or "tuck in" the child part of Self within the Safe Place with the Higher Power figure prior to ending the guided imagery.
- Encourage the client to repeat small pieces of the nurturing dialogue with the Child part of Self from home. Remind the client to use an adult competency memory, posture, or cue word. Suggest adding a short set of slow butterfly taps at home to deepen the positive affect.
- The strengthened True Parent and the Competent Adult aspects of the Adult Self over time evolve into the healthiest version of the adult, the Authentic Self.

TROUBLESHOOTING

- **If the client reports they are stuck in negative feelings toward the Child part of Self...**
  The clinician should remain supportive and avoid conveying a sense of urgency or judgment. Normalize the client's response. Suggest the client place a hand over their heart and visualize a time they felt compassion toward another child to access the nurturing aspect of themselves. Additionally, suggest the Adult part of Self ask a Resource Team member or the child's Higher Power/Caregiver figure for assistance in accessing compassion for their Child part of Self (see Protocol Scripts 5, 6, and 7).
  If the response remains negative, pause the activity and check whether the client is operating from a time-oriented Competent Adult state. *Say...* "And how old do you feel inside right now?" If a "Velcro Kid" of any age is activated, repeat the grounding and time orientation exercises.
  If the client still reports negative feelings toward the Child/Adolescent part of Self, *say...* "Sometimes it's easier for individuals to begin developing a nurturing relationship with the Newborn part of Self. All infants are born innocent and new. They've just crossed over from a higher plane of existence, with nothing but a natural desire to give and receive love." If the Newborn part of Self does not have a Safe Place with a Higher Power/Caregiver, create a Newborn Safe Place (see Protocol Script 5). Then return to the *Corrective Attachment Experiences Between the Child/Adolescent and True Parent Parts of Self* protocol for the Newborn part of Self.
  Alternatively, give the client permission to pause the work for today. *Say...* "If you'd rather, you can just observe the Higher Power providing the nurturing care for today."
- **If the client reports that the Child/Adolescent part of Self is distancing due to lack of trust in the Adult part of Self...**
  Encourage the Adult part of the client to honor the feelings of the Child/Adolescent part of Self. Guide the client in stepping back from the younger part, validating the feelings, and taking a pause in the work or continuing slowly.

Remind them that by doing so, they are providing reassurance, comfort, and care. Role model an accepting attitude without urgency for change.

- **If the client reports that the Child/Adolescent part of Self is resistant due to the part's low self-worth or lack of experience receiving affection or care...**
  Encourage the Adult part of Self to invite the Child part's Higher Power or another resource figure to support and encourage the Child part of Self in allowing the Adult part to provide affection.

- **If the Adult part of Self has difficulty holding onto differentiation from the Child part during the activity...**
  When there is a high level of enmeshment between the Adult part of Self and the Child part of Self or the client is on the higher end of the spectrum of dissociation, it may be difficult for the Adult part of Self to maintain differentiation. For example, one client reported that she sensed a shift to the perspective of the Child part of Self as soon as she stepped into the Safe Place house. After re-accessing her most Adult part of Self, we made a plan. Instead of stepping into the house, she gave the Child part of Self nurturing and reassuring messages through the open window of the house. This physical boundary allowed her to maintain differentiation so she could provide the Child part with nurturing experiences from her Adult part.

- **If the client insists that the therapist speak directly to the Child part of Self...**
  In this situation, *say...* "You and I have a trusting adult-to-adult relationship, and I value that. I know, however, that it is not effective for me to have a direct relationship with that Child/Adolescent part(s) of you. The time for getting needs met from outside adults was in childhood. I don't have the power to fix what happened in the past, and anything I would do or say directly would ultimately lead to disappointment and even stronger seeking of needs by younger parts of you. Only through working with your internal system will we be able to assist the younger parts of you with feeling genuinely worthy and safe. But remember, I am here to help the Adult part of you with meeting the needs of the younger parts of you. I have an unshakable belief that you do have what you need inside of you to provide healing on the inside, with just a little assistance from me."

PAUSE AND REFLECT FOR THE THERAPIST

Have paper and pen ready for making notes as you read this *Pause and Reflect* activity. Think about your work and a client relationship that has left you unsettled. What are the emotions? Anxiety? Fear? Resentment? Irritation? Frustration? Powerlessness? How old do you feel when you are experiencing the emotions? Is there something in the relationship with your client that reminds you of a childhood relationship? Is it activating stored emotions, perceptions, or sensations related to a Child/Adolescent part of Self?

Access the True Parent part of you to give reassurance to the Child/Adolescent part(s) of you. Use the adult body posture, memory, or cue word to access your most Competent Adult part of Self to begin. Place a hand over your heart and think of your most nurturing and protective aspects. Visualize peeking into or stepping into the Safe Place of the younger part of you. Reach out in a loving way toward the Child/Adolescent part through touch or by looking into the eyes of the younger part. Invite a Higher Power or Resource Team member for assistance as needed. Reassure the younger part that they don't have to worry about adult work or adult relationships. Reassure the younger part of you that the Adult part of you will find adult supports, that the younger part deserves to relax and let go of Adult life. Reassure the younger part of you that they are good and lovable just as they are, and that they don't have to change a thing. Pay attention to your body. Is there a positive shift? Apply 4 or 5 repetitions of slow BLS through alternating taps to deepen the shift.

USEFUL TERMS AND DEFINITIONS

AFTT-A: Attachment-Focused Trauma Therapy for Adults

AIP: adaptive information processing

BLS: bilateral stimulation

EMDR: Eye Movement Desensitization and Reprocessing

PROTOCOL SCRIPT 9. CORRECTIVE ATTACHMENT EXPERIENCES BETWEEN THE CHILD/ADOLESCENT AND TRUE PARENT PARTS OF SELF

Adapted from Bradshaw, J. (1990). *Homecoming: Reclaiming and healing your inner child*. Bantam Publishing; and Potter, A. E. (1994). *Inside out: Rebuilding self and personality through inner child therapy* (therapist manual and client workbook). Accelerated Development, Inc.

1. Introduce the Activity. *Say...* "Strong feelings stored in the 'Kid Part' of the brain are easily triggered in adult life, often by adulthood relationships. It's very common for the activated Child/Adolescent part(s) of Self to carry feelings of anxiety, vulnerability, rejection, anger, hurt, or abandonment from the past into present-day relationships. It's also not unusual for the Child/Adolescent part(s) to try to get old unmet needs met through adulthood relationships, which creates problems due to the activated 'Kid Brain.' However, you have everything you need inside of you to bring healing to the Child/Adolescent part(s) of you. You can create corrective attachment experiences between the more nurturing, True Parent part of you and the Child/Adolescent part(s) of you. You'll be providing feelings of contentment and worthiness to the Child/Adolescent part(s) of you, and you'll be strengthening the True Parent part of you for healing the Child/Adolescent part(s) through this protocol. Would you be willing to do some guided imagery with me and see how it goes?" _____ *(If the client is not ready, accept where the client is at and don't proceed with the activity at this time.)*

2. Time-Orient by Grounding the Client in the Present-Day Adult Part of Self. *Say...* "To begin, let's make sure you're grounded in present time. Just notice the feeling of your feet on the floor and notice colors and objects in the office here. Notice the age of your hands and your grown-up size. Do you feel oriented to present time right now?" (*If the answer is no, continue with grounding and time orientation.*) _____ "Okay, great. Let's access your Competent Adult memory now. Can you think of it now?" _____ "See if you can shift your body posture to help you step into the Competent Adult part of you. How does that feel to you?" _____ "Now, it's very important for you to know that we're not going back in time or even thinking about past memories. We'll work through memories later on in therapy. Right now, we're going to work with the Child/Adolescent part(s) of Self you carry within you now, in *present-day time*. The Child/Adolescent part(s) within you reside in the here-and-now just as you do."

3. Identify the Child/Adolescent Part(s) of Self With Which to Begin The Activity. *Say...* "We've developed a Safe Place and Higher Power/Caregiver figure for your Child/Adolescent part(s) of Self, age _____." (**See Protocol Script 5.**) "What age is the Child/Adolescent part of Self who most needs reassurance and connection?" _____ "Okay, this gives us a good place to start. Remember that we can stop at any point during the imagery. You can just hold up your hand as a stop signal."

4. Initiate the Guided Imagery and Dialogue. *Say...* "If it's okay with you, place a hand over your heart and just think about the nurturing and protective aspects of yourself you would like to bring to this work today. I'll give you a minute, and just tell me when you're ready to continue." (*Pause.*) "Okay, great. Picture, if you can today, the Child/Adolescent part of you in their Safe Place with the Higher Power/Caregiver." (***Either Higher Power or Caregiver term can be used. Vivify the imagery for the client with details that you know.***) "Tell me what else you see or hear there, today."

_____

_____

"As your grounded, competent, present-day self, take just a step into the Safe Place with the Child/Adolescent part. Ask the Child/Adolescent part of you if it's okay for you to stay for a bit." (*Pause.*) "How is the Child/Adolescent part of you responding?"

_____

_____

5. Encourage the Adult Part of Self to Reach Out in Some Way. *Say...* "If you can, you might reach out and connect physically, perhaps with a light touch on the Child/Adolescent's hand or by looking into the Child/Adolescent's eyes, or with a hug if it seems okay. (*Pause.*) What are you noticing?" _____ (*If the response is positive, strengthen the positive affect with a short set of slow BLS.*)

6. Get Assistance If Needed. *If the client reports feeling uncomfortable or negative towards the Child/Adolescent part, say...* "See if you can ask the Child/Adolescent part's Higher Power/Caregiver for help with reaching out to the Child/Adolescent part. Or you may bring in a Resource Team member to help you. Whatever you think might work. Take your time and let me know how it goes when you're ready."

_____ (*If the response is positive, strengthen the positive affect with a short set of slow BLS.*)

7. Begin Providing the Nurturing Messages (With Continuous Slow BLS Throughout). *Say…* "I'll guide you with nurturing and reassuring messages for the Child/Adolescent part of you; however, feel free to change or add anything *you* want to say. Feel free to dialogue silently and internally, or to speak aloud; either way is fine. I'm only making suggestions; feel free to change or add to anything I suggest. Remember to let me know or signal me any time you want to pause to check in with me or if you want to stop for now. I'll be adding slow BLS throughout the dialogue." (***Check in with the client if you have any concerns during the dialogue activity.***)

Begin slow BLS and say…

"To begin the dialogue, let the Child/Adolescent part of you know that it's okay to stay in the Safe Place with the protective and nurturing figure and just be a kid. There's nothing they have to do now and nowhere they have to go. Let the Child/Adolescent part know they don't have to worry about a thing in the Safe Place. There's no need to be watchful or vigilant. Remind the Child/Adolescent that the Adult you is managing adult life. The Child/Adolescent part of you is not responsible for anyone or anything in your adult life today, or any day.

"Let the Child/Adolescent part of you know they are protected and safe; they are part of your body and you are an adult now. The events of Childhood/Adolescence are over. Those difficulties are in the past. Anything that happens in your adult life will be handled by the Adult part of you and nothing in adulthood will have any consequence to them. This is their time to relax.

"Let the Child/Adolescent part of you know that they are lovable and valuable, just as they are. They are exactly who they are supposed to be. They were born with a Spiritual Essence at the core that is perfect and unchangeable. No one can be perfect, and they don't have to be perfect to be valuable and worthy. They are worthy just as they are. They don't have to do anything different or be any different.

"Let the Child/Adolescent part of you know that they belong. They are a part of you. You and the Child/Adolescent part of Self are connected.

"Add anything else that comes to you that you might want to say to the Child/Adolescent part of you."

8. Check in Regarding the Feelings of the True Parent and Child/Adolescent Part and Reinforce a Positive Shift With Slow BLS. *Say…* "How does it feel to be that True Parent for the Child/Adolescent part of you today?" _____
"What is your sense regarding the feelings of the Child/Adolescent part of you right now?" _____ (*If the response is positive, reinforce with a short slow set of BLS.*)

9. Create the Magical Cord of Love/Light of Love (Apply Slow BLS Throughout the Dialogue). *Say…* "If it feels okay to do so, I would like to create some imagery to increase the internal sense of secure, healthy connection between the Child/Adolescent part and that True Parent aspect of you. I'm going to add the BLS throughout this guided imagery." (***Start slow BLS.***) "Let the Child/Adolescent part of you know that you and the Child/Adolescent are eternally connected through a beautiful, magical cord of love, made of a glittery, shimmery light, that runs heart-to-heart, from your heart (the heart of the Adult part of you), to the heart of the Child/Adolescent part of you. Take a moment to picture this beautiful light of love. Remind the Child/Adolescent part that the light and the love are continuous and unconditional and that even when the Adult part of you engages in present-day adult life, the loving connection between the True Parent and Child/Adolescent parts of you will remain. Take a moment, now, to picture another beautiful, magical cord of love between the Child/Adolescent part of Self and the Higher Power/Caregiver figure (or any additional figures that have been placed within the Child/Adolescent part's Safe Place). The loving connection with the Higher Power is also unconditional, and it is eternal." *Stop BLS and say...* "How did that go?"_____ "What are you noticing in your body?" _____ (*Strengthen positive sensations with a short set of slow BLS.*)

10. Closure. *Say...* "Enfold the Child/Adolescent part of you along with the Higher Power/Caregiver safe and sound in the Safe Place inside your heart. Remember that the cord of love will allow the Child/Adolescent part of you to feel the loving connection with this True Parent aspect of you, even while you return to managing your adult life. What are you noticing as you return to this room right now?" _____
(*Strengthen positive sensations with a short set of slow BLS.*)

11. Home Practice. *Say...* "To further deepen the positive messages for the Child/Adolescent part of Self, you can continue to repeat small pieces of this activity, even if only briefly. For example, when you wake up in the morning or when you're falling asleep, you might dialogue internally and remind the Child/Adolescent part of you that they're worthy, and that they're safe and sound in the Safe Place and that there's no need to be concerned with your grown-up life. You can even add a little bilateral stimulation with what is called the 'butterfly hug' by crossing your arms like a hug across your chest and slowly, gently tapping just 3 or 4 times slowly, back-and-forth."

REFERENCES

Bradshaw, J. (1990). *Homecoming: Reclaiming and healing your inner child*. Bantam Publishing.

Fisher, J. (2017). *Healing the fragmented selves of trauma survivors: Overcoming internal self alienation*. Routledge.

Forgash, C. (2008). Integrating EMDR and ego state treatment for clients with trauma disorders. In C. Forgash & M. Copeley (Eds.), *Healing the heart of trauma and dissociation with EMDR and ego state therapy* (pp. 1–55). Springer Publishing Company.

Fraser, G. A. (2003). Fraser's "Dissociative Table Technique" revisited, revised: A strategy for working with ego states in dissociative disorders and ego-state therapy. *Journal of Trauma and Dissociation*, 4(4), 5–28. https://doi.org/10.1300/J229v04n04_02

Gonzales, A., & Mosquera, D. (2012). *EMDR and dissociation: A progressive approach* (1st ed., revised). Self-Published.

Knipe, J. (2015). *EMDR toolbox: Theory and treatment of complex PTSD and dissociation*. Springer Publishing Company.

Martin, K. (2018, April). *Mastering the treatment of complex trauma: Transforming theory into practice*. Presentation, Omaha, Nebraska.

Parnell, L. (1999). *EMDR in the treatment of adults abused as children*. W. W. Norton & Company.

Paulsen, S. (2009). *Looking through the eyes of trauma and dissociation*. The Bainbridge Institute for Integrative Psychology.

Phillips, M. (2008). Combining hypnosis with EMDR and ego state therapy for ego strengthening. In C. Forgash & M. Copeley (Eds.), *Healing the heart of trauma and dissociation with EMDR and ego state therapy* (pp. 91–116). Springer Publishing Company.

Potter, A. E. (1994). *Inside out: Rebuilding self and personality through inner child therapy* (therapist manual). Accelerated Development, Inc.

Schmidt, S. J. (2020). *Ego state therapy interventions to prepare attachment-wounded adults for EMDR*. DNMS Institute LLC.

Schwartz, R. C. (1995). *Internal family systems therapy*. Guilford Press.

Twombly, J. H., & Schwartz, R. C. (2008). The integration of the internal family systems model and EMDR. In C. Forgash & M. Copeley (Eds.), *Healing the heart of trauma and dissociation with EMDR and ego state therapy* (pp. 295–310). Springer Publishing Company.

Watkins, J. G., & Watkins, H. H. (1997). *Ego states: Theory and therapy*. W. W. Norton & Company.

Wesselmann, D., Schweitzer, C., & Armstrong, S. (2014). *Integrative team treatment for attachment trauma in children: Family therapy and EMDR*. W. W. Norton & Company.

CHAPTER 13

Parts' Work: Negotiating New Roles for Parent and Adult Parts of Self in Attachment-Focused Trauma Therapy for Adults

INTRODUCTION

Imagine a client's personality as a family-owned corporation, OA, Inc. (Optimal Attachments, Inc., ha!). The company's values and culture are drawn from the family's deep belief in people's goodness and worth and in their responsibility to care and stand up for themselves and each other. The corporation is structured so that work is divided among departments, employing people who have the skills and abilities to perform the tasks necessary for the company to accomplish its goals. Departments coordinate and cooperate with each other. The corporation and each department have leaders. Leaders are accountable to the family owners and their employees. Employees work in teams and their input and participation are regarded as essential to the company's good reputation. The corporation works hard at fostering and maintaining strong relationships both within the company and with other companies.

Next, imagine a different client's personality as a family-owned corporation, NOA, Inc. (Nonoptimal Attachments, Inc.). The corporation was founded on the family's belief that people are bad, cannot be trusted, and should only look out for themselves. Work is divided into departments, but the employees are expected to do their job without the necessary skills or training. Departments work in isolation and are competitive with each other for the leaders' attention and approval. If something goes wrong in one department, another department is blamed for the problem. The family owners and corporation leaders are either distant and uninterested (as long as the job gets done) or micro-manage employees with belittling and demeaning reactions. Employees are discouraged to give input into how the corporation is managed or suggest changes that could improve how the company runs.

Now, imagine that corporation OA is going to buy out and take over company NOA. Decisions need to be made about whether employees of the old corporation will have jobs in the new company. The OA family pledges to include as many employees from the old company as possible even if they don't have exactly the right skills or training. Their priority is finding employees who are committed to joining the OA team and willing to abide by the rules based on the company's values. They use a hiring committee to interview employees from the old company and evaluate their commitment to becoming a part of the OA corporation. NOA employees are thanked for their years of service to the old company. They are given the choice to become a part of the new company. The hiring committee tells them that their job descriptions in the new company will be a little different or there may be different expectations about how the employees do their jobs in the new company and asks for a commitment to make the changes to be a part of this new corporation—to be willing to consider the possibility of changing. They aren't automatically let go. They aren't expected to already know how to do their new job. They are just asked for a commitment to change.

Like employees of the NOA company, clients who were raised in nonoptimal or invalidating environments got messages about being bad, defective, or not good enough and that what they felt or thought wasn't important. Expectations of them were either unrealistically high or low. They were not taught or modeled the skills they needed to navigate adult life and relationships. As a result, the inner personality system development was stunted and ended up with under- and overdeveloped parts, weak or rigid boundaries among parts, parts with negative self-beliefs and affect, a lack of strong and fair leadership by the Competent Adult part of Self, and insufficient teamwork among parts.

The Attachment-Focused Trauma Therapy for Adults (AFTT-A) model details clients' internal organization through the Parent-Adult-Child (P-A-C) diagrams (see Figures 7.2 and 7.3). Specifically, attachment trauma leaves Child/Adolescent parts vulnerable and distorts the Parent and the Adult parts of Self. The Parent part intended to offer clients self-nurturing and inner protection develops into the Critical Parent part that relies on disapproval and blame to control clients' emotions, thoughts, and behaviors. The Adult part of Self aimed at providing leadership to the internal personality system and managing clients' present-day lives morphs into either the Emotion Controller-Regulator (emotion overcontrol) or a little "a" part (emotion under-control).

Up to this point, AFTT-A therapists aided clients to reconstruct the internal personality system in a step-wise approach by:

- explaining how the development of inner personality systems is impacted by either validating or invalidating childhood environments (see Protocol Scripts 1, 2, and 3);
- accessing and reinforcing the clients' belief in the positive cognition, "I'm okay no matter what," by installing a Safe Place and Higher Power (see Protocol Script 4);
- differentiating, protecting, and nurturing Child/Adolescent parts by giving them Safe Places and Higher Powers (see Protocol Script 5);
- connecting clients to an Inner Resource Team which supports self-beliefs of "I have everything I need" and "I am not alone anymore" (see Protocol Scripts 6 and 7);
- tapping into and fortifying the fledgling Competent Adult part's abilities and confidence through the *Strengthening the Competent Adult Part of Self* protocol (see Protocol Script 8); and
- activating the inherent nurturing and protective qualities in the True Parent part in the *Corrective Attachment Experiences Between the Child/Adolescent and True Parent Parts of Self* protocol (see Protocol Script 9).

13. PARTS' WORK: NEGOTIATING NEW ROLES FOR PARENT AND ADULT PARTS OF SELF

In the next protocol, *Negotiating New Roles for Parent and Adult Parts of Self*, therapists use the elements of reconnection and integration to continue the transformation of the Critical Parent into the True Parent part and the Emotion Controller-Regulator/little "a" into the Competent Adult part of Self. The newer versions of clients' parts of Self provide clients with essential qualities and skills so they are equipped to become members of their Resource Teams.

Typically, clients come to therapy with Critical Parent and Emotion Controller-Regulator/little "a" parts of Self that are not oriented to time and still operate under the assumption that clients' younger parts are in the same kind and level of danger they experienced during childhood. The parts believe that their past ways of protecting clients are still crucial for clients' survival. *Negotiating New Roles for Parent and Adult Parts of Self* protocol corrects misinformation the Critical Parent and the Emotion Controller-Regulator/little "a" parts were taught by attachment figures in childhood. The protocol reframes the reality that the parts themselves aren't bad but the information and rules they were taught by real-life attachment figures in childhood were faulty and the protective measures they subsequently developed helped clients survive but are not helpful or useful in present-day life.

STEPS

Prior to beginning the protocols steps, review with clients the Critical Parent and Emotion Controller-Regulator/little "a" parts of P-A-C diagrams. In Protocol Script 10, *Negotiating New Roles for Parent and Adult Parts of Self*, provided at the end of the chapter, therapists use Figure 7.2 *P-A-C Diagrams: Validating Childhood Environment* and Figure 7.3 *P-A-C Diagrams: Invalidating Childhood Environment* to refresh clients' memories about development of the internal personality system within both the context of validating and invalidating childhood environments. They emphasize the impact of attachment trauma on maturing personality parts. The *Negotiating New Roles for Parent and Adult Parts of Self* protocol focuses on negotiating changes with Critical Parent and Emotion Controller-Regulator/little "a" parts of Self.

Critical Parent and True Parent Parts of Self

The AFTT-A model reminds clients that, as children, they absorbed and internalized messages from real-life attachment figures and, as a result, the nurturing part of their Parent part of Self underdeveloped and whose messages were often unsupportive or had conditions or obligations. The protective quality of the Parent part whose messages were intended to keep clients safe from harm overdeveloped or morphed into a distorted version called the Critical Parent whose derogatory and disapproving messages became clients' negative cognitions or core beliefs.

AFTT-A therapists believe that the Critical Parent part did not intend to hurt clients, had clients' best interests at heart, and did the best it could with what it was given from real-life adults. The inner Parent's job was to take in and internalize messages from attachment figures, which they did. So, the problem wasn't inherent to the Parent part of Self but rather with the negative messages received from real-life attachment figures and the impact on the part's development. The negative external messages sabotaged the Parent part's ability to internalize a sense of caring and safety in healthy and helpful ways.

Clients are also reminded that the AFTT-A process assists them in transforming from the Parent part's past version (Critical Parent) to the new version (True Parent) so, as adults, they can tap into messages of self-caring and security whenever needed. They reflect on the sense of their developing True Parent part from the *Corrective Attachment Experiences Between the Child/Adolescent and True Parent Parts of Self* protocol.

Emotion Controller-Regulator/Little "a" and Competent Adult Parts of Self

The AFTT-A model explains to clients how their "Adult Brain" or "Thinking Brain" develops as they move into adolescence and adulthood. Clients raised in an invalidating environment didn't get the encouragement and the age-appropriate learning experiences needed to learn the cognitive skills to reason; consider alternatives; set goals; make and follow through with plans; solve problems; and understand and regulate emotions, thoughts, and behaviors. As a result, clients' brains either overdeveloped into the Emotion Controller-Regulator, remained in an immature state called little "a," or bounced back and forth between over- and under-control.

The Emotion Controller-Regulator aspect of the "Adult Brain" is basically stuck in one function; to avoid and control emotions. This overcontrolled version of the Adult part of Self was formed because clients had to figure out on their own during childhood how to cope with intense emotions, chaotic situations, and unfathomable harm. Their nervous systems were forced to cycle between being hypervigilant and braced for danger in the sympathetic part of the autonomic nervous system (ANS) or overwhelmed, frozen, and numb in the dorsal vagal channel of the parasympathetic ANS. As a result, the Emotion Controller-Regulator became overprotective and defensive by shutting down feelings that made clients feel vulnerable or by pushing people away.

Little "a" is the underdeveloped version of the Adult part of Self and appears when clients' brains remain in an immature state that defaults to allowing Child/Adolescent parts to "run the show" in clients' adult lives. Clients who function from little 'a' have intense emotions and often have addictions, chaos in relationships and jobs, and even legal problems.

Again, AFTT-A therapists teach clients that the old versions of the Adult part of Self had their best interests at heart but were thwarted in doing their intended jobs of mediating and balancing internal parts as well as responding in competent and authentic ways to situations and relationships in adult life. Unfortunately, the Emotion Controller-Regulator part often leads clients to be distant and aloof in attachment relationships and have difficulty experiencing and expressing emotions as well as asking for help from their therapist as they work through adverse memories. The little "a" part may be overly dependent on their therapist.

Clients are also reminded that the AFTT-A process assists them in transforming the Adult part of Self from the past versions (Emotion Controller-Regulator and little "a") to the new version (Competent Adult) so, as adults, they handle present-day challenges with confidence and competence. They reinforce the positive qualities and affect from the experience of the emerging Competent Adult part in the *Strengthening the Competent Adult Part of Self* protocol (see Chapter 11).

1. Discuss Goals for Resource Team Meeting.
The ultimate goal for clients, their newly formed Resource Team, and the older and newer versions of their Parent and Adult parts of Self is for the Critical Parent and the Emotion Controller-Regulator/little "a" parts to work with the newer versions of their parts and for those parts to become members of clients' Resource Teams. Clients work with their Resource Team members to aid the Critical Parent and True Parent parts in joining and working together, the Emotion Controller-Regulator/little "a" and the Competent Adult parts in joining and working together, and both sets of parts in becoming members of the Resource Team.

2. Convene the Meeting With Resource Team Members: Reinforce Positive Affect With Short Sets of Slow Bilateral Stimulation
Clients formed and installed their Resource Team (see Chapter 10) with bilateral stimulation (BLS) that reinforced the positive affect associated with accessing and strengthening links to their inner resources such as positive attributes and helpful qualities. Before calling the Resource Team meeting to order, therapists want to double-check that their clients still have positive affect connected to their team and to meeting with their team. Any negative thoughts, emotions, or sensations that emerge as the client reconvenes their Resource Team can be set aside in the container already linked to the Resource Team and Meeting Place. If negative affect persists, the therapist brainstorms and resolves issues interfering with the client reconnecting with their Resource Team by reworking the protocols for *Brainstorming Internal Resource Team Members* and *Installing the Internal Resource Team*.

3. Explain the Purposes of the Meeting to Resource Team Members
Resource Team members are willing and able to help clients with any challenge. The client's Resource Team serves as the hiring committee previously mentioned in the Introduction. Their main tasks for the meeting are to assist clients in:

- assessing the willingness of old and new versions of the Adult and Parent parts to change and to assume new roles in clients' lives;
- encouraging the old and new versions to learn to work together as they continue to integrate into the competent and confident Adult part of Self; and
- evaluating the readiness of the versions to become Resource Team members.

Resource Team members are open and objective through the interview process, and at the same time, are familiar with the Critical Parent and Emotion Controller-Regulator/little "a" parts and their impact on clients' lives. The Resource Team knows their job history.

4. Make a Team Decision About Which Old and New Versions of Parts to Bring to the Meeting First: Critical Parent and True Parent Parts or Competent Adult and Emotion Controller-Regulator/Little "a" Parts
AFTT-A therapists have and portray an unshakable belief that clients have whatever they need to act in their own best interest. Consequently, they rely on the client and their Resource Team to decide jointly which set of parts to bring into the Meeting Place first. Clients sometimes need to be reminded that they are not making the decision by

themselves but with their team's input and support. My clinical experience is that most clients bring in the Critical Parent and True Parent parts first.

5. Describe the Visual Aspect of Parts of Self

Clients often don't have a visual image of their Critical Parent/True Parent parts or of their Emotion Controller-Regulator/little "a"/Competent Adult part. Clients might describe a voice they hear inside their head, a body sensation they have, an overwhelming feeling, or an absence of feelings or body sensations. They may describe a loud, sharp voice giving them hurtful messages. They might feel an overwhelming sense of shame, fear, or anger but not know what caused the emotion. They may report body sensations such as tension in their chest and throat or an overall numbness and emptiness.

For the purposes of the Resource Team meeting in *Negotiating New Roles for Parent and Adult Parts of Self* protocol, therapists encourage clients to imagine a figure, being, animal, object, or force of nature that visually embodies their experience of the old and new versions of their Parent or Adult part of Self. Therapists help clients visualize the images of the old version of Parent and Adult parts by asking them to talk about the messages they get from that old version of themselves. What might the part look like that gives them those messages? What do they think right before they feel overwhelming shame and how can that thought be envisioned? What emotion goes with the tension or numbness, what started the emotion, what does the part look like that started that emotion? What thought precedes the numbness or emptiness?

Therapists help clients imagine their True Parent part of Self by revisiting what they experienced in the *Corrective Attachment Experiences Between the Child/Adolescent and True Parent Parts of Self* protocol (see Chapter 12). They assist clients to visualize their Competent Adult part by connecting to images from the *Strengthening the Competent Adult Part of Self* protocol (see Chapter 11).

BOX 13.1 CLIENT EXAMPLE: VISUALIZING THE CRITICAL PARENT PART OF SELF

Therapist: What I'd like for us to do today is talk to those parts, the Critical Parent and the True Parent parts of you, and see if they're willing to negotiate new ways of doing their jobs with you, to work together and take a place around the campfire as members of your Resource Team. How does that sound?

Client: That would be great!

Therapist: How about if we do some work with those parts and see what they have to say? See if they're willing to work together and do their job in ways that would be more helpful to you.

Client: Okay.

Therapist: What are some of the messages that critical voice gives you?

Client: Well, nothing I ever do is good enough, people will hurt me, there's something wrong with me.

(continued)

BOX 13.1 CLIENT EXAMPLE: VISUALIZING THE CRITICAL PARENT PART OF SELF (*continued*)

Therapist: When you hear those messages, what do you notice about the voice saying them?

Client: A real mean voice.

Therapist: Male? Female?

Client: Female. Like a witch.

Therapist: If you imagine, what would that voice look like?

Client: Actually, like a witch. You know, the Wicked Witch from the Wizard of Oz?

Therapist: I like that! What we want to do now is convene a meeting of you and your team and invite these two parts in for an interview about whether the Critical Parent is willing to consider the changes it needs to make, if they're willing to work together, and ready to become a part of your team. Like I said before, we want to reassure them that they don't already have to know how to do the job just make a commitment to do their jobs differently. How does that sound?

Client: Good!

6. Invite Parts Into a Meeting With Resource Team Members

Clients sometimes describe a sense of being "called on the carpet" or "called to the principal's office" when they are first introduced to the idea of bringing the old versions of their Parent and Adult parts of Self into a Resource Team meeting to discuss whether the parts are ready and willing to become team members. Deep down, the Critical Parent and the Emotion Controller-Regulator/little "a" parts know that the roles they played and the ways they did their jobs were hurtful to clients in the long run. They know that they were intended to play roles to nurture, protect, regulate, and balance, but they couldn't because they didn't know how. They weren't taught how. Shame and inadequacy lie underneath the appearances of defensiveness, arrogance, helplessness, fragility, or justifications. The old versions of the Parent and Adult parts of Self literally "did the best they could with what they had." Their best efforts helped clients survive their childhoods but backfired when clients needed to feel competent and confident navigating adult life and relationships.

One way to normalize the Resource Team meeting and make it less threatening is to compare the gathering to a job interview as described in this chapter's introduction. The past versions of the Parent and Adult parts of Self are likened to employees of a company that was been taken over by another company and the new company wants to determine if employees of the old company are willing to join the new company. The Resource Team understands that the older versions didn't get the training and experience they needed to do their intended jobs and shows appreciation for the job they did at the old company. The Resource Team genuinely wants them to become team members, as long as they are willing to consider the possibility that they can change and that they are willing to work with the newer version of their part of Self to learn their new roles and how to do their jobs in more helpful and useful ways.

> **BOX 13.2 CLIENT EXAMPLE: INVITING CRITICAL PARENT PART OF SELF TO THE RESOURCE TEAM MEETING**
>
> **Therapist:** How do you and your team want to invite the Critical Parent and True Parent parts to join you?
>
> **Client:** The Secret Service guy lets them onto the rock with the camp fire.
>
> **Therapist:** Imagine doing that. (Pause.) What do you notice?
>
> **Client:** The team is welcoming but watchful too. The True Parent seems excited but I don't think they're going to let the Critical Parent get away with too much! (Laughs.) She doesn't seem too happy to be there.
>
> **Therapist:** How so?
>
> **Client:** She knows something is up!

7. Discuss the Parts' Role(s) in the Client's Life

Since clients have just started accessing the True Parent and Competent Adult parts, most of the Resource Team meeting is spent talking about the roles the Critical Parent and Emotion Controller-Regulator/little "a" played in clients' lives. They were intended to play nurturing, protective, balancing, and regulating roles but the client, Resource Team, and parts explore what functions and responsibilities they had instead.

8. Explore Both the Positive and Negative Impacts the Old Version of Part Had on the Client's Life, Thank Part for How It Helped Client Up to Now, Reinforce the Positive Affect With Short Sets of Slow BLS

Clients often realize during the Resource Team meeting that they would not have survived or be where they are now if it weren't for the Critical Parent and Emotion Controller-Regulator/little "a" taking over responsibility for helping them at some point(s) during childhood. Acknowledging both the negative and positive effects on clients is equally important. Two points are helpful to make during the parts' job interviews with the Resource Team:

- The part was developed during childhood, so it represents a young and immature state that has child-like thinking and ways of reacting based on what was modeled for them and taught to them.
- The part is not oriented to time, so it reacts to current events as if the past danger is still present.

9. Discuss the Old and New Versions of Parts' Feelings About and Reactions to Each Other: Reinforce Positive Affect with Short Sets of Slow BLS

Clients often don't realize that their past versions of the Parent and Adult parts of Self have already made an initial commitment to change into the True Parent and Competent Adult parts and have experienced thoughts, emotions, and behaviors that reflect the positive movement toward change. In the two previous protocols, clients accessed and strengthened the natural or intrinsic abilities of the Parent part to nurture, protect, and connect with the Child/Adolescent part of Self as well as the Competent Adult part of

Self to balance, regulate, coordinate, and orchestrate what's needed in a challenging present-day situation. The preliminary shifts toward becoming the healthier form of their parts facilitates the conversation between the old and new versions.

10. Explain the Need for Parts to Work Together to Become a Resource Team Member(s): *If the Old and New Versions Are Not Ready to Integrate With Each Other,* **Discuss How They Will Work Together**

Parts need information about what changes will be expected from them to work together and to become Resource Team members. They need reassurance that they don't already have to know how to do their new jobs. The Resource Team and the newer version of the part will help them to learn to play their roles in more constructive or beneficial ways. They only need to make a commitment to consider the possibility of trying something new.

Overdeveloped parts might protest that they can't try something new because they might make a mistake or look foolish. Underdeveloped parts may claim that they can't possibly change because they are too fragile or too overwhelmed. The good news is that everything they need to play a new role or to do their job in a different way already exists within the Resource Team.

Clients and the Resource Teams take parts' skill levels and needs into consideration and seem to instinctively know how to integrate parts as team members. One client's Resource Team may accept parts as team members during the first interview. Others may give them a conditional acceptance with a probationary period to assist parts to gain the necessary skills and to observe how team members do their jobs. For example, one of my clients was a nurse and used their experience as a mentor to student nurses as their model for incorporating the Parent and Adult parts of Self into their Resource Team. Like student nurses at the hospital where my client worked, parts were initially allowed only to observe Resource Team members doing their jobs. When the parts started practicing new roles, the Resource Team members supervised them until they were certain the parts demonstrated proficient skills. Finally, the parts were permitted to act independently within the Resource Team.

BOX 13.3 CLIENT EXAMPLE: NEGOTIATING NEW ROLES WITH THE CRITICAL PARENT AND TRUE PARENT PARTS OF SELF

Therapist: How would you like to start the discussion?

Client: Well, the True Parent seems pretty comfortable. Mrs. T. is explaining to the Critical Parent why she's with us. Mrs. T. has this really calm and patient way of talking so she doesn't seem to feel threatened.

Therapist: What is Mrs. T. saying?

Client: That we understand that she has done the best she can with what she was given, that I wouldn't be where I am today if she hadn't been with me along the way but also that she needs to change. That she won't be allowed to talk to me the way she has in the past.

Therapist: How does it seem your Critical Parent is responding to that?

(continued)

> **BOX 13.3 CLIENT EXAMPLE: NEGOTIATING NEW ROLES WITH THE CRITICAL PARENT AND TRUE PARENT PARTS OF SELF** (*continued*)

Client: She's not happy at all. She's afraid I'll get hurt if she doesn't do her job.

Therapist: What does she need to hear to know that no one's telling her she needs to stop doing her job, that she just needs to agree to consider the possibility that she can still protect you but in a different way?

Client: I'm telling her that and that I know she wants the best for me.

Therapist: How does your Critical Parent seem to feel about that?

Client: She looks less upset but is still uncertain.

Therapist: How can your team help with that?

Client: They're telling her that she doesn't have to figure out how to do her new job by herself. That the True Parent and the whole team will help her.

Therapist: How does your Critical Parent feel about that?

Client: She's actually relieved. She says she knows she has hurt me but didn't know how to do anything different. She really wants to do a good job.

11. Gain the Commitment of Part(s) to Work Together and With the Resource Team: Reinforce the Positive Affect With Short Sets of Slow BLS

Resource Team members offer guidance and direction in the commitment step of the *Negotiating New Roles for Parent and Adult Parts of Self* protocol. They built rapport and trust with parts as potential team members. They are nonjudgmental in their approach to parts. They convey their commitment to help parts become team members. In return, the Resource Team expects commitment from the Parent and Adult parts of Self to be willing to consider the possibility of change, of playing different roles, and of doing their jobs in more useful and helpful ways.

> **BOX 13.4 CLIENT EXAMPLE: REINFORCING THE POSITIVE AFFECT CONNECTED TO PARTS' AND THE RESOURCE TEAM'S COMMITMENT TO CHANGE**

Therapist: And how do you feel as you experience the conversation with your team and the Parent parts?

Client: Relieved, too. And more hopeful.

Therapist: Where do you notice feeling the relief and hope in your body?

Client: A warm feeling in my heart. An easing of tension kind of all over.

Therapist: Any positive cognition that would go with this experience?

Client: We can do this together!

Therapist: So, hold the Meeting Place scene, the relief and hope, the warmth and easing, and the thought, "We can do this together," and feel the tones.

(Slow, short BLS sets to strengthen the client's positive affect as they connect to their new Resource Team.)

12. Discuss the Resource Team's Suggestions and Concerns Before Accepting New Team Member(s): Strengthen and Reinforce the Positive Affect With Short Sets of Slow BLS

The last step in the parts' job interview/Resource Team meeting is to open the discussion to any kinds of comments, concerns, and doubts, so that the client, team, and parts have the opportunity to brainstorm solutions to potential barriers or difficulties before accepting parts as new Resource Team members.

(Repeat the protocol with old and new versions of the second part, starting with Step 5.)

POINTS TO REMEMBER

- Remind clients to practice meeting with and using their Resource Team between sessions.
- Use intuition/mindful awareness when clients are talking about their lives/time in between sessions to notice "red flags" that Critical Parent or Emotion Controller-Regulator/little "a" parts have separated from their newer versions (True Parent and Competent Adult) and relapsed into old protective patterns.
- In session, note changes in voice, body posture, facial expression, eye contact, getting stuck in negative cognitions, looping during BLS sets as signs old versions of Parent (Critical Parent) and Adult (Emotion Controller-Regulator/small "a") parts of Self have reverted to old thought and behavior patterns.
- Appeal to the core of the parts' original purpose and role in the client's life; they were meant to help and they had the client's best interests at heart.
- Remind client, parts, and Resource Team that there was nothing wrong with the parts themselves; the parts aren't defective. The parts' limitations to help were due to the dysfunctional messages and strategies they learned from real-life attachment figures.
- Balance kind compassion with firm insistence that the Critical Parent needs to follow through with its agreement to work with its newer version, the True Parent, and that Emotion Controller-Regulator/little "a" parts need to uphold their commitment to work with their newer version, the Competent Adult. Remind them of their commitment to do their jobs differently as part of the Resource Team.
- Remind parts that they don't already have to know how to do their job differently; they only need to make a commitment to consider the possibility of changing.
- Use time orientation to help the Critical Parent or Emotion Controller-Regulator/little "a" parts remember that the danger is past (Martin, 2012). Differentiate between "now" and "back then," keeping in mind that old ways of helping the client are no longer needed or helpful. They have a newer version that will mentor and support them.

TROUBLESHOOTING

- If the client has strong emotional reactions to the Critical Parent or Emotion Controller-Regulator parts, check to see if a Child/Adolescent part is "hiding out" in the Meeting Place and needs to be tucked into their Safe Place. Time orientation is helpful to ensure that the client's Competent Adult part of Self is at the negotiation table.

- If the client's Critical Parent, Emotion Controller-Regulator, or little "a" parts voice reluctance or refusal to consider the possibility of change, they may not be oriented to time; they still believe that the danger from childhood is real and they need to continue to play their old roles or do their jobs in old ways to protect the client from danger. Again, time orientation helps clients discern the difference between "now" and "back then" so client's parts of Self are free to make changes based on adulthood needs in the present moment.

PAUSE AND REFLECT FOR THE THERAPIST

> **BOX 13.5 DEB'S STORY: NEGOTIATING NEW ROLE FOR THE CRITICAL PARENT PART OF SELF WITH RESOURCE TEAM**
>
> Ann and I did a demonstration at a live training that ended up helping me in creating a new role for the Critical Parent part of me. When I invited my Critical Parent part of Self to meet with my Resource Team and me, the part came into the meeting space looking like Boo Radley in the movie *To Kill a Mockingbird*, the way Boo appears when he first shows up. He was hiding in the shadows, and he seemed big and a little scary. The Boo in my meeting space transformed the way Boo did in the movie when he stepped out of the shadows and we found out that he'd protected Scout and carried her to safety. As I began speaking to the Boo Radley part of me, I discovered that this self-critical part of me that seemed so threatening was actually attempting to protect me from outside criticism by keeping the critical voice going on the inside. In the end of the exercise, my Boo Radley part agreed to become a gentle and nurturing True Parent figure on my Resource Team.

At this point, take some time to reflect on your experiences with your challenging client. Think about how messages from your Critical Parent or Emotion Controller-Regulator part interfere with your work with your client. Brainstorm ways you could negotiate with your Critical Parent or Emotion Controller-Regulator/little "a" part to develop a new role or a different way of playing their role that will be helpful to you in working with the client.

USEFUL TERMS AND DEFINITIONS

AFTT-A: Attachment-Focused Trauma Therapy for Adults

BLS: bilateral stimulation

P-A-C-diagram: Parent-Adult-Child diagram

PROTOCOL SCRIPT 10. NEGOTIATING NEW ROLES FOR PARENT AND ADULT PARTS OF SELF

Adapted from Berne, E. (1964). *Games people play: The basic handbook of transactional analysis.* Random House; Fraser, G. A. (1991). The Dissociative Table Technique: A strategy for working with ego states and dissociative disorders and ego-state therapy. *Dissociation: Progress in the Dissociative Disorders*, 4(4), 205–213; Fraser, G. A. (2003). Fraser's "Dissociative Table Technique" revisited, revised: A strategy for working with ego states in dissociative disorders and ego-state therapy. *Journal of Trauma and Dissociation*, 4(4), 5–28. https://doi.org/10.1300/J229v04n04_02; and Potter, A. E. (1994). *Inside out: Rebuilding self and personality through inner child therapy* (therapist manual and client workbook). Taylor and Francis Group.

Prior to start of the protocol, review with the client the Critical Parent and Emotion Controller-Regulator/little "a" personality parts in Parent-Adult-Child (P-A-C) diagrams. Discuss parts using Figure 7.2 P-A-C Diagrams: Validating Childhood Environment and Figure 7.3 P-A-C Diagram: Invalidating Childhood Environment. Review the True Parent part of Self from the Corrective Attachment Experiences for the Child and New Parent Parts of Self-Visualization and the Competent Adult part of Self from the Strengthening the Competent Adult Part of Self-Imagery.

1. Review Goals for Old and New Versions of Parts. *Say...* "The ultimate goal is for both the Critical Parent and the Emotion Controller-Regulator/little 'a' parts to work with the newer versions of their parts and to become members of your Resource Team. To accomplish that, our next steps help the Critical Parent and the True Parent parts work together, the Emotion Controller-Regulator/little 'a' and the Competent Adult parts to work together, and both sets of parts to become members of your Resource Team."

2. Discuss Goals for the Resource Team Meeting. *Say...* "Let's call a meeting with your Resource Team and talk with them about how the Critical Parent and Emotion Controller-Regulator/little 'a' parts of yourself were formed by childhood attachment trauma and how they need to continue to grow and change into the newer versions of their parts so they can be more helpful to you and they can become members of the team. The ultimate goal is for the Critical Parent and the Emotion Controller-Regulator/little "a" parts to work with the newer versions of their parts and for those parts to become members of your Resource Teams. To accomplish that, our next steps help the Critical Parent and True Parent parts join and work together, the Emotion Controller-Regulator/little"a" and the Competent Adult parts join and work together, and both sets of parts to become members of the Resource Team. After you and your team talk, you all will interview the Critical Parent and Emotion Controller-Regulator/little 'a' parts along with their healthier versions to see if they're willing to play their roles in your life in more helpful ways and join the team."

3. Convene a Meeting With the Resource Team Members. *Reinforce positive affect related to the client reconnecting with the Resource Team with short sets of slow BLS with tappers or butterfly taps. Practice container for setting aside the negative affect if needed.*

4. Explain the Purposes of the Meeting to the Resource Team Members. *Say...* "I invite you to talk to your team about the purpose of your meeting. They already know about your parts of Self and how they were impacted by your childhood. You want to let them know that you need their help in bringing these parts of you into the meeting, assisting your parts to recognize the need to change what role(s) they played or job(s) they did for you in the past, and deciding if the parts are ready to become members of the Resource Team."

5. Make a Team Decision About Which Old and New Versions of Parts to Bring to the Meeting First: Either Critical Parent and True Parent Parts or Emotion Controller-Regulator/Little "a" and Competent Adult Parts.

6. Describe Visual Aspect of Old and New Versions of Part of Self. *Say...* "Sometimes people already have an image or a visual depiction of the (*name the parts the client and team decided to meet with first*) and sometimes they hear it as a voice or see it as a message. For the purposes of your meeting today, we want to get an idea of what (*name parts*) look like so they can be brought into the Meeting Place for their job interview. *Ask...* "How do you imagine the (*name parts*) look?"

_____
_____

7. Invite the Old and New Versions of the First Part Into the Meeting With Resource Team Members. *If the client reports negative affect, ask...* "How can your team help with that?" *Once a positive affect is elicited, reinforce with short, slow sets of BLS with tappers or butterfly taps. Practice the container for setting aside the negative affect if needed.*

8. Discuss Parts' Role(s) in the Client's Life. *Ask...* "Who on your team needs to explain to (*name parts*) about the reason why they've been asked to join you in the meeting?"_____

Ask... "What is important for (*name parts*) to know about the purpose of the meeting?"

_____
_____

Say... "Perhaps, (*name old version of part*) can tell the team when they came into your life, why they thought they needed to help you, and what they've done for you over the years."

_____
_____

9. Explore Both the Positive and Negative Impact the Old Version of Part Had on the Client's Life. Thank the Part for How It Helped the Client Up to Now. Reinforce Positive Affect With Short Sets of Slow BLS. *Ask...* "How do (*name old version of part*) feel about how they've affected your life so far? What's been positive and what has been not so positive? How do you feel about what they said?"

_____
_____

If the client reports negative affect, ask... "How can your team help with that?" *Elicit positive affect. Strengthen and reinforce with BLS.*

13. PARTS' WORK: NEGOTIATING NEW ROLES FOR PARENT AND ADULT PARTS OF SELF

Say... "I think it's important for (*name of old version of part*) to know that you and the team understand they had your best interests at heart and did the best they could with the information they were given by the adults in your life as you were growing up." *Say...* "Let's have you or someone on the team give the information to that part of you." *Ask...* "How does that part of you feel? What do you notice as you listen to it?"

___

___

If the client reports negative affect, ask... "How can your team help with that?" *Elicit positive affect. Strengthen and reinforce with BLS.*

10. **Discuss the Old and New Versions of Parts' Feelings About and Reactions to Each Other.** *Say...* "Next, we ask (*name parts*) to talk together with the help of the team about what they think of and feel about each other. Since they are different versions of the same part of you, we want them to continue to transform into one part or a unit that will play the most helpful roles they were intended to play on your team and in your life." *Elicit and reinforce positive affect with short sets of slow BLS.*

11. **Explain the Need for Parts to Work Together to Become a Resource Team Member(s).** *If the old and new versions are not ready to integrate with each other, discuss how they will work together. Say...* "Use your Resource Team to help (*name parts*) figure out how they are going to work together."

___

___

12. **Gain the Commitment of the Part(s) to Work Together and With the Resource Team.** *Say...* "Sometimes your parts think they should already know how to do their new jobs or play their new roles. It's important for them to know that no one expects them to know how to do their new job yet. Right now, they're just making a commitment to consider the possibility that they can change. Their newer version and the Resource Team will teach them and show them everything they need to know about their new job. See what (*name parts*) think about that."

___

Ask... "How do you feel about what (*name parts*) said?"

___

___

If the client reports negative affect, ask... "How can your team help with that?" *Elicit and reinforce positive affect with short sets of slow BLS.*

13. Discuss the Resource Team's Suggestions and Concerns Before Accepting New Resource Team Member(s). *Say...* "Before you end the meeting, I'd like you to invite your Resource Team members to share any ideas, concerns, or suggestions before you decide if (*name parts*) will become a Resource Team member." *Ask...* "How does the Resource Team feel about (*name parts*) becoming a member?"

_____

_____

Reinforce the positive affect with short sets of slow BLS. Ask... "How do you feel about (*name parts*) joining your Resource Team?"

_____

_____

If the client reports negative affect, ask... "How can your team help with that?" *Reinforce positive affect with short sets of slow BLS. Ask...* "Is there anything else that needs to be said or done before you complete the scene?"

_____

_____

Reinforce positive affect with short sets of slow BLS.

*REPEAT PROTOCOL WITH OLD AND NEW VERSIONS OF SECOND PART OF SELF, STARTING WITH STEP 5.

REFERENCES

Berne, E. (1964). *Games people play: The basic handbook of transactional analysis.* Random House.

Fraser, G. A. (1991). The Dissociative Table Technique: A strategy for working with ego states and dissociative disorders and ego-state therapy. *Dissociation: Progress in the Dissociative Disorders,* 4(4), 205–213.

Fraser, G. A. (2003). Fraser's "Dissociative Table Technique" revisited, revised: A strategy for working with ego states in dissociative disorders and ego-state therapy. *Journal of Trauma and Dissociation,* 4(4), 5–28. https://doi.org/10.1300/J229v04n04_02

Martin, K. M. (2012). How to use Fraser's dissociative table technique to access and work with emotional parts of the personality. *Journal of EMDR Practice and Research,* 6(4), 179–186. https://doi.org/10.1891/1933-3196.6.4.179

Potter, A. E. (1994a). *Inside out: Rebuilding self and personality through inner child therapy* (therapist manual). Accelerated Development, Inc.

Potter, A. E. (1994b). *Inside out: Rebuilding self and personality through inner child therapy* (client workbook). Accelerated Development, Inc.

CHAPTER 14

Parts' Work: Tucking Child/Adolescent Parts of Self Into Their Safe Places in Attachment-Focused Trauma Therapy for Adults

INTRODUCTION

So far in the Attachment-Focused Trauma Therapy for Adults (AFTT-A) process, clients have learned about parts of Self and how their personality structure is developed in both validating and invalidating environments through the Parent-Adult-Child (P-A-C) diagrams. They have created and installed Safe Places and Higher Powers for their Adult and Child/Adolescent parts of Self to differentiate among personality parts, strengthened their internalized sense of nurturing and protection, and began to experience corrective attachment relationships among parts of their internal personality system. They have accessed and reinforced positive links to a team of inner resources that foster clients' beliefs that they have everything they need within themselves and they no longer have to be or feel alone. They have strengthened the competent and confident aspects of their Adult part of Self and provided healthy attachment experiences between their Adult and Child/Adolescent parts. Lastly, they have renegotiated new roles and jobs for the Critical Parent and Emotion Controller-Regulator/little "a" parts to integrate them as members of the newly formed Resource Team.

Clients with a history of attachment trauma often have Child/Adolescent parts blended or enmeshed with their Adult part of Self. As a result, clients go through their present-day life with their attention divided between their efforts to fulfill their adulthood needs for love, connection, respect, meaning, and belonging and their Child/Adolescent parts' attempts to get unmet childhood needs met through present-day relationships. Even though Child/Adolescent parts are given Safe Places and Higher Powers so they could experience getting all their needs met in the present moment, these needs can get triggered when clients say or do (or don't say or do) something Child/Adolescent parts interpret as dangerous, potentially getting them hurt or into trouble or thwarting their efforts to get attention, acceptance, or protection through clients' current relationships.

I (A.P.) learned over the years as a therapist that clients' Child/Adolescent parts can be *very, very* determined in their quest to get unmet childhood needs met through clients' current lives. Children up to a certain age have magical thinking as a part of their ego-centric perspective of themselves in relationship to what transpires in their lives; they believe that they cause what happens to them and around them. Children's ego-centric thinking leads to the mistaken belief that they cause situations and others' behaviors and reactions. This child-like thinking impacts children's development of self-regard and self-esteem. Consequently, if good things happen to them and around them (they receive messages of encouragement, acceptance, and protection), they are good. Conversely, if bad things happen to them and around them (they are abused and/or neglected and receive messages that they are not good enough or they can't trust adults to love and protect them), they are bad (Erikson, 1993; Piaget & Inhelder, 1969)

> **BOX 14.1 ANN'S STORY: CHILDREN'S EGO-CENTRIC AND MAGICAL THINKING**
>
> I got angry at my mom one morning before I left for school when I was in second or third grade. I remember muttering to myself as I walked to school, stomping on every sidewalk crack that I could find because I believed the saying, "Step on a crack and break your mother's back." Yes, I know, how horrible! I really felt justified in getting back at her for whatever she had done that I thought was unfair or unreasonable. Well…I had the whole day at school to stew about the fact that I had really broken my mother's back and she was alone and helpless at home. So, I made I deal with God on the way home from school: I would avoid every crack in the sidewalks between school and home and my mom's back would be fixed. Of course, when I got home, my mom's back was just fine. Now, I didn't ask her, "Mom, was your back broken sometime today and then it was unbroken?" I knew if I said that to her, she would know that I had caused her injury and she would know what a terrible child I was. Instead, I just figured since I had avoided stepping on all the cracks on the way home, God has kept His part of our bargain. Whew!

Clients with a history of attachment trauma carry child-like thinking into their adult relationships. Inner Child/Adolescent parts of Self are either hopeful that their needs will finally be met or are petrified their needs will never be met. They think, "If I just act a certain way or if I stop doing a certain behavior, if I am more this way or less that way, then I will finally get my needs met"; "If I can get this person to love me then I am good enough and worthwhile or if I can't, then I am bad and unworthy"; "I just need to try harder, do more"; or "I give up!" As a result, Child/Adolescent parts' motives for adult relationships are often at odds with the goals of the Competent Adult part of Self. For example, a client who is acting out of their Competent Adult part may want to be in a relationship that offers a balance between closeness and respect for each partner's individuality but their Child/Adolescent part may want to be taken care of and have no responsibilities; thus, feeling threatened if the client is in a relationship in which a partner has their own friends or wants time to themselves.

Clients acting from the Competent Adult part of Self have choices about their actions and reactions. They take in and consider information from all inner parts of Self as well as from others in their lives and current situations. They reason through what options are best for themselves and others. However, clients whose Adult and Child/Adolescent parts are enmeshed bring old childhood beliefs and patterns of behavior into their adult relationships. Their Child/Adolescent parts attempt to get their unmet childhood needs met through present-day relationships but ultimately, clients end up not getting *either* their childhood *or* adult needs met. The following scenarios are examples of how the learned behaviors of enmeshed Child/Adolescent parts impact adult attachment relationships:

- Clients gained approval during childhood for taking care of the adults in their life or for parenting their own parents. In present-day relationships, they over-function but don't get the appreciation they think they deserve from others and develop resentments.
- Clients were given attention during childhood under the condition that they deny their needs and take care of themselves. They end up in relationships in which they are aloof and distant, angry if their partners have any expectations of them, perhaps even showing disdain for closeness and their partner's needs.
- Clients' attachment figures had unrealistically high expectations, overemphasized achievement, and were very critical. Some clients internalize the overly high expectations and critical messages and become very perfectionistic, overfocusing on work and accomplishments. Other clients with a similar upbringing may rebel against rules and expectations and under-function or underachieve in their adult life, expecting others to pick up their slack or clean up their messes.

The AFTT-A model approaches work with inner Child/Adolescent parts of Self and the reconstruction of the internal personality system in a unique manner. AFTT-A therapists do not want to develop close relationships with clients' younger parts. Instead, they facilitate direct communication between clients and their Child/Adolescent parts of Self and among the parts themselves so inner parts develop healthy attachments with each other, the internal personality system, and the client. The therapist's role in parts' work is to ensure that the Competent Adult part of the Self is participating in discussions with parts and clients have the information and the skills needed to communicate effectively and continue to form corrective inner attachment relationships with their personality system.

AFTT-A therapists attune to the presence of clients' younger parts in therapy sessions and in their lives between sessions. Therapists are often trained not to start sessions with questions like "How did your week go?" or "How are you doing?" and to see those questions as more of a waste of time. I (A.P.) begin sessions with general and open-ended questions so clients choose how they initially open up in therapy, what they want to talk about, and how deeply they want to talk about their initial topics. As a therapist, I view clients' preliminary report as an opportunity to listen for, become aware of, and attune to the presence of clients' Child/Adolescent parts of Self and their involvement in clients' lives since the last session. Did a younger part sneak out of their Safe Place and try to hijack a relationship? I also pay attention to the possibility that other parts of Self like the old Critical Parent or Emotion Controller-Regulator/little "a" have reneged on their commitment to change. Did the Critical Parent part relapse into old patterns of disapproval and blaming? Did the Emotion Controller-Regulator decide to take a trip to the Bahamas, leave the little "a" in charge, and the client ended up overwhelmed with intense emotions? I use my impressions and intuition about clients' reports or topics as a springboard for the subsequent work to be done in the session.

Up to this point in the AFTT-A process, therapists assisted clients in forming healthy bonds between parts of Self and their Higher Powers (see Protocol Scripts 4 and 5), with members of the Inner Resource Team (see Protocol Scripts 6 and 7), between the True Parent and Child/Adolescent parts (see Protocol Script 9), and between the Resource Team and the reworked Critical Parent (True Parent) and Emotion Controller-Regulator/little "a" (Competent Adult) parts (see Protocol Script 10). Protocol Script 11, *Tucking the Child/Adolescent Part of Self Into the Safe Place*, focuses more closely on the relationship between the Competent Adult, True Parent, and Child/Adolescent parts of Self; how younger parts are involved with and impact clients' current lives; and how to resolve issues like time disorientation that interfere with maintaining healthy boundaries between the Child/Adolescent parts and clients' adult lives (see Protocol Script 11 at the end of this chapter).

STEPS

1. Discuss Child/Adolescent Part's Involvement on and Impact on the Therapy Session or Present-Day Life

We coined the term "Velcro Kids" to describe Child/Adolescent parts that are blended or enmeshed with the Competent Adult part of Self. They are so tangled up with client "Adult Brains" that separating them from the more adult aspects of the personality might sound like strips of Velcro being torn apart. One client described their very ingrained Child/Adolescent parts as "Super Glue Kids." As a result of parts' enmeshment, clients manage their present-day lives while simultaneously struggling to respond to feelings, demands, and reactions from Child/Adolescent parts. As stated in the chapter's introduction, the motives and the intentions of clients' Adult and Child/Adolescent parts are often at odds, thus leaving clients torn between getting adulthood needs met and the futile attempts by Child/Adolescent parts to make up for what happened or didn't happen in childhood.

Therapists begin with clients by reviewing information gained from earlier protocols related to parts of Self and the P-A-C diagrams (see Figures 7.2 and 7.3). Since the foundation of differentiating and reconnecting parts was started in previous protocols, therapists continue the groundwork of distinguishing between parts; separating out Child/Adolescent parts to be tucked back into an internalized sense of nurturing and safety while freeing the Competent Adult part of Self to orchestrate the internal system and adult relationships and situations. They brainstorm with clients the ways their adult lives and relationships have been affected by the involvement of their younger parts.

Next, therapists help clients familiarize themselves with signs that the Child/Adolescent and Adult parts are enmeshed, and their younger part is running the show. The following behaviors and reactions offer clues to Child/Adolescent part involvement in adult life:

- The therapist observes the client's presentation in session; for example, changes in voice, body posture, facial expression, eye contact, getting stuck in negative cognitions, looping during bilateral stimulation (BLS) sets.
- The therapist notes their own reactions to the client's presentation in session; for example, body sensations, emotions, thoughts, judgments, intuitions.
- The client reports old behavior patterns, relationship issues, negative core beliefs.
- The client shows or reports emotional reactions out of proportion for situations, experiencing the same emotion regardless of the situation and/or getting stuck in emotions.

- The client has difficulty completing protocols in session or assignments between sessions.
- The client comes late to sessions, frequently cancels sessions, or doesn't show up for sessions.

2. Identify the Child/Adolescent Part in Session or Through the Client's Description of Events Between Sessions

Once clients identify behaviors, reactions, and feelings associated with their Child/Adolescent part of Self, therapists assist them in pinpointing the age of the younger part that is eavesdropping on clients' adult life. Questions helpful for finding a Child/Adolescent part's age are "How old did you feel when that was happening?" "How old do you feel as you talk about this?" "Tell me about a time you felt this way when you were younger." Therapists then ascertain the physical location of the younger part; for example, in the therapy room, waiting for the client outside of the therapy room, or hanging out at the clients' house or place of work.

Note: If the identified Child/Adolescent part does not already have a Safe Place and Higher Power, return to the Safe Place and Higher Power for Child/Adolescent Parts of Self protocol (see Protocol Script 5). If the younger part already has a Safe Place and Higher Power, continue with this protocol.

BOX 14.2 CLIENT EXAMPLE: ENMESHED ADOLESCENT PART IN A PRESENT-DAY SITUATION

Therapist: How about if we maybe look at that conversation with your dad over the weekend in light of what we've talked about so far related to parts of Self: "Adult Brain"/"Kid Brain." Would that be okay?

Client: Sure.

Therapist: As you look back at that conversation with your dad over the weekend, what do you notice about how you felt?

Client: I felt like I always do with my dad—I'm never going to measure up. He's disappointed in me.

Therapist: What feelings did you have as you had those thoughts?

Client: Sad. Hopeless.

Therapist: When you look back at that conversation, how old did you feel?

Client: I'm not sure I know what you mean.

Therapist: Well, I understand that you felt sad and hopeless having that conversation with your dad where he seemed disappointed in you. Sometimes, your emotions are just about what's happening in the present moment, and sometimes, they can come from the present moment and the past if the situation brings up those same feelings from your past relationship with your dad. Like we've talked about before, that younger part of you sometimes "eavesdrops" on your adult life, gets mixed up about time, and you end up experiencing

(continued)

> **BOX 14.2 CLIENT EXAMPLE: ENMESHED ADOLESCENT PART IN A PRESENT-DAY SITUATION** (continued)
>
> that Child/Adolescent part's feelings. You were triggered by what happened with your dad last weekend on top of the feelings that you as an adult had. Does that make sense?
>
> Client: Yeah, I get it now. I remember thinking to myself, "Why do I still get so upset when my dad talks to me that way?" So maybe a little of both.

3. Invite the Client to Talk to the Child/Adolescent Part With Their Higher Power Figure

As mentioned in the Introduction, the AFTT-A model encourages clients to develop healthy bonds with their inner parts since they will be empowered to take responsibility for their internal personality system as well as their relationships in their present-day life. To that end, therapists support direct communication between clients and their parts. Child/Adolescent parts of Self are not invited into the therapy room or into a visualization to develop a relationship with the therapist but, rather, to develop a relationship with the client through their Competent Adult part, with the therapist as mentor and coach.

AFTT-A therapists apply a variety of techniques to invite the Child/Adolescent part and their Higher Power into a therapy session and to help clients familiarize themselves with their younger part; for example, guided imagery, visualization, and sand tray work. The *Tucking the Child/Adolescent Part of Self Into the Safe Place* protocol combines visualization with BLS to reinforce positive affect accessed during the protocol. Once the client's younger part is introduced to the Competent Adult and True Parent parts and the therapist notes at least a basic level of comfort or ease, clients dialogue with the Child/Adolescent part that felt the need to leave their Safe Place and interject themselves into the client's present-day life.

4. Find Out Reasons for the Child/Adolescent Part Getting Triggered/Sneaking Out of Safe Place

Child/Adolescent parts still intervene in clients' adult lives even after they were installed in their own Safe Place with a Higher Power. They believe they have a good reason for leaving their Safe Place; in their minds, they have something essential to tell the client or something urgent to do for the client. Clients' younger parts need to learn to trust the Competent Adult part of Self to be able to handle present-day life. They need reassurance that even if the client makes mistakes or messes something up in their present-day life, nothing bad will happen to the Child/Adolescent part and the Competent Adult part can access and activate whatever resources and connect to whatever people they need to be able to navigate challenges, disappointments, hurt, and loss. Becoming oriented to time is a process for younger parts and, especially early in therapy, they are often triggered to leave their Safe Place. The following list includes common reasons Child/Adolescent parts get triggered back into clients' adult life:

- The aspect of Safe Place and/or Higher Power/Caregiver needs to be tweaked/adjusted.

- A present-day life event or circumstances triggers a sense of danger. The younger part loses orientation to time, becomes mixed up between "now" and "back then," and thinks danger is real in the present moment.
- A present-day life event or circumstance triggers hope that an unmet childhood need might be satisfied in an adult relationship or situation. The Child/Adolescent part loses orientation to time, becomes mixed up between "now" and "back then," and thinks getting an unmet childhood need met in present life is urgent.
- The client and the Competent Adult part of Self need information that the younger part holds.
- The adult part is missing or grieving loss of the relationship with the Child/Adolescent part or loss of what role(s) the Child/Adolescent part played in their current life.
- The Child/Adolescent part is missing or grieving the loss of the relationship with the Adult part or loss of what role(s) they played in client's present-day life.

5. Link the Child/Adolescent Part's Cognitions and Behavior With Past Roles, Beliefs, and Fears

The Child/Adolescent parts are not oriented to time when they are triggered in clients' adult lives (Martin, 2018). They have the brain development, the experiences, the beliefs, the learned patterns of behavior, and the feelings of the client at that age. As a result, clients and their Child/Adolescent parts often have conflicting motives and goals in adult situations. AFTT-A therapists educate clients about the reality of Child Adolescent parts when they are "eavesdropping" on clients' current lives. Let's say a client has an 8-year-old Child/Adolescent part. The 8-year-old part doesn't know it's the present moment and the client is an adult. They don't have an adult perspective and can't be objective or reason through feelings or understand that they were not responsible for what happened to them. The 8-year-old Child/Adolescent part believes that the past *is* the present moment, the danger *is* real, their needs are *not* being met, and all the bad things they were told about themselves *are* true. Even though the Child/Adolescent part was given a Safe Place and a Higher Power so that all their needs are met in the present moment, they lose time orientation when they leave their Safe Place. They revert back to their 8-year-old reality.

Now let's say the client asks for a raise in an assertive manner from their boss. The Adult part views their firm and confident way of interacting with their boss as positive, perhaps even progress. They deserve to give themselves a pat on the back! However, the Child/Adolescent part in their 8-year-old brain who was taught not to have any needs or to bother anyone with their needs perceives the Adult part's actions as dangerous. Their experience is that if they have needs, they will be rejected. They will be seen as a nuisance. The client's feelings are now ambivalent because their Child/Adolescent part's reality is triggered into the current situation with their boss.

At first, the client feels proud of the way they requested a raise. They begin to feel a little nauseated and anxious. They worry that their boss is angry at them for asking for a raise. The boss might even fire them for being so demanding! The client's 8-year-old part insists that the client goes back and apologizes to the boss for being so needy. The client doesn't recognize that their Child/Adolescent part is out and needs to be tucked back into their Safe Place, so they go back to apologize for asking for a raise, maybe even makes a case against being given a raise. In the end, the client not only doesn't get a raise but their sense of competence and confidence in being assertive when asking for what they want is undermined.

Let's look at the same scenario but with a client who has an Adolescent part: a 16-year-old part who is angry and defiant. The 16-year-old part learned from relationships with attachment figures that adults in their life were not capable of caring for them and developed beliefs that needing love and caring meant they were weak and pitiful. The 16-year-old learned that keeping people from getting close was a sign of strength and power. So, imagine this client also asking their boss for a raise in an assertive way. Again, they feel proud of themselves for approaching their request with self-assurance and skill. Yet, the teen part in their 16-year-old brain interprets the client's actions as insecure and wimpy. The client whose Competent Adult part of Self is enmeshed with the time-disoriented 16-year-old brain reverts back to beliefs about how they always need to be on guard and suspicious because people can't be trusted and only want to take advantage of them. As a result, the client starts to question what they said and did and begins to feel angry, thinks they should have asked for more, even a promotion. After all, the boss never really appreciated them or saw their potential.

This client also doesn't realize that their Adolescent part is out and needs to be tucked back into their Safe Place, so they go back to tell their boss how lucky they are to have them as an employee, that they are the one who holds the place together, and their boss needs to finally show their gratitude for all the client has done for them by offering a bigger raise or a much-deserved promotion. Again, not only does the client not get a raise but they have now alienated their boss, and the old beliefs about others are reinforced.

In both scenarios, therapists use the information they gain from clients about current situations and listen for cognitions, emotions, and behaviors that sound more like they belong to a younger part rather than someone acting from their Competent Adult part of Self. They help clients detect what the younger part was taught to believe about themselves and others, the Early Bonding Contract rules they might still follow (see Table 15.1: Early Bonding Contract Rules and Possible New Rules in Chapter 15), the roles they played in their families, and what they are afraid might happen (or not happen) in the client's life if they fail to intervene. As clients step back to observe their younger part's involvement in their adult life, they begin to separate the "Velcro Kid" from their Competent Adult part of Self and, through the *Tucking the Child/Adolescent Part of Self Into the Safe Place* protocol, reinforce boundaries between the Competent Adult and Child/Adolescent parts of Self, thus, regaining an adult perspective and tools and skills to effectively handle present-day situations.

> **BOX 14.3 CLIENT EXAMPLE: TALKING TO ADOLESCENT PART WHO "SNUCK OUT" OF THE SAFE PLACE**
>
> Therapist: So, that's an example of your kid part coming out of their Safe Place and you trying to have that conversation with your dad at least in part from your "Kid Brain."
>
> Client: I can see that.
>
> *(continued)*

BOX 14.3 CLIENT EXAMPLE: TALKING TO ADOLESCENT PART WHO "SNUCK OUT" OF THE SAFE PLACE (*continued*)

Therapist:	Let's have a chat about that with that younger part of you. Would that be okay?
Client:	Yeah.
Therapist:	Where do you think we'd find that younger part of you?
Client:	(Laughs.) Right here.
Therapist:	Here with you in my office?
Client:	Yep.
Therapist:	I'd like you to ask that younger you in your mind what happened over the weekend that made it seem necessary to leave their Safe Place.
Client:	I needed help because I was making the situation worse and my dad was going to get really mad.
Therapist:	So, you couldn't handle the situation by yourself and you needed help?
Client:	(Laughs.) I guess so.
Therapist:	What do you think that teenage part of you needs to hear from you about that?
Client:	Well, like when I created the Safe Place in the first place, so there are no worries for the younger part of me about having Dad mad ever again. That's in the past and now that part of me can be on the soccer field with the team and the coach.
Therapist:	How does it feel when you tell your younger self that?
Client:	True but not true.
Therapist:	So, that teen part of you is a little mixed up still between now and back then.
Client:	Yes.
Therapist:	Would it be okay to help you with that?
Client:	Yes.
Therapist:	As we've done before, I want you to look around. You're in my office with me. You and I have only known each other for a few months. I didn't know you when you were younger. Look at your hands. Notice that they are the hands of an adult. And the clothes you're wearing. You bought them as an adult. As you do that, what do you notice?
Client:	I feel better. Less anxious, more sure of myself.
Therapist:	Where do you feel that in your body?
Client:	Across my shoulders, chest, and back.
Therapist:	What sensation do you notice?
Client:	Strength. Calm.

(Do slow, short sets of BLS to reinforce the positive affect with the Competent Adult part of Self.)

6. Thank the Child/Adolescent Part for Giving Information to and Bringing the Issue to the Attention of the Client and Therapist

Child/Adolescent parts (in whatever age brain they have) truly believe that clients need them in their adult lives to stay safe, to get ahead, to keep from being hurt, or to be loved and accepted. They believe that the only way to help is to convince clients that the past is present and if the client would just follow the old Bonding Contract rules and go back to old behaviors, then everything will be fine and unmet needs will finally be met. The *Tucking the Child/Adolescent Part of Self Into the Safe Place* protocol assists clients to see how younger parts have helped them so far in their lives. Clients develop compassion for and acceptance of their younger parts when they understand how Child/Adolescent parts can only think, believe, feel, or act in the way the client did at that age. Clients express their appreciation for their younger parts' positive motives and attempts to protect them and get unmet needs met in their adult life.

At times, clients dislike or are angry at their Child/Adolescent parts. They believe the lies they were told during their childhood; they were bad and caused or deserved the abuse or neglect. Clients then turn those beliefs against their own Child/Adolescent parts, viewing them through the lens of those who harmed them. Clients express regret to their younger parts for buying into abusers' lies and turning against them. The compassion and acceptance clients gain for their younger parts invalidate the old beliefs and continue the therapeutic work toward a healthy attachment relationship among the Competent Adult, True Parent, and Child/Adolescent parts of Self.

7. Reset Boundaries With the Child/Adolescent Part by the Competent Adult Part

Anyone who has children, has babysat children, or been around children at bedtime knows what it's like when they don't want to go to bed. They will try anything—another story, a trip to the bathroom, a snack, a glass of water, a check for monsters, a favorite stuffed animal (no, not the giraffe, the teddy), the light needs to be left on or turned off, or the door needs to be open or closed (no, open just a little). The bottom line is they need to go to bed because it's good for them to get enough sleep. Setting boundaries with younger parts of Self is very similar to putting children to bed even when they don't want to go. Setting boundaries with very young Child parts is comparable to having a toddler who has learned to crawl or pull up and walk. If the house has stairs, parents install a baby gate to keep the toddler safe. Setting boundaries with older Child parts is also likened to a couple who needs to have a conversation about family finances. They don't sit their children at the table to read the bank statements and create a budget. Instead, they shoo their children out of the room to play while they, as the adults, take care of the "grown-up" business.

Child/Adolescent parts were installed in a Safe Place with a Higher Power (see Chapter 9) so that all their needs for love and safety are met in the present moment. When they leave their Safe Place, the Competent Adult and True Parent parts of Self act as nurturing and protective parents; they tuck the younger parts back into an internalized sense of care and security with kindness *and* firmness.

14. PARTS' WORK: TUCKING CHILD/ADOLESCENT PARTS OF SELF INTO SAFE PLACES

BOX 14.4 CLIENT EXAMPLE: TUCKING THE ADOLESCENT PART OF SELF INTO THE SAFE PLACE

Therapist: I'd like you to go back and talk to the younger part of yourself about going back to the Safe Place—the soccer field with the team and coach. I'd like you to say that no matter what happens between you and your dad now, that teenage part inside of you is going to be okay. How does that feel?

Client: Less anxious and worried.

Therapist: Anything else that's needed before the younger you gets tucked back into the Safe Place?

Client: That I'm going to be okay.

Therapist: What do you need to say about that?

Client: Well, I can't promise I'll always be okay.

Therapist: True.

Client: I don't know.

Therapist: Give yourself a minute.

Client: I can say that even if I'm not okay now, I have people who can help me. I have my own Safe Place and Higher Power. And the kid part of me can still be okay and not feel like they need to take care of me anymore.

Therapist: What does that younger part of you think of that?

Client: Seems to believe me. I said it wasn't the fault of that younger me that Dad was so unhappy, and now everyone's on the soccer field with the coach. The coach has his hand on the shoulder of my younger part.

Therapist: How does that younger part of you seem to be feeling?

Client: Not even paying attention to me anymore.

Therapist: Oh good! How do you feel as you as you sit here in my office?

Client: I feel proud of myself. More capable.

Therapist: Where do you notice that in your body?

Client: Same places as before.

Therapist: Hold in mind feeling proud and capable with the strong calm sensations across your shoulders, chest, and back. Feel the tones and notice what happens.

(Do slow, short sets of BLS to reinforce the positive affect.)

8. Reinforce the Truth About Unmet Childhood Needs and Losses

One of Freud's defense mechanisms is termed "repetition compulsion" (Freud, 1990). We humans want to finish what is unfinished and make whole what is incomplete. Child Adolescent parts want to rectify what was wrong and fulfill what was left undone.

Unfortunately, Child/Adolescent parts have limited abilities and skills to accomplish such changes but will try the same methods over and over no matter how unsuccessful, thinking they will get a different result. Repetition compulsion involves magical thinking; if I just try this over and over, I'll *finally* get those unmet childhood needs met. Repetition compulsion serves to protect clients from the reality of their childhoods and the grief over their losses. If they keep hope that they can get their childhood needs met, they don't have to admit that the time for getting those needs met is over and, no matter what they do, those needs will never be met through relationships in their adult lives.

After the Child/Adolescent part is tucked back into their Safe Place, their Higher Power and the Competent Adult and True Parent parts of Self continue to set boundaries by telling them the truth about the probability of getting their unmet childhood needs in the client's present-day life. I (A. P.) tell clients, "There's good news and there's bad news. Which would you like first?" In actuality, the good news and the bad news are the same: No matter what Child/Adolescent parts try to do in present-day life, their childhood needs will never be met. Younger parts can get their needs met in the present moment in their Safe Places with their Higher Powers and clients can get their adulthood needs met, but the time to get childhood needs met is over. The attachment figures in their life screwed up and blew the chance to meet their needs so the opportunity to have their childhood needs met has been lost.

Child Adolescent parts learn they no longer need to play the roles and do the jobs they had in childhood. The only job they have from now on is to stay in their Safe Place with their Higher Power and the only role they need to play is to be a child at whatever age they are. Clients through their Competent Adult part of Self and with the help of their own Higher Power and their Resource Team are responsible for resolving the past, doing their grief work, and taking charge of the internal personality system as well as their present-day lives. Clients have the resources and support they need to come through hard times, make mistakes, and deal with loss and disappointment while the Child/Adolescent parts of Self are insulated from any consequences from the clients' adult lives.

9. Reassure the Child/Adolescent Part That the Danger Is in the Past

Child/Adolescent parts are triggered from their Safe Places when circumstances or situations in a client's adult life are similar enough to the past that they get disoriented to time and believe that the danger from childhood is still real in present-day life. In other words, current situations trigger the cluster of neural networks that contain memories and associated beliefs, scenes, feelings, and body sensations. The neural network clusters are parts of what the AFTT-A model views as Child/Adolescent Parts of Self or "Kid Brain" and are disconnected from the adaptive information processing (AIP) system in the part of the brain that AFTT-A refers to as "Adult Brain" so when the network clusters are tapped into, time disorientation occurs and the past traumatic event or circumstances feel like they are happening now (Martin, 2018). The AFTT-A model believes that what happens to the clients in the context of their primary attachment relationships in childhood (in addition to discrete abusive and neglectful incidents) is also contained in the neural networks in the "Kid Brain" and that flashbacks are considered the result of a Child/Adolescent part being triggered. The client who experiences a flashback has a time-disoriented younger part in charge.

Time orientation is an essential element of the *Tucking the Child/Adolescent Part of Self Into the Safe Place* protocol. When time-disoriented younger parts of Self are "out" in a client's adult life, they are reluctant and even defiant or terrified to return to their Safe Places. They think that something very bad will happen to them and/or the client if they don't play the role they did in the past. Their magical thinking leads them to believe that the old behaviors and patterns are the only answers to the current situation in adult life.

Therapists teach and coach clients to reassure their Child/Adolescent parts through use of time orientation. Therapists model for their clients the unshakable belief that clients in their Competent Adult part of Self have the necessary inner resources and support to help younger parts know they are safe and loved in the present moment and the danger is past. The Competent Adult part of Self accesses and activates the True Parent part in the internal personality system to soothe and comfort the Child/Adolescent parts.

10. Review the Child/Adolescent Part's Safe Place and Higher Power to Ensure Their Nurturing and Protective Qualities Meet the Younger Part's Needs

Make sure that the Higher Power knows how to be reassuring and protective when the Child/Adolescent part has the urge to eavesdrop in the client's adult life. If not, rework with the Safe Place and Higher Power for Child/Adolescent Parts of Self *protocol.*

Safe Places and Higher Powers for both Adult and younger parts of Self are not "etched in stone" as clients are told early in the AFTT-A process. Therapists consider the possibility that Child/Adolescent parts were able to sneak out of their Safe Places because their places and/or caregivers did not meet their needs for care and/or safety. Therapists guide clients to enlist the Competent Adult part of Self to talk to their younger parts about their experiences so far in their Safe Places with their Higher Powers. Sometimes, the place isn't protective enough and might need walls, force fields, or other types of enclosures to strengthen the safety aspect of the previously chosen place. Other times, the Child/Adolescent part's Higher Power wonderfully represents the qualities of love, acceptance, and encouragement but doesn't have the ability to set and maintain firm boundaries, to say "no" when it's time to tuck in. If the therapist or their client finds a weakness in either/both the Child/Adolescent part's Safe Place and Higher Power, they revisit the *Safe Place and Higher Power for Child/Adolescent Parts of Self* protocol illustrated in Chapter 9 to rework and strengthen the protective aspects of the previously installed Safe Place and Higher Powers.

11. Set Up a Plan for Communication Between the Adult and Child/Adolescent Parts While the Younger Part Remains in the Safe Place

Child/Adolescent parts in the AFTT-A model do not participate in Resource Team meetings and are not in charge of the subsequent phases of Eye Movement Desensitization and Reprocessing (EMDR) therapy. However, younger parts have information for clients and their therapists that is essential to completing the tasks of phases 3 to 8 of EMDR. They have traumatic memories and associated affect encapsulated in the neural networks of "Kid Brain" that need to be connected to and reprocessed through the AIP system in "Adult Brain." AFTT-A encourages clients to talk with Child/Adolescent parts while they are in their Safe Places with their Higher Powers. When younger parts are connected to a sense of nurturance and protection in the present moment, the likelihood decreases that time disorientation, flooding, or abreaction will occur.

The last step in the *Tucking the Child/Adolescent Part of Self Into the Safe Place* protocol is setting up a strategy for the younger part to use in communicating with the client's Competent Adult part of Self while remaining in their Safe Place without having to be present for or participate directly in Resource Team meetings or to take charge of reprocessing adverse events. Sometimes, a previously installed Resource Team member takes on the responsibility of being the Child/Adolescent part's intermediary. A new team member might be added to serve as the spokesperson or representative of younger parts; for example, guardian ad litem. Other times, devices are installed to facilitate the Child/Adolescent part's ability to share information necessary for clients to complete phases 3 to 8 of EMDR therapy.

POINTS TO REMEMBER

- Use intuition/mindful awareness when clients are talking about their lives/time in between sessions to notice "red flags" about the Child/Adolescent part being "out" or "eavesdropping" in present-day life. Be brave!
- In session, note changes in voice, body posture, facial expression, eye contact, getting stuck in negative cognitions, or looping during BLS sets as evidence of a younger part out of their Safe Place. Be brave!
- Young "Kid Brain" has magical thinking that "if only..." the client does this or that, their unmet childhood needs would be met in adult life. This helps avoid deep grief related to childhood losses.
- The dialogue is between the Adult and Child/Adolescent parts of Self, facilitated by the therapist, not between the parts and the therapist whether in room or with imagery.
- Teach and model kind compassion with firm insistence that Child/Adolescent part needs to return to the Safe Place. Use the example of putting a child to bed.
- Time orientation helps the Child/Adolescent part and Adult Self know the danger is past and differentiate between back then and now and good news/bad news.
- Rework the Child/Adolescent part's Safe Place and/or Higher Power if needed.
- Use short sets of slow BLS to reinforce the positive affect of the client sitting in the office, *not* of the Child Adolescent Part.

TROUBLESHOOTING

BOX 14.5 CLIENT EXAMPLE: ATTUNING TO THE CHILD PART OF SELF "SNEAKING" INTO A RESOURCE TEAM MEETING

I worked with a client who had difficulty using their Resource Team with their Competent Adult part of Self in present-day life. When they reported a situation between sessions when the Resource Team could have been involved but wasn't, we called a meeting with the Resource Team in their Meeting Place.

As the team meeting progressed, Resource Team members seemed to be saying all the right things, but something felt off to me. One of the Resource Team

(continued)

14. PARTS' WORK: TUCKING CHILD/ADOLESCENT PARTS OF SELF INTO SAFE PLACES

> **BOX 14.5 CLIENT EXAMPLE: ATTUNING TO THE CHILD PART OF SELF "SNEAKING" INTO A RESOURCE TEAM MEETING (continued)**
>
> members was a lizard from a C. S. Lewis story about redemption and resurrection that represented the transformed addict brain or the spiritual component of their addict part. While the client and the Resource Team were brainstorming ways they could connect in between sessions, I had a brief visual image of the lizard. Only my image showed a child-size pair of sneakers sticking out from under the lizard, like it was a costume rather than an actual reptile. I told the client about what I saw (yes, I was brave!) and they realized a younger part had disguised itself as the real lizard team member, insisting on being a part of the team and the team meeting. We used the *Tucking in Child/Adolescent Parts of Self* protocol to tuck the client's younger part, lizard costume and all, back into their Safe Place. Once my client had only adults on the Resource Team, they were able to access and apply inner resources to challenges in adult life.

- If the client has difficulty identifying triggered Child/Adolescent parts in their present-day life, normalize by giving examples of other clients' experiences, use stories mentioned in the chapter, or review Figure 7.3 P-A-C diagrams: Invalidating childhood environment.
- If a younger part of Self is reluctant to return to their Safe Place, suggest the client ask the part if there's something else they think is important for the client and/or therapist to know; review Child/Adolescent part's Safe Place and Higher Power to see if changes need to be made so the part's needs will be better met; or examine the relationship between the Adult and younger parts of Self to see if the client has become dependent on the Child/Adolescent part for the role that they have played and is reluctant to let the part return to their Safe Place.

PAUSE AND REFLECT FOR THE THERAPIST

At this point, take some time to think about a challenging client with whom you work, perhaps someone who has difficulty following through with assignments, is stuck and doesn't seem to be able to move forward, seems to need more than you can offer, or is critical of you as a therapist. Instead of focusing on the client, consider your own feelings and thoughts about and reactions to the client. Consider the possibility that at some point in sessions, a Child or Adolescent part tugs at your therapist brain wanting attention, getting angry or impatient, or panicking. Dividing your attention between your younger part and what's happening in the therapy session interferes with your capability to be present with the client. If that's true, go through the steps of the *Tucking the Child/Adolescent Part of Self Into the Safe Place* protocol, with your Competent Adult part of Self dialoguing with the Child/Adolescent part of you triggered by therapy with your client.

Notice the ways you can tell that your Child/Adolescent part is "out." Become aware of how the younger part responds to being tucked back in. Observe how you feel when that younger part of you is tucked in. Prior to your next session with the client, check on your Child/Adolescent part to make sure they're in their Safe Place. If not, take a few moments to tuck that Child Adolescent part back into their Safe Place, reassuring them that you as a therapist have what you need to handle the therapy session and that even if you make a mistake, nothing bad will happen to them.

USEFUL TERMS AND DEFINITIONS

"Adult Brain": The parts of the brain that house EMDR's adaptive information processing (AIP) system and include higher cognitive processes such as learning, problem-solving, decision-making, language, understanding of emotions, and narrative memory.

AFTT-A: Attachment-Focused Trauma Therapy for Adults

AIP system: adaptive information processing system

BLS: bilateral stimulation

DID: dissociative identity disorder

"Kid Brain": The neural network clusters in the emotional/social part of the brain that store unprocessed memories of adverse events and are disconnected from a sense of time and from the parts of the brain capable of processing memories and transferring them into narrative memory. AFTT-A views the neural networks as encapsulating more than memories of adverse events and includes the experiences, cognitive development, learning during a particular client age.

P-A-C diagram: Parent-Adult-Child diagram

PROTOCOL SCRIPT 11. TUCKING THE CHILD/ADOLESCENT PART OF SELF INTO THE SAFE PLACE

Adapted from Berne, E. (1964). *Games people play: The basic handbook of transactional analysis.* Random House; Bradshaw, J. (1990). *Homecoming: Reclaiming and healing your inner child.* Bantam Publishing; Fraser, G. A. (1991). The Dissociative Table Technique: A strategy for working with ego states and dissociative disorders and ego-state therapy. *Dissociation: Progress in the Dissociative Disorders,* 4(4), 205–213; Fraser, G. A. (2003). Fraser's "Dissociative Table Technique" revisited, revised: A strategy for working with ego states in dissociative disorders and ego-state therapy. *Journal of Trauma and Dissociation,* 4(4), 5–28. https://doi.org/10.1300/J229v04n04_02; Martin, K. (2018, April). *Mastering the treatment of complex trauma: transforming theory into practice.* Presentation, Omaha, Nebraska; and Potter, A. E. (1994). *Inside out: rebuilding self and personality through inner child therapy* (therapist manual and client workbook). Taylor and Francis Group.

1. Discuss the Child/Adolescent Part's Involvement in and Impact on the Therapy Session or Present-Day Life. Say… "We've talked about parts of your internal personality system especially when we looked at the *Parent-Adult-Child (P-A-C)* diagrams and about how your experiences growing up affected the way those parts of you developed, the way you think and feel about yourself and others, and how you look at and react in relationships in your life today. We're going to focus on the Child/Adolescent part of you today, learn how that part of you still impacts your adult life, and how to separate your younger part from your Adult part and life. We want to free that Competent Adult part of Self to be in charge of the choices you make in current situations. As we've said before, Child/Adolescent parts of Self have unmet needs from childhood and have the mistaken idea—from that child-like magical thinking—that they can somehow get those unmet childhood needs met in your present-day relationships. You, in your Competent Adult part of Self, know that's not possible but the Child/Adolescent parts don't realize that. As a result, you often are trying to manage your life today while, at the same time, trying to respond to the Child/Adolescent parts' feelings and demands. You end up feeling torn between getting your needs met as an adult and trying to placate the younger part of you who has very different motives than you do in your current relationships.

"The first step in helping the Adult part of you get back in charge of your internal system as well as your present-day life is to identify when a younger part of you has 'snuck out' of their Safe Place and is 'eavesdropping' on your adult life, thinking they need to step in and help you with whatever is going on in the moment." *Ask...* "What signs have you identified so far that clues you into the possibility that a younger part of you is involved in your feelings?"

___

___

2. Identify the Child/Adolescent Part in Session or Through the Client's Description of Events Between Sessions. *When you note a possible Child/Adolescent part in session or the possibility of a Child/Adolescent part's involvement in the client's adult life as they report about their time between sessions, ask...* "I wonder how you were feeling?" or "What came up for you?"

___

___

Ask... "How old do you feel when you describe (*repeat client's clue to Child/Adolescent part's involvement*)?"

___

___

If the identified Child/Adolescent part does not already have a Safe Place and Higher Power, return to the Safe Place and Higher Power for Child/Adolescent Parts of Self *protocol. If the Child/Adolescent part already has a Safe Place and Higher Power, continue with the protocol. Say...* "It seems like that younger part of you thinks they needed to leave their Safe Place. Where do you think we would we find your Child/Adolescent part?"

___

___

3. Invite the Client to Bring Forward Their Competent Adult and True Parent Parts of Self to Talk to the Child/Adolescent Part With Their Higher Power Figure. *Say...* "Let's talk about how you can approach your Child/Adolescent part so that they can get tucked back into their Safe Place. Who do you think needs to go with you to talk to the younger part of you?"

___

___

Say... "How does your Child/Adolescent part need to be approached so they can feel as safe and comfortable as possible?"

_____
_____

Say... "Imagine going up to your Child/Adolescent part." *Ask...* "How does the younger you seem to feel about meeting you?"

_____
_____

Ask... "How do *you* feel as you talk to your Child/Adolescent part?"

_____
_____

Access and reinforce the client's positive affect with short sets of slow BLS with tappers or butterfly taps. Practice the container for setting aside the negative affect if needed.

4. Find Out Reasons for the Child/Adolescent Part Getting Triggered/"Sneaking Out" of Safe Place. *Say...* "Child/Adolescent parts usually think they have pretty good reason for coming out of their Safe Places. How about asking that younger part if it would be okay to talk about why they needed to leave their Safe Place? I'd like to invite you to ask the younger part of you what they thought was important to tell you."

_____
_____

5. Link the Child/Adolescent Part's Cognitions and Behavior With Past Roles, Beliefs, and Fears. *Say...* "The younger part of you doesn't know that it's 'now' and not 'back then' anymore. They don't know that the danger is past. They only have the experiences, the beliefs, the learned patterns of behavior, and the feelings that you had at that age." *Invite the client to talk to the Child/Adolescent part about what they need to hear to feel reassured. Access and reinforce client's positive affect with short sets of slow BLS.*

_____
_____

6. Thank the Child/Adolescent Part for Giving Information and Bringing Issue to the Attention of the Client and Therapist. *Say...* "The Child/Adolescent parts of Self really believe that people need them in their adult lives to stay safe, to get ahead, to keep from being hurt, or to be loved and accepted. Your Child/Adolescent part believes that the only way you'll be okay and everything will be fine is if you follow the old Bonding Contract rules and use old behaviors just one more time." *Invite the client* to talk with and thank the Child/Adolescent part about how they tried to help the client in their life.*

Access and reinforce the client's positive affect with short sets of slow BLS.

7. Reset Boundaries With the Child/Adolescent Part by the Adult Part of Self. *Say...* "I'd like you to tell your Child/Adolescent part that it's time for them go back to their Safe Place with their Higher Power." *Ask...* "What does that younger part of you need to hear so they can get tucked back into their Safe Place?"

Ask... "How do you feel about being able to tuck the younger part of you back into their Safe Place with their Higher Power? How do you feel when you see your Child/Adolescent part get reconnected to the sense of nurturing and protection?"

Access and reinforce the client's positive affect with short sets of slow BLS.

8. Reinforce the Truth About Unmet Childhood Needs and Losses. *Say...* "So, there's good news and there's bad news. The *bad* news is that no matter what your Child/Adolescent part tries to do in your present-day life, your childhood needs will never be met. The adults in your life blew the chance to meet your needs when you were that age so the time to get childhood needs met is over. The *good* news is that no matter what your Child/Adolescent part tries to do in your present-day life, your unmet childhood needs will never be met! Instead, your younger part gets all their needs met in the present moment when they stay in their Safe Place, and *you* are able to meet your adulthood needs with the help of your Competent Adult part of Self, your Resource Team, and your Higher Power. From now on, the only job your Child/Adolescent part has is to stay in their Safe Place with their Higher Power and be whatever age they are." *Access and reinforce client's positive affect with short sets of slow BLS.*

9. Reassure the Child/Adolescent Part That the Danger Is in the Past. *Say...* "When your Child/Adolescent part sneaks out of their Safe Place and into your adult life, they're stuck in the past and really believe that something bad will happen to them or to you if they don't warn or help you like they always have." *Ask...* "How can you soothe and reassure your younger part that they are safe and loved in the present moment and that the danger is past?"

Ask… "How does your Child/Adolescent part feel about what you said?"

_____

_____

Ask… "How do you feel to be able to calm and reassure the younger part of yourself?"

_____

_____

Access and reinforce the client's positive affect with short sets of slow BLS.

10. Review the Child/Adolescent Part's Safe Place and Higher Power to Ensure Their Nurturing and Protective Qualities Meet the Child/Adolescent Part's Needs. Make Sure That the Higher Power Knows How to Be Reassuring and Protective When the Child/Adolescent Part Has an Urge to Eavesdrop in the Client's Adult Life. *Say…* "Let's look at the Safe Place and Higher Power we gave your Child/Adolescent part." *Ask…* "Is there anything about them that needs to be changed to be more protective and reassuring to your younger part?"

_____

_____

If yes, rework with Safe Place and Higher Power for Child/Adolescent Parts of Self *protocol. If no, continue with the protocol.*

11. Set Up Plan for Communication Between the Adult and Child/Adolescent Parts While the Child/Adolescent Part of Self Remains in the Safe Place. *Say…* "We've talked about how we don't have Child/Adolescent parts involved in Resource Team meetings, running your present-day life, and being in charge of reprocessing traumatic memories in therapy. So, let's find a way for the Child/Adolescent part of you to communicate with you and your Resource Team without having to leave their Safe Place. Let's brainstorm with your Resource Team the best ways for your younger part to pass on important information while staying in their Safe Place with their Higher Power."

_____

_____

Ask… "What does the younger part of you think of the ideas? Is there anything that needs to be changed?"

_____

_____

Say… "Imagine practicing the new way of communicating with your Child/Adolescent part so they can share information with you and/or your Resource Team." *Ask…* "How does the younger part of you seem to feel about what you've set up?"

_____

_____

Ask... "How do *you* feel about the new way of communicating with your Child/Adolescent part?"

_____

_____

Access and reinforce the client's positive affect with short sets of slow BLS.

Ask... "Is there anything that needs to be said or done to complete the scene?"

_____

_____

Strengthen and reinforce the positive affect with short sets of slow BLS.

REFERENCES

Erikson, E. (1993). *Child and society* (2nd ed.). W. W. Norton & Company.

Freud, S. (1990). *Beyond the Pleasure Principle*. W. W. Norton & Company.

Martin, K. M. (2012). How to use Fraser's Dissociative Table Technique to access and work with emotional parts of the personality. *Journal of EMDR Practice and Research, 6*(4), 179–186. https://doi.org/10.1891/1933-3196.6.4.179

Martin, K. (2018, April). *Mastering the treatment of complex trauma: Transforming theory into practice*. Presentation, Omaha, Nebraska.

Piaget, J. & Inhelder, B. (1969). *The psychology of the child*. Basic Books, Inc.

CHAPTER 15

Revising the Early Bonding Contract Rules in Attachment-Focused Trauma Therapy for Adults

INTRODUCTION

Infants are born with an innate knowledge that they need closeness and connection with their parents to survive. Any threat of disconnection from their parents naturally triggers a fear response. When young children sense their parents' love and commitment, their fear is replaced with feelings of security and safety. Infants soon discover that their behaviors can impact parents' interactions with them, either negatively or positively. By the time they are toddlers, they've adapted their behaviors to maximize closeness with their parents.

Not all parents respond similarly to the job of caring for an infant. Infants and young children learn through trial and error what works and what doesn't work to keep their parents close. What works and doesn't work is different depending on the background of the parents. Parents usually intend to do the best they can, but they are naturally impacted by patterns that developed even during their own childhood attachment relationships. Parents who are uncomfortable with infants' range of emotions and with the intimacy of caring for an infant get more distant when the infant expresses emotions and needs. Their infants learn to suppress their feelings and needs to keep their parents staying closer. The infants learn to exhibit minimal emotions, even when distressed.

Some parents are comfortable with closeness and affection but get overwhelmed with their own frequent feelings of distress. Subsequently, their responsiveness to their infants' needs is intermittent and depends upon the parents' emotional state. By the time they are toddlers, the infants have learned to express their needs and emotions with volume and intensity to get the attention they need.

Children are wired for survival, and their strategies feel to them as necessary as breathing. Other common strategies that may work or be added as children get older include becoming ill or helpless to elicit caregiving from a parent or becoming a caregiver or pseudo-partner for the parent. Some children learn that being a high achiever earns the closeness they want, and other children discover staying in conflict with a parent keeps them close. The unconscious rules that children develop may work for their specific situations growing up, but the strategies definitely become obstacles to healthy relationships in adulthood.

The term *Early Bonding Contract* (Cramer, 1992; Wildwind, 1992) refers to the unconscious rules or strategies that young children adopt for keeping their parents close or *bonded* in whatever way is possible for the situation. It's an unspoken contract that feels immutable from a very young age.

ATTACHMENT PATTERNS THROUGH THE LENS OF THE EARLY BONDING CONTRACT

One way to look at attachment categories of infancy and childhood is through the lens of the Early Bonding Contract. Already, at 12 to 18 months of age, patterns of attachment can be identified by observing toddlers' behaviors with their mothers during the Strange Situation assessment (Ainsworth & Bell, 1970). During the Strange Situation assessment, the toddler is stressed by steps in the procedure involving the parent leaving and the stranger entering the room. The most significant moment in the assessment is the reunification with the parent. The toddler's behaviors upon the parent's return can be categorized as secure attachment or nonsecure attachment. The two nonsecure responses include the ambivalent/resistant pattern and the avoidant pattern. Ambivalent/resistant and avoidant patterns are strategies that help the infant keep the parent as close as possible. In addition to one of the three primary categories, the infant may show signs of attachment disorganization. Disorganization is not a strategy, but a sign that strategies have failed and the infant is experiencing fear (Liotti, 2004; Lyons-Ruth & Jacobvitz, 2016).

Secure toddlers of secure parents go immediately to the parent upon the parent's return at the end of the Strange Situation assessment. They are easily soothed by the parent. The secure parent is comfortable with the toddler's needs and with providing comfort through physical closeness, eye contact, and soothing words. The toddler has developed an Early Bonding Contract that gives them permission to seek comfort and closeness when needed from the parent. The parent is responsive and doesn't pull away, which lowers the toddler's anxiety about getting their needs met from the parent. The Early Bonding Contract rules allow secure children to have healthy relationships into adulthood.

Nonsecure, avoidant toddlers have learned that direct expression of needs is not helpful. Their parent, influenced by their own attachment experiences, pulls away in response to their child's cries, leaving the toddler in more distress. The toddler learns to repress their needs and turn off their cries for greater success with keeping the parent nearby. Later, as an adult, the Child parts of Self continue to repress emotions and needs for emotional closeness. Any attempts to change the avoidance in favor of shared emotional intimacy will trigger anxiety for the Child parts of Self. In adulthood, the strategy becomes the dismissive attachment pattern.

Nonsecure, ambivalent/resistant toddlers have learned that their parent is responsive and affectionate some of the time and unresponsive at other times. The parent's response is unpredictable. The strategy for the toddler is to up their game for getting their needs met. The Early Bonding Contract is all about making the demands louder and longer, as any amount of attention, if not affection, is better than no attention in that moment. In adulthood, the Child parts of Self remain vigilant about keeping others close and getting their needs met. Attempts to relax and let go of the relationship vigilance paradoxically raises anxiety for the Child parts of Self. In adulthood, the strategy becomes the preoccupied attachment pattern.

There's a caveat to the continuity of avoidant or ambivalent/resistant strategies. Sometimes, cultural pressures in adolescence create a shift in strategies. For example, an adolescent who loudly makes demands for attention or assistance from others may be looked down upon by peers who view independence as more acceptable and "cool." By shutting down their feelings and stepping into a persona of independence and autonomy to match their peers, they can keep their peers closer. However, in adulthood, either the bonding rules of the avoidant Adolescent part of Self or the earlier bonding rules of the resistant-ambivalent younger Child part of Self may be triggered, depending upon the circumstances and the relationship.

The disorganized pattern is observed in a smaller percentage of toddlers. Main and Solomon (1990) observed toddlers covering their head with their hands, twirling, walking, or crawling backward, flapping their arms or looking disorganized in other ways when the mothers re-entered the room. In long-term studies, as disorganized toddlers reach preschool age, they become either controlling/caregiving or controlling/punishing toward their parent. As they reach adolescence and adulthood, the disorganization raises their risk for dissociative disorders (Lyons-Ruth & Jacobvitz, 2016). In adulthood, the Child parts of Self hold anxiety and disorganization, interfering with developing trust in adulthood relationships.

OBSTACLES IN ADULTHOOD

In adulthood, younger parts that abide by a nonsecure or disorganized Early Bonding Contract will likely be triggered by present-day partner, friendship, work, and parent/child relationships. Dismissive attachment patterns can cause a partner to feel a lack of emotional intimacy. Preoccupied patterns in adulthood can lead to frustration and conflict. Disorganization can lead to triggers and intense reactions that are confusing to partners and others.

Direct attempts to help adult clients change their patterns in relationships may be met with conscious or unconscious resistance. For the Child parts of Self, the rules of the Early Bonding Contract feel necessary to survival. Adulthood attempts to change the old rules to something healthier may trigger anxiety for the younger parts because they perceive the old rules as the only way to avoid getting hurt.

OVERVIEW OF STEPS FOR REVISING THE EARLY BONDING CONTRACT

The Attachment-Focused Trauma Therapy for Adults (AFTT-A) *Revising the Early Bonding Contract Rules* protocol utilizes dialogue between the Adult part of Self and the Child part of Self and a modification of the Eye Movement Desensitization and Reprocessing (EMDR) Future Rehearsal to calm anxiety and allow the development of healthy interpersonal patterns. The first step involves a collaboration between therapist and client to identify the client's Bonding Contract early rules and desired new rules for the future. The therapist facilitates messages from the Adult part of Self to younger parts of Self that provide reassurance that it's okay to change. A Future Rehearsal, adapted from Popky's (2005) future state protocol within his

DeTUR model, is implemented that takes place "at some point in the future" when all associated anxiety is resolved. Slow bilateral stimulation (BLS) is used to reduce anxiety and deepen positive affect. Paradoxically, permission not to change the rules often leads to changing the rules. Following are the steps for the *Revising the Early Bonding Contract Rules* protocol (see Protocol Script 12 at the end of this chapter).

STEPS FOR REVISING THE EARLY BONDING CONTRACT

1. Explanation
Explain the purpose of the Early Bonding Contract and the reason the relationship patterns are so difficult to change. Emphasize that the client's patterns in interpersonal relationships may have been effective for getting needs met the best they could when they were young. Explain that some measure of proximity, some type of bond, and some amount of attention feels better to young children than feeling all alone.

2. Brainstorm the Early Bonding Contract Rules
Make sure the client is in their Competent Adult part of Self by shifting their body into a posture associated with the positive state, using their cue word, or using a competency memory. Once the client is operating from their Competent Adult part of Self, suggest they reflect upon their childhood relationship patterns and how their behaviors may have helped reduce their anxiety about rejection or abandonment. Next, suggest they reflect upon the way in which those patterns may show up in adulthood. The clinician shows the client Table 15.1 "Common Early Bonding Contract Rules and Possible New Rules" to help. Note that the Early Bonding Contract rules are negative cognitions (NCs) that involve interpersonal behaviors clients may feel compelled to carry out during their interpersonal relationships.

3. Brainstorm Hypothetical New Rules
Remind the client that this next step does not involve changing any behaviors. Suggest the client think about rules for behaving in relationships that would lead to healthier interactions at some point in the future when they no longer fear the changes. Make a list of the client's preferred new rules. Note that new rules are positive cognitions (PCs) that involve healthy interpersonal behaviors. Refer again to Table 15.1 to help.

4. Facilitate a Dialogue Between the Adult Part of Self and the Child/Adolescent Part of Self
Ask the client how old they usually feel when they get anxious about their relationships. It's fine if more than one Child part is identified. Ask the Competent Adult part of Self to visualize the Child part of Self in their Safe Place (see Protocol Script 5). Encourage the Adult part to dialogue with the Child part and reassure the younger part there will be no repercussions for them related to any changes the adult client makes in the future. Furthermore, the younger part won't have to do anything at all. Facilitate reassuring dialogue with other young parts as needed. Add slow BLS throughout the guided imagery and the reassuring dialogue to reinforce and deepen the internal messages. Afterward, ask the client to notice the felt sense and reinforce with a short, slow set of BLS.

Table 15.1 Early Bonding Contract Rules and Possible New Rules

Common Early Bonding Contract Rules	Possible New Rules
I must...	Now I can...
watch your face to anticipate what you need.	let go of watching your face.
change myself to make you happy with me.	make my own decision about what to change.
be perfect and not make mistakes.	make mistakes.
achieve and perform for you.	achieve when it's important to me.
not make waves.	voice my opinions and disagree.
tolerate mistreatment.	stop tolerating mistreatment.
keep from being noticed.	call attention to myself in a positive way.
be silent.	be as loud as I want to be.
take care of my own needs by myself.	allow others to know what I need.
take care of all of your needs.	both give and receive support.
stay at a distance.	be close to someone when it's right for me.
not ask for help.	ask for help.
not show or ask for affection.	show or ask for affection.
not trouble you with my needs or feelings.	go to those I trust and share what I need or feel.
not show vulnerability.	experience vulnerable feelings.
not get angry.	feel and express anger appropriately.
hide my talents.	let my talents show.
not be successful.	enjoy my successes.
not be happy or playful.	be happy and playful.
be a clown.	be myself.
be sick/helpless to get attention.	find connections when I'm healthy.
act out to get attention.	ask for what I need, even when I'm quiet.
have meltdowns to get attention.	find healthy reciprocal relationships.
be in control of you.	let others be.
take care of you to be connected to you.	develop closeness with healthy others.
be loud and demanding so you will listen.	find others who can listen when I'm quiet.
stay in conflict with you to remain connected.	find healthy others for positive connections.
denigrate you to feel safe and in control.	find others with whom I feel safe and in control.
hurt you when I feel hurt to feel in control.	treat others well and find reciprocal relationships.

Source: Adapted from Cramer, B. G. (1992). *The importance of being baby: The scripts parents write and the roles babies play.* Addison-Wesley; and Wildwind, L. (1992). *Treating chronic depression.* EMDRIA Conference, Sunnydale, California.

5. Run the Future Movie on a Screen While Applying Slow BLS

Identify present-day relationships that present challenges for the client. These relationships may include a partner, parent, child, friend, supervisor, or coworker. Ask the client to choose one individual for the exercise. Explain they will be viewing themselves, as an adult, at some point in the future when all anxiety is resolved and they are ready to adopt the new rules. Explain that they will see themselves in a room with the individual on a movie screen. They won't need to visualize any interactions or behaviors or "do anything" in particular during the mental movie Suggest the client observe their body posture, facial expression, or voice tone on the movie screen. Ask permission to add slow BLSs throughout.

Initiate the visualization of the movie on the screen while you read slowly through the chosen "new rules" and apply a set of slow BLS throughout to help lower anxiety and internalize the new rules. Stop the BLS and check in regarding what the client is feeling. If the response is positive or neutral, suggest they "just notice that" and add another slow, short set of BLS. If the client reports any anxiety during the mental movie, direct the client to fast forward the movie farther into the future when their anxiety is resolved.

6. Step Into the Movie and Deepen the Positive Shift With Slow BLS
Repeat the movie exercise, but with directions to step into the future movie and experiment with how it feels instead of being an observer. Remind the client that this is only an experiment and that it is taking place in the future when all anxiety has been resolved. There is nothing they need to change in the present day. Suggest the client notice how their body feels, how their face feels, and how their voice feels during the future mental movie. Next, read the new rules and apply slow BLS. Check in as to any emotions or sensations. If the client reports positive emotions or sensations, deepen the experience with a short set of slow BLS.

> **BOX 15.1 CLIENT EXAMPLE: CHANGING THE EARLY BONDING CONTRACT RULES**
>
> When this client first entered therapy, they stated that they wanted to work through grief over their father's death. The client claimed their relationship with their partner was positive but admitted they had never felt safe in their relationship with their mother. Over time, I (D.W.) discovered that the client was excessively pleasing toward both their mother and their partner. The client became disorganized and disoriented when discussing early negative experiences with their mother. I hypothesized that the client had an unresolved/disorganized attachment pattern related to their early relationship with their mother. After the client worked to strengthen their Competent Adult part of Self and build a safe and nurturing system for their younger parts of Self, they identified their Early Bonding Contract as, "I must continually change to be who you want me to be," "It's my job to keep you happy," and "I have to set aside my own needs and feelings." The client identified possible new rules might be: "It's my job to keep myself happy," "I can decide what to change," and "My needs and feelings are also important." I facilitated some dialogue between the Adult and the Child parts. The client's Adult part of Self reassured their Child part of Self that there would be no consequences for the Child part if they were to do some things differently. I applied a short set of slow tactile BLS to deepen the positive shift. I then read the client's new rules while they visualized themselves with their mother "at some point in the future when all their anxiety was resolved." Slow BLS was added throughout. We conducted the imagery a second time, but this time the client imagined themself with their partner as I read through the new rules. Soon after we worked on revising the client's Early Bonding Contract, the client revealed longstanding serious abuse by their partner. Soon after that, they started steps toward divorce. The client is now married and living happily in a healthy, mutually supportive marriage. According to the client, their relationship with their mother has improved to the point that they are enjoying their time together.

POINTS TO REMEMBER

- The Early Bonding Contract rules develop because they have worked or partially worked at some point in early childhood for achieving some measure of connection or decrease in anxiety about rejection. Even though the Early Bonding Contract rules create problems in satisfaction with present-day relationships, attempts to change the rules trigger fears of rejection or abandonment held by one or more Child parts of Self.
- Clients with preoccupied patterns will tend to choose Early Bonding Contract rules to demand, cling, control, or fix others in their relationships. Clients with avoidant patterns tend to choose Early Bonding Contract rules that reduce vulnerability through keeping others at a distance, derogating some others, idealizing some others, or avoiding feelings.
- Child parts of different ages may operate with different bonding rules, in which case clients may use some combination of the two types of patterns in their present-day relationships.
- The protocol should be presented as an experiment to see how it might feel to adopt the new rules at some future time when it feels fine to do so.
- The future mental movie is nondirective. The protocol gives clients permission to take their time and to envision it their own way.
- Ensure that the client is operating from the most Competent Adult part of Self to conduct the protocol. The Child part(s) are reassured and tucked into their Safe Places to reduce triggering childhood fears.

TROUBLESHOOTING

If the client reports anxiety, you can say…

- "Use your cue word and your body posture and make sure you are in your Competent Adult part of Self."
- "Check inside. Are all Kid parts tucked into Safe Places? Are all kid parts aware that this is your adult life and your adult body?"
- "I'd like you to push the movie farther into the future—a distant future when anxiety is resolved."
- "Invite your Child part to look through your eyes at your hands and notice that these are grownup hands. Notice the rings you now wear. Look through your eyes at your feet. They are grownup feet. Take your time."
- "Are there other younger parts who need to be tucked in before we continue this exercise?"

PAUSE AND REFLECT FOR THE THERAPIST

- Look over the lists of Early Bonding Contract rules and preferred new rules and reflect on what helped you in your relationship with your parents in your earliest years. Think of the clients you have identified as most personally challenging. How might your old rules be getting in the way of providing secure responses to nonsecure behaviors or statements by your clients? What are the new rules that you would like to adopt for yourself? Write them down.

- Use your body posture, cue word, or competent adult memory to step into your Competent Adult part of Self. Visualize your Child part of Self in the Safe Place with your Higher Power/Caregiver. Dialogue internally and let your Child part of Self know that any changes you make are inconsequential for the child.
- See yourself on the movie screen in the future, in your office, with one of your clients. This is a future time when you have no anxiety about adopting the new rules. Notice your body, your face, your voice.
- Step into the movie and notice how it feels in your body. If you notice any positive emotions or sensations, deepen the response with some slow self-tapping. If you have a negative response, shift into a posture associated with your Competent Adult part of Self and move the movie farther into the future, when you have the capacity to adopt the new rules. Notice any positive shift and deepen it in with a short set of slow BLS.

USEFUL TERMS AND DEFINITIONS

AFTT-A: Attachment-Focused Trauma Therapy for Adults

BLS: bilateral stimulation

EMDR: Eye Movement Desensitization and Reprocessing

NC: negative cognition

PC: positive cognition

RDI: Resource Development and Installation

PROTOCOL SCRIPT 12. REVISING THE EARLY BONDING CONTRACT RULES

Adapted from Cramer, B. G. (1992). *The importance of being baby: The scripts parents write and the roles babies play.* Addison-Wesley; Popky, A. J. (2005). DeTUR, an urge reduction protocol for addictions and dysfunctional behaviors. In R. Shapiro (Ed.), *EMDR solutions: Pathways to healing* (pp. 167–188). W. W. Norton & Company; and Wildwind, L. (1992). *Treating chronic depression.* EMDRIA Conference, Sunnydale, California.

1. **Explanation.** *Say...*"I'd like to talk about something called the Early Bonding Contract today; is that okay with you?"

"Before we start, you might want to make sure you're fully in your Competent Adult part of Self, perhaps by shifting your body posture (see Protocol Script 11). Does that feel okay to you?" _____ "I think of the Early Bonding Contract as a set of rules that young children adopt to get their parents to bond with them or meet their needs as best as they can. Babies are born with an innate sense that they'll die without closeness to the parent. They're born with a fundamental need to love and be loved and a fear of being unloved and abandoned. All parents, of course, have vulnerabilities or off days that lead to occasional misattunement with their infants or young children. Difficulties start when parents have mood problems or carry attachment issues from their own upbringing that get in the way of meeting their child's needs with consistency. The good news is that babies and toddlers are resilient and learn the best ways to seek comfort and attention that get them more of what they need, at least in some way. Through trial and error, young children find what works best to keep their parents nearby or showing attention in some way or other. These relationship patterns make up the 'Early Bonding Contract' rules. The patterns or rules are linked to survival, so they're hard to give up and tend to carry over into adulthood relationships later on.

"Unfortunately, the rules usually don't work well in adult relationships, but attempts to change the patterns trigger panic in the Child/Adolescent part of the brain. The Child/Adolescent part believes *'I have to follow these rules, or I'll end up all alone.'* Do you think it's worth exploring whether you might be operating from some old Early Bonding Contract rules?"

_____

_____

2. Brainstorm the Early Bonding Contract Rules. *Say…*"Make sure you're in your most Competent Adult part of Self, perhaps by getting into your Competent Adult posture, so you can consider your Early Bonding Contract rules from your present-day adult perspective. Keep in mind that I'm not going to ask you to change anything today. Perhaps you can think a bit about how you were with your parents as a young child. What were the things you did that might have helped you get their attention or helped you avoid rejection?" (*The clinician shows the client Table 15.1 "Early Bonding Rules and Possible New Rules"*). "If you had some healthy methods for getting the closeness or attention you needed, we'll discuss those, too." (*On a separate paper, write down the rules that resonate for the client.*)

"I'd like you to look at these old rules and reflect on which of them might be getting in the way in your present-day adult relationships. I'll make an asterisk beside the rules that are causing present-day problems. I can also add any relationship rules you think of that you may have added on in your adult life. I can note 'sometimes' next to the ones that come up for you only occasionally."

3. Brainstorm Hypothetical New Rules. *Say…*"Let's look at the list of Early Bonding Contract rules. There's no need to make any changes to your rules right now, but at some point in the future, when it feels okay to change the way you respond in your adulthood relationships, which rules would you keep and which would you let go?"

"Let's look at the chart again." (*Together, look at Table 15.1 again.*) "Which of these new rules would you like to adopt? You might also think of some that aren't on this list." (***Write down preferred new rules.***) "Again, there's no need to change anything in your adult relationships right now."

4. Facilitate a Dialogue Between the Adult Part of Self and the Child/Adolescent Part of Self.
Say... "Check once again to make sure you're in your Competent Adult part of Self, right now. Now, see if you can let yourself touch on the anxiety that comes up when you think of making changes in the way you interact with others. How old does that make you feel?" _____ "Now, shift your body posture to make sure you're solidly back into your Competent Adult part of Self. Let me know when you feel grounded in your Adult state." (*Pause.*) "I'll guide you in some reassuring dialogue with the Child/Adolescent part of you, if that's okay with you." (*Pause.*) "I'll add a little slow BLS to reinforce the reassuring messages." (***Add slow BLS while guiding the client's inner dialogue.***) "See your Child/Adolescent part of Self in the Safe Place." (*See Protocol Script 5.*) "Remind the Child/Adolescent part of you to stay safe and sound in the Safe Place with the loving Higher Power/Caregiver figure. Reassure the Child/Adolescent part of you that although you might make some changes in the way you interact with others in the future, the Child/Adolescent won't have to make any changes, and the Child/Adolescent won't have any consequences because of changes you make." (*Stop BLS.*) "How did that go?"

5. Run the Future Movie on a Screen While Applying Slow BLS.
Say... "What are some present-day relationships that you find at least somewhat challenging?"

"As an experiment, I'd like you to choose just one of these relationships—one that is a little challenging but not highly distressing—for a little imagery exercise. Who would you like to pick?" _____ "I'm going to ask you to see yourself in a room with that person, not doing anything in particular, while I read through the new rules. I'd like you to just notice your body posture, facial expression, and possibly voice. I'll add slow BLS throughout if it's okay with you." _____ "Okay, now, create the movie screen and see yourself on the screen in the same room with (*chosen individual*). This is taking place in the future—down the road, when you've already adopted the new rules and feel no anxiety about the changes. You don't need to visualize saying or doing anything specific. You might just be curious about your body posture, your facial expression, and possibly voice tone in the movie. While you look at the future movie, I'll read through your chosen new rules and add slow BLS to deepen the effects." (*Add slow BLS while reading through the client's preferred new rules.*) "Take a pause. How did that go?" _____ "Did you notice anything about your body posture, your expression, or your voice?"

_____

_____

If the client reports anxiety during the mental movie, say… "Check your posture and use your cue word to make sure you are in your most Adult part of Self. Next, check inside and make sure all Child/Adolescent parts are tucked in. Next, fast forward the movie on the screen farther into the future, all the way to a distant future when your anxiety is resolved and we'll try it one more time, just briefly." (*Repeat guided imagery.*)

6. Step Into the Movie and Deepen the Positive Shift With Slow BLS.
Say… "This time, I'd like you to experiment with stepping into the movie instead of watching the movie. You're just trying it out. The movie is still taking place in the future. You're still in the room with the chosen individual, and you don't have to *do* anything at all. Just be curious about how your body and face and voice *feel* in this future scene. I'll read through the new rules and add a slow set of BLS." (*Add slow BLS while reading the new rules again.*) "How do you feel? What do you notice?"_____ *If positive, say…* "Let's deepen that." (*Add a slow, short set of BLS.*)

REFERENCES

Ainsworth, M. D., & Bell, S. M. (1970). Attachment, exploration, and separation: Illustrated by the behavior of one-year-olds in a strange situation. *Child Development*, 41(1), 49–67. https://doi.org/10.2307/1127388

Cramer, B. G. (1992). *The importance of being baby: The scripts parents write and the roles babies play*. Addison-Wesley.

Liotti, G. (2004). Trauma, dissociation, and disorganized attachment: Three strands of a single braid. *Psychotherapy: Theory, Research, Practice, Training*, 41(4), 472–486. https://doi.org/10.1037/0033-3204.41.4.472

Main, M., & Solomon, J. (1990). Procedures for identifying infants as disorganized/disoriented during the ainsworth strange situation. In M. T. Greenberg, C. Dante, & E. M. Cummings (Eds.), *Attachment in the preschool years: Theory, research, and intervention* (pp. 121–160). University of Chicago Press.

Popky, A. J. (2005). DeTUR, an urge reduction protocol for addictions and dysfunctional behaviors. In R. Shapiro (Ed.), *EMDR solutions: Pathways to healing* (pp. 167–188). W. W. Norton & Company.

Lyons-Ruth, K., & Jacobvitz, D. (2016). Attachment disorganization from infancy to adulthood: Neurobiological correlates, parenting contexts, and pathways to disorder. In J. Cassidy & P. Shaver (Eds.), *Handbook of attachment: Theory, research, and clinical applications* (3rd ed., pp. 667–695). Guilford Press.

Wildwind, L. (1992). *Treating chronic depression*. EMDRIA Conference, Sunnydale, California.

CHAPTER 16

EMDR Therapeutic Story Method in Attachment-Focused Trauma Therapy for Adults

INTRODUCTION

The Adult Attachment Interview (AAI) is a structured interview that is scored to identify secure, nonsecure preoccupied, nonsecure dismissive, or unresolved/disorganized categories of attachment in adult subjects. The unresolved/disorganized attachment pattern is evident during the AAI (Main & Hesse, 1990) when discussion related to unresolved loss or childhood abuse triggers disorientation and disorganization in the subject's use of language. For example, the subject may confuse pronouns, become confused about the sequence of events, or irrationally blame themselves for getting abused. In therapy, the mental disorganization may be evident during history taking or a general discussion related to traumatic events, or when the therapist refers to a person or event that is triggering. Outside of therapy, the mental disorganization may show up anytime the traumatic event is triggered by conscious or subconscious reminders during interactions with children, partners, parents, or others. Outside of situations that trigger the abuse or loss memories, the client may exhibit either secure or nonsecure patterns.

RATIONALE FOR USE OF THE THERAPEUTIC STORY

Lovett (2007, 2015) developed the Therapeutic Story as a modification for implementing Eye Movement Desensitization and Reprocessing (EMDR) trauma reprocessing with children who are too young to articulate what happened and who need an adult perspective of events. Often, young children are affected by events related to infancy or birth, and the story helps children understand what happened and access sensations and emotions related to the non-remembered events for reprocessing. Additionally, telling children what happened through a story allows the therapist to provide helpful, adaptive information for children who don't have the knowledge they need to make sense of what happened due to their developmental age. The story approaches the trauma gently by using a third-person point of view, keeping descriptions of events brief and at first leaving out mention of any emotions, which can be elicited in subsequent readings. The child chooses a method and speed of tactile bilateral stimulation (BLS) that is comfortable for them. The therapist or parent reads the story, and the BLS is applied throughout the reading. This begins the desensitization process and helps the child begin internalizing the adaptive information.

Writing the story with adults gives the therapist the opportunity to clarify their case formulation and provide their patient with a path toward trauma resolution and momentum toward healthy functioning. In the case of adults with unresolved/disorganized attachment patterns, the overall goal of the use of the Therapeutic Story is to help them achieve an "earned secure" and organized status as evidenced by the ability to discuss their loss or abuse memories while remaining organized in their thinking (Main & Hesse, 1990). While unresolved/disorganized adults may initially confuse sequence, pronouns, and assignment of responsibility for abuse, the Therapeutic Story is written with clear sequence and appropriate identification of who did what and who is responsible.

Just as Lovett (2007, 2015) applies the Therapeutic Story method as a gentle and safe way to approach traumatic events with vulnerable child clients, the Therapeutic Story method can be a gentle, safe way for disorganized adult clients to begin addressing and reprocessing their memories due to the third-person narrative and the brevity with which the events are described. Further safety is provided by the inclusion of adaptive information grounded in a present-day perspective.

For many adults with a history of attachment trauma, unprocessed preverbal trauma drives triggered emotions and/or sensations even though the preverbal events are not consciously remembered. The Therapeutic Story for adults as well as children can include preverbal events along with hypothesized beliefs. When the Therapeutic Story is read aloud and paired with BLS for adults in Attachment-Focused Trauma Therapy for Adults (AFTT-A), the story accesses emotions and sensations related to the unremembered trauma and the BLS begins the process of desensitization, integration of the adaptive information, and creation of mental organization. After reading the story one or more times, I (D.W.) often invite the client to add emotions or other aspects of the story that may have come to mind as the story was read.

Flexibility of Timing and Time Period

The Therapeutic Story is not necessarily written for every AFTT-A client, but it's an effective way to begin addressing the traumas with adult clients who demonstrate significant disorganization in response to discussion of traumatic events. Writing the story gives the therapist the opportunity to clarify their case formulation and provide their patient with a path toward trauma resolution and momentum toward healthy functioning.

There is flexibility regarding when to write a story and regarding the period of time being addressed. The story may address any part of the client's growing up years, depending upon what stage or age included the most traumatic events. In the AFTT-A protocol, a Therapeutic Story can include two or three of the client's worst memories. It is read aloud with BLS as a gentle way to transition to standard EMDR reprocessing. The story can be written and read aloud with BLS after EMDR reprocessing of several traumas for the purpose of bringing the events together in an organized, sequential way and through the present-day, positive perspective. For clients with a very complicated history and many traumatic events over a long period of time, a simple story can be written for each "chapter" in the client's early life. For example, the therapist and client may write the infant chapter and complete the infant chapter before moving on and writing the toddler/preschooler chapter.

The story may be written by the therapist alone, the patient alone, or the therapist and the patient together. If the therapist alone writes the story, they can present it as their understanding, and they can ask the patient to help them make the story more accurate, eliciting input from the patient's adult self. If the patient alone writes the story, the therapist can ask questions and request clarification, requiring input from the patient's adult self. Writing the story together, over several sessions, gives the patient a re-do of their experience with the reassuring presence of a calm, competent adult.

A Therapeutic Story may be written and read aloud to address the unremembered infant or toddler part of the client's story after reprocessing the remembered events. Reading aloud the preverbal part of the story with BLS often activates emotions and sensations consistent with what happened and allows the client to reprocess those unremembered events through the reading of the story.

Overview of the Therapeutic Story Protocol in AFTT-A

The first step to writing a Therapeutic Story in AFTT-A is to decide upon a timeframe for the story. The story may be written around adolescence, elementary school, or toddlerhood, depending upon when the most traumatic events happened. Next, the therapist and client create a timeline that sequences positive and negative events by jotting the events along the timeline. While creating the timeline, the therapist and client can begin discussing beliefs, both positive and negative, that may have developed during various events and jotting them down on the timeline (Wesselmann, Schweitzer, & Armstrong, 2014). From there, the therapist can use the Therapeutic Story outline as a guide and collaborate with the client in writing the story in session. A sample story is provided to assist with understanding regarding the story-writing concepts.

After the story is written, the client chooses the type of tactile BLS (such as alternating taps on the backs of the client's hands or holding alternating electronic tactile pulsars) and a speed that is the most comfortable. The therapist reads the story and adds the BLS throughout the reading to begin the desensitization and integration of adaptive information.

The story may be read multiple times. Often the client's comfort level with their story as a whole and their sense of organization around the story continues to increase with each reading. As with children (Lovett, 2007, 2015), the adult client can be asked what the child in the story thought, felt, wondered, wanted, needed. BLS can be used to process each, with imagined reparation, such as the presence of a protective adult, along with cognitive interweaves. Once the story has been read two or more times, the therapist can ask the client to raise a hand and let them know when they have reached a portion of the story that retains some strong emotions, and then apply phases 3 through 8 for that portion of the story. After reprocessing the individual incident, the therapist can bring out the story again to find any remaining points of disturbance. In this way, the story can become a roadmap for EMDR therapy.

Even preverbal trauma can be reprocessed with standard EMDR phases 3 through 8. Identify the target image by asking, "As I re-read this preverbal part of the story, notice what image comes into your mind." If an image doesn't come to mind, they can be asked to imagine what a child might feel in that situation. Then proceed with the other EMDR phase 3 questions and reprocess with standard EMDR procedures.

STEPS FOR WRITING THE THERAPEUTIC STORY

For more information, see Protocol Script 13 at the end of the chapter.

1. Describe the Rationale

Explain to the client that you would like to write a Therapeutic Story about a portion of their early years that is sequential and organized and includes negative beliefs as well as helpful information. Explain that later you will read the story aloud and apply BLS through tapping or tactile pulsars to help them begin reducing distress and internalize helpful information. Explain that the story as a whole will help their brain make sense of things and remain organized and calm when they are reminded of their past.

2. Create a Timeline

Make sure the client is grounded in the Competent Adult part of Self to begin this step. Explain to the client that you need to determine the time period for the story, and that it could focus on infancy, early childhood, later childhood, or adolescence. Ask the client what part of the growing up years seems the most difficult to address, and then ask if it's okay to focus on that period of time.

Draw a line on a piece of paper. Consider using butcher paper or two pieces of paper taped together horizontally to provide more space. Draw a horizontal line with slash marks to represent each year.

Explain that you will be noting both positive and negative events on the timeline. Begin by noting on the timeline where the client lived, with whom, and when. Next, with the client's help, note any positive memories or positive known events. Then note negative memories that come to the client's mind, reminding the client to use a stop signal if they get overwhelmed. Don't discuss the events, only make notations. Pace the creation of the timeline with the tolerance of the client. It may be necessary to work in small increments to complete the activity over multiple sessions. Finally, brainstorm the negative beliefs and positive beliefs that may have developed at various points on the timeline, jotting them down in the appropriate places.

3. Write the Story

With the client's permission, the therapist begins filling in the Therapeutic Storytelling Outline found in Exhibit 22.13, making suggestions, but asking the client to contribute thoughts and ideas or change things. (See Exhibit 22.13 in Chapter 22 or access the form online through Springer Publishing Connect: Use the code on the opening page of this book to access the digital product and select Chapter 22.) Write the story in third person and allow the client to decide whether to include their first name in the story. Don't include too many events or details about events. Use the timeline to help provide basic facts and beliefs. If it's easier, the therapist can write most of the story outside of therapy, leaving blank spaces for the client to help fill in the child's beliefs during the session. Leave out emotions during the initial writing of the story. Emotions and sensations that come up during the reading of the story can be desensitized with BLS. Description of the emotions can be added to the story later, if desired.

Following the outline, the story should begin by grounding the client in present time with ample positive information about the client and what they enjoy in present-day life. The first past event should be a positive one, such as "They were born good and lovable like every other baby in the world." This is followed by a brief identification of a negative event and what the child believed, followed by helpful, adaptive information. To provide helpful information, the story outline suggests saying, "The (Competent Adult part of the client/the therapist/caring others) wants the younger part(s) of the client to know that…."

Additional positive and negative events are identified in the story. Be sure to include what was confusing for the client as a child as well as adaptive information that addresses the confusion. To conclude the story, identify what the client is still struggling to do or believe and any positive beliefs or behaviors the client is working to adopt.

The outline is meant to be a suggestion. Feel free to adapt the outline as needed.

4. Read With BLS

Allow the client to choose a speed that is comfortable. The story can be read one, two, three, or more times with the BLS to bring down overall disturbance and help integrate the adaptive information.

5. Later, Reprocess Individual Events

After one or more times reading the story, over multiple sessions if needed, ask the client to identify individual events from the story that retain an emotional charge. Process those events individually, applying EMDR phases 3 through 7. The story can become a roadmap, helping the therapist and client identify relevant targets for reprocessing.

BOX 16.1 CLIENT EXAMPLE: THERAPEUTIC STORY

An adult with many positive qualities, such as kindness and caring for the well-being of others, enjoys learning new things and spending time with a friend. They live in an apartment downtown. They have inside and outside resources, including an inside Resource Team of angels, an outside friend who is trustworthy, and a therapist they see on a regular basis.

Like everyone else in the world, the adult experienced both positive and difficult events/situations in their life. One positive event was that they were born good and lovable, with a predisposition to be healthy and strong.

One difficult situation took place before they were born. Their mother was going through some tough times, and the developing baby was bathed in stress hormones, and that was uncomfortable for the developing baby. The Competent Adult part of them wants every part inside of them to know that they were safe, they did develop into a healthy baby, and their mother was doing the best they could for their situation.

(continued)

> **BOX 16.1 CLIENT EXAMPLE: THERAPEUTIC STORY** (continued)
>
> Another difficult thing was the mother believed some of the teachings of the time. The mother held the baby sometimes but also left the baby to cry alone in their crib in their own separate room without picking them up many times. If the baby could talk, the baby might have said, "I'm afraid I will die. I can't do this by myself." The Adult part of them wants every part inside to know that the baby should not have had to do it by themself. However, the baby was strong and healthy and they survived. They were lovable and good. And their mother was doing the best they could with what they knew at the time.
>
> A positive thing was that, as life continued, the toddler developed their own ways to cope. They played and developed a fun imagination. As they grew, they played out in nature and enjoyed the trees and the bugs. When they were out in nature, the little child thought, "I'm fine as I am." They felt happy playing and skipping.
>
> Another difficult thing was when the little child's father was mean and hit their brother and them. They were confused as to why their mother didn't help them. They thought, "I can't trust anyone," and "Maybe there is something wrong with me." The Competent Adult part of them wants every part inside to know that they were good. They deserved good care, and they deserved to be safe, like all children in the world. Their father didn't know how to raise children and their mother didn't know how to protect them. The little child was lovable and strong, and they did survive through those tough times.
>
> Another positive thing was that they got involved in dance as they got older, and they found joy in dancing. They were talented, and they felt good about themself when they danced.
>
> They are older now, and sometimes they still struggle to believe it is safe to trust others, and they still struggle with knowing in every part of them that they are a good and lovable person. But with the help of their inside and outside resources, they have found some people who are trustworthy. They have begun to understand that it is safe to trust some people and that they are a good and lovable person who deserves to have good people in their life. They work hard in therapy to continue to heal, and they are learning to take very good care of themself.

POINTS TO REMEMBER

- Begin with a simple timeline. Include positive and negative events and note positive and negative beliefs that developed during those events. There is no need to include emotions on the timeline.

- The Therapeutic Story can be written in session, but the therapist can begin writing the story outside of session if it's helpful to do so. The *Therapeutic Storytelling Outline* (see Exhibit 22.13 in Chapter 22 or access the form online through Springer Publishing Connect: Use the code on the opening page of this book to access the digital product and select Chapter 22) can be helpful for organizing the story. Adapt the outline as needed.

- To decrease the intensity of emotions for the client, write the Therapeutic Story in third person. Allow the adult to choose whether to include their name. The events in the story should not include details. Leave out description of emotions, at least in the initial writing and reading of the story. The story should stay simple and focus on just one difficult portion of the client's life. Make sure there is ample positive information included in the story.

- The Therapeutic Story is read aloud, adding tactile BLS throughout the reading of the story. Allow the client to choose the type of tactile BLS and a speed that feels comfortable for using throughout. Repeat the story until the client reports it is less disturbing overall.

- Desensitize emotions that arise during the reading of the story. Add cognitive interweaves as needed. Return to the story to identify specific events that need to be reprocessed with EMDR phases 3 through 7.

TROUBLESHOOTING

- If the client has a great deal of trauma from infancy to adulthood and it's impossible to highlight one part of the growing up years as the most difficult, you can write the client's story in two, three, or more chapters. For example, you might write the infancy story, the early childhood story, the later childhood story, the preteen story, the adolescent story, and perhaps the young adult story. Each chapter concludes with adaptive information. Work with each chapter separately. This prevents the activity from becoming too overwhelming.

- If the client has tremendous difficulty identifying positive events, explore relationships with any peers, teachers, neighbors, or even pets that the client felt good about or any skills or abilities that the client learned or discovered while growing up. You can also look for mastery experiences such as academic successes or early job successes.

PAUSE AND REFLECT FOR THE THERAPIST

Was there a part of your growing up years that was especially troubling to you? Consider writing an adult perspective on a portion of your growing up years. Begin by creating a simple timeline of that portion of your life. Include both positive and difficult events or situations, noting what happened when and noting negative and positive beliefs associated with the events. Begin writing the story using the outline. Seek your own therapeutic support if this feels overwhelming. To conclude your story, you can include positive, adaptive beliefs and behaviors that you are working to adopt in your personal life as well as in your professional life as a therapist.

USEFUL TERMS AND DEFINITIONS

AAI: Adult Attachment Interview

AFTT-A: Attachment-Focused Trauma Therapy for Adults

BLS: bilateral stimulation

EMDR: Eye Movement Desensitization and Reprocessing

TFCBT: Trauma-Focused Cognitive Behavioral Therapy

PROTOCOL SCRIPT 13. CREATING THE THERAPEUTIC STORY

Adapted from Lovett, J. (2007). *Small wonders: Healing childhood trauma with EMDR.* Free Press/Simon & Schuster; Lovett, J. (2015). *Trauma-attachment tangle: Modifying EMDR to help children resolve trauma and develop loving relationships.* Routledge/Taylor & Francis Group; and Wesselmann, D., Schweitzer, C., & Armstrong, S. (2014). *Integrative team treatment for attachment trauma in children: Family therapy and EMDR.* W. W. Norton & Company.

1. Describe the Rationale. *Say…* "I'd like to work with you to create a Therapeutic Story related to a part of your life that holds some challenging memories. For example, you might choose early childhood, later childhood, or adolescence. The purpose of writing the story is to help organize your memories and make sense of them. Later, I'll read your story aloud while you hold the tappers to help reduce distress and help your brain start to integrate the helpful information. We'll work together to write your story. To make it easier, we'll write it in the third person and name the difficult events only briefly. We'll include positive events or situations, too, and we'll include negative beliefs but also helpful thoughts and ideas. Are you okay with this plan?"
_____ (*If yes, continue. If no, table the activity for a later date.*) "What part of your life is especially challenging to think about?"

_____

_____

2. Create a Timeline. *Say…* "The first step is to create a timeline for the time period we've chosen by placing events in appropriate sequence on the timeline." (*The therapist draws a line and makes marks to represent ages.*) "Help me identify where you lived at different points on the timeline." (*The therapist and client work together to note places where the client lived. Different colors can be used to designate various places where the client lived.*) "Take your time and see if you can name some positive events during this time period. Either you or I can write the positive events on the timeline. Events might be related to family, but might also be related to friends, hobbies, or school events." _____ (*Positive events are noted on the timeline.*) "Take your time and see if you can name some negative events or situations with just a word or two, and you or I can write those on the timeline." _____ (*Negative events are noted on the timeline.*) "What positive thoughts or beliefs might you have had at the time of each of these positive events?" _____ (*Note the thoughts or beliefs at the appropriate places on the timeline.*) "Can you think of any thoughts or beliefs that you might have had at the time of each of these negative events?" (*If this last part is too difficult, let it go for now.*)

_____

_____

3. Write the Story. *Say…* "Would you be okay with us working on your Therapeutic Story today? We can pace the writing according to your comfort level, stopping at any point you want to stop." _____ (*If yes…*) "I'd like to make sure you're operating from your most adult self as we start the story. Can you make sure your body posture is one that puts you in your most adult state?" _____ (*If yes, the client shifts body posture as needed.*) "Great, how does that feel?" _____ (*The therapist gives assistance through mastery imagery or grounding skills if the client struggles finding the adult state.*) "We'll use the timeline along with this outline to help us." (*Refer to the outline provided in this chapter.*) "I can start us off, but please jump in at any point with the words you want me to use. If I use words that don't fit, please correct me. We're going to write this in third person, but we can use your name in the story, or we can leave your name out of the story. Which would you prefer?" _____ "Okay, that's fine. Now let's go to the first paragraph, which starts us off with some positive thoughts about present day." (*Continue by working together to fill in the outline. Refer to Exhibit 22.13: Therapeutic Storytelling Outline.*)

4. **Read With BLS.** *Say…*"Now, with your permission, I'd like to read the story through today, adding the bilateral stimulation at a speed of your choosing. Is it okay with you if we do this next step today?" _____ (*If yes…*) "Let me know which speed, intensity, and type of bilateral stimulation makes you feel the most comfortable, today." (*Proceed with trying out speed and intensity of the BLS through alternating taps on the backs of the client's hands and/or use of alternating tactile pulsars.*) "Before I begin reading, can you shift your body posture or use an adult competency memory and let me know when you feel like you're operating from your most adult state?" _____ "I'll begin reading now, but at any point you can share with me something that has come up for you that you want me to know about, and at any point we can stop reading for today, just let me know. Otherwise, I'll just read it all the way through, while applying the bilateral stimulation." (*The therapist reads the story all the way or partially through depending on the client's preference, while the client holds the tactile pulsars.*)

5. **Later, Reprocess Individual Events.** (*After two, three, or four times reading the story over two, three, or four sessions, return to individual events from the story that retain an emotional charge and process those events with EMDR standard protocol.*) *Say…*"Today, I'll start reading the story without adding BLS. You hold your hand up when I get to a place in the story that still holds some emotional charge." (*Implement EMDR phases 3 through 7, targeting the identified event.*)

REFERENCES

Lovett, J. (2007). *Small wonders: Healing childhood trauma with EMDR*. Free Press/Simon & Schuster.

Lovett, J. (2015). *Trauma-attachment tangle: Modifying EMDR to help children resolve trauma and develop loving relationships*. Routledge/Taylor & Francis Group.

Main, M., & Hesse, E. (1990). Parents' unresolved traumatic experiences are related to infant disorganized attachment status: Is frightened/frightening parental behavior the linking mechanism? In M. T. Greenberg, D. Cicchetti, & E. M. Cummings (Eds.), *Attachment in the preschool years: Theory, research, and intervention* (pp. 161–182). University of Chicago Press.

Wesselmann, D., Schweitzer, C., & Armstrong, S. (2014). *Integrative team treatment for attachment trauma in children: Family therapy and EMDR*. W. W. Norton & Company.

CHAPTER 17

The Emotionally Corrective Therapeutic Relationship in Attachment-Focused Trauma Therapy for Adults

INTRODUCTION

Adults who were raised in an emotionally neglectful, rejecting, or abusive environment frequently develop nonsecure attachment patterns that continue into adulthood. Adults with dismissive patterns tend to be avoidant of emotional closeness and negative emotions. Adults with preoccupied patterns tend to be insistent about getting their emotional needs met through close relationships, and they experience emotions strongly. Adults with unresolved/disorganized attachment patterns with respect to a history of unresolved childhood abuse or loss experience mental disorganization when memories are triggered (Hesse, 1999).

Some adults with a difficult childhood have experienced at least one emotionally corrective relationship that led them to a new perspective and an emotional shift so profound that their attachment pattern shifted from nonsecure to "earned" secure (Cohen, 2005; Saunders et al., 2011). Attachment-Focused Trauma Therapy for Adults (AFTT-A) therapists provide attuned, secure-based responses to nonsecure client behaviors and words (Wesselmann & Potter, 2019). The therapeutic relationship is a powerful component of AFTT-A for improving clients' attachment patterns (Figure 17.1).

If clients carry nonsecure and/or disorganized attachment patterns, a certain look or tone of voice from the therapist or a moment of misattunement can activate Child parts of Self holding mistrust, fear, anxiety, anger, or other childhood emotions experienced in close relationships. Clients' nonsecure relationship patterns and associated defense mechanisms may be especially activated in the therapy office when childhood traumas are addressed (Laliotis, 2017). It's vital for therapists to stay grounded in their most therapeutic adult state and remain mindful and attuned when clients are triggered.

CREATING AN EMOTIONALLY CORRECTIVE THERAPEUTIC RELATIONSHIP

The AFTT-A therapist effectively uses the therapist's Self for positive therapeutic change by providing attunement and secure-based responses to clients' words and behaviors. The emotionally present therapist doesn't judge clients' emotions or attempts to "control" or "fix." The therapist listens and reflects upon the clients' words or actions, even when they appear out-of-proportion to the situation. Secure-based responses include, "Tell me more about…" "It sounds like you're feeling/thinking…. Do I have that right?" The AFTT-A therapist's body posture and facial expression

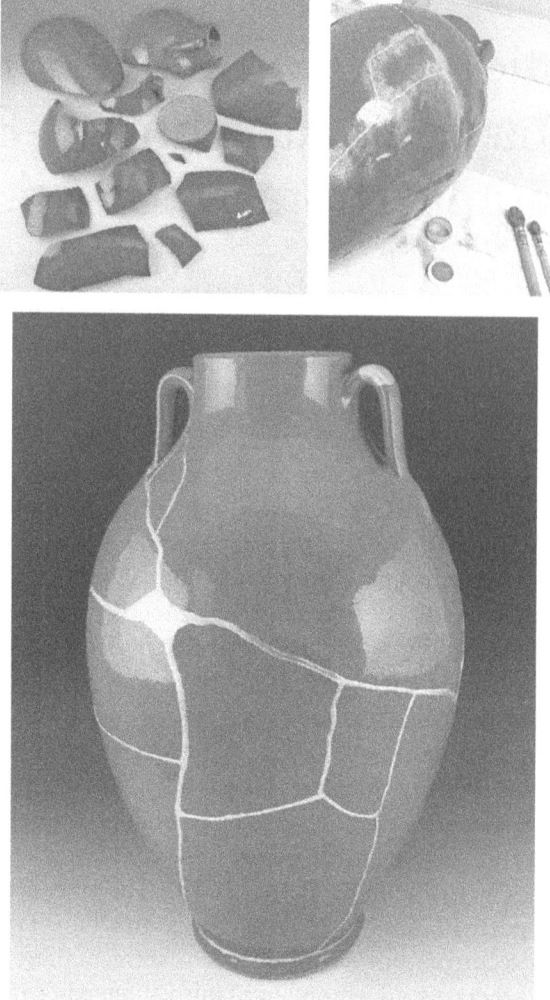

FIGURE 17.1 Client transformation process through Attachment-Focused Trauma Therapy for Adults: Kintsugi process analogy.

Source: Courtesy of Morty Bachar, Lakeside Pottery Studio, https://www.lakesidepottery.com.

show a calm demeanor. The therapist applies interventions only when clients' feel heard and understood.

Acknowledging Therapist Triggers

Providing a healthy, emotionally corrective therapeutic relationship can be challenging. In the presence of clients with strong nonsecure defense mechanisms, it's easy to lose perspective. Even the therapist with a secure or earned secure attachment may be triggered unexpectedly by clients' nonsecure words or behaviors.

Therapists may also have unresolved abuse or loss memories. Activation of traumatic memories by clients' discourse in therapy can activate therapists' sympathetic nervous system, interfering with attunement. If an anxious Child part of Self is activated for the therapist, it can overwhelm the therapeutic Adult part of Self, and the therapeutic relationship will fail to be a source of safety for the client in that moment. To minimize breeches in the therapeutic relationship, the therapist remains mindful of activated Child parts of Self, intentionally tucking them back into a Safe Place and reconnecting fully with the therapeutic Adult part of Self.

If we observe our responses and identify a pattern of triggers, it's important to bring those triggers back to consultation, peer consultation, or to personal therapy and look at childhood to identify associated childhood situations or events. This can be a wonderful opportunity for a breakthrough in our own self-growth. Through doing our own work, we increase our capacity to operate from our most therapeutic Adult part of Self. From a strengthened, therapeutic adult state, we have greater capacity to provide secure-based responses to clients' nonsecure words or actions (Wesselmann & Potter, 2019).

Considering Therapist Beliefs

None of us gets through childhood without some unfortunate events. Most of us can identify at least some negative beliefs carried from childhood that have the potential to catch us off guard and negatively impact our therapeutic presence.

For example, we may have internalized judgmental or critical thoughts from a parent or significant other who was judgmental and critical. If we hold the bar too high for ourselves due to internalized judgments, we are likely to hold the bar too high for others as well, including our clients. From an activated internal Critical Parent part of Self, we may be telling ourselves that our client *should* behave a certain way: "My client should follow my suggestions and directions/make steady progress/never get angry with me/agree with me/manage their emotions during the session/be grateful for any accommodations I make for them." The Critical Parent part is not honoring the client's traumatic past and the natural struggles caused by unprocessed traumatic memories. The judgmental thoughts trigger frustration and irritation, interfering with our most therapeutic Adult part.

Table 17.1 compares negative cognitions (NCs) about self and client that might be present for therapists with dismissive, preoccupied, and disorganized tendencies. The table also describes useful positive cognition (PC) goals for therapists.

By staying mindful of our negative thoughts, we can step back and choose not to respond from the negative perspective. The AFTT-A therapist develops an emotionally corrective relationship through active listening, attunement, and secure-based responses.

Secure-Based Responses to Clients' Anger

Clients' Adolescent or Child parts of Self may carry unprocessed anger related to childhood traumatic events. Activation of Child parts carrying anger may be evident in clients' sudden and unexpected angry words and behaviors in therapy. Clients' expressions of anger may activate a Child part in the therapist. The therapist may experience fear, anxiety, or anger in response.

Consider the client with a dismissive, derogatory status who carries childhood negative beliefs that it's not safe to trust others. The client's anxiety regarding an intervention in session may trigger an activated Adolescent part leading to the

Table 17.1 Therapist Attachment Tendencies: Negative Cognitions and Positive Cognitions

Therapist Attachment Tendencies	Negative Cognitions about...	Goals for Positive Cognitions about...
Dismissive	**Self**: I can't be vulnerable. I have to be right. I can't lose. I have to be in control. I already know everything I need to know. **Client**: My client is being difficult/resistant. My client shouldn't need me so much. My client isn't working hard enough. My client's emotions are unnecessary.	**Self**: I can be vulnerable. It's okay to be wrong. I don't have to win. I can let go of control. I can learn from my work with my client. **Client**: My client is doing the best they can. My client's needs make sense in the context of their past experiences. My client is moving at the pace that is right for them. My client's emotions are natural.
Preoccupied	**Self**: If my client backslides, I'm not worthy/good enough. I should already know everything I need to know. I need to convince my client to do what I think they should do. **Client**: My client should be more cooperative with me. My client is supposed to be happy with me.	**Self**: I'm worthy, even when my client doesn't respond as I'd hoped. I can continue to grow as a clinician. I can offer help and my client can choose how to respond. **Client**: My client is doing the best they can. I can listen and attune when my client is unhappy with me.
Unresolved/Disorganized	**Self**: My memories aren't safe. My emotions are bad. I can't handle this. I'm powerless. I'm not capable. I have to protect myself. **Client**: My client's memories aren't safe. My client's emotions are bad. My client is fragile. My client is safe in the present moment.	**Self**: My memories are just memories. My emotions are just emotions. I can handle this. I have choices. I'm capable and I have resources. I'm not in danger. **Client**: My client's memories are just memories. My client's emotions are just emotions. My client has what they need to handle this. They are not in danger in the present moment.

Source: Adapted from Hesse, E. (1999). The Adult Attachment Interview protocol, method of analysis, and empirical studies. In J. Cassidy & P. R. Shaver (Eds.), *Handbook of attachment: Theory, research, and clinical applications* (pp. 552–598). Guilford Press; and Main, M., Kaplan, N., & Cassidy, J. (1985). Security in infancy, childhood, and adulthood: A move to the level of representation. *Monographs of the Society for Research in Child Development.* 50(1/2), 66–104. https://doi.org/10.2307/3333827.

statement, "This therapy's really stupid." If the therapist appears distant, shut down, or irritated in response to the client's statement, the client's negative perception that others can't be trusted is strengthened.

Consider the client who struggles with trust and avoids vulnerability with preoccupied, angry words or actions. In the initial session, the client complains loudly about the fees and policies regarding missed appointments. Changing the policies in response to the client's words reinforces the client's nonsecure behaviors, while responding with irritation reinforces the mistrust.

By consciously remaining mindful of our own inner state and staying firmly grounded in the perceptions and thought processes of our most therapeutic Adult part of Self, we can provide a secure-based, emotionally corrective response to clients' anger or irritation. If we can stay mindful and recognize activation of clients' younger parts as well as taking good care of our own, the secure-based response will come more readily.

Following are brief examples of nonsecure and secure-based responses to clients' anger:

Nonsecure therapist response: "Settle down, your behavior is childish." "You're behaving irrationally, you need to stop." "I don't know what you're upset about."

Secure-based therapist response: "You're really frustrated with me right now. Tell me more; I'm going to just listen and try to understand. Then we'll work together to problem-solve."

Secure-Based Responses to Clients' Vulnerable Emotions

Clients' expressions of vulnerable emotions such as sadness or anxiety can also trigger strong emotions in us during therapy. If our tendency is toward the dismissive defenses, we may have an automatic reaction of feeling "burdened" by clients' expressions of emotions. Without self-awareness, we may automatically respond by distancing from our clients' emotions and minimizing their emotional experience. For example, we might provide logical reasons why they shouldn't feel what they feel or offer solutions to "fix" their situation. We may even revert to "talk therapy" about superficial topics to avoid activating any emotions at all. We may have internal judgments to help us achieve more emotional distance, such as, "They should be able to handle that" or "They're making a bigger deal of it than they need to. It's not that bad."

Avoidance of emotions is self-protective but diminishes our therapeutic presence. We may show our judgments through facial expressions or through body posture. Clients will naturally sense our judgments and feel uncomfortable and defective in response, which likely deepens their negative self-beliefs.

If we have a preoccupied tendency and our client is experiencing vulnerable emotions, we may experience our own vulnerable emotions front and center, showing anxiety in our face, voice, or posture and escalating anxiety for the client. On the other hand, we may attempt to "parent" the client, further activating the client's Child part of Self with soft, overly comforting, nurturing words. Our anxiety slows or halts our client's progress.

If we can stay mindful of our dismissive or preoccupied tendencies, we can notice the automatic tendencies and then mentally step back into our most therapeutic Adult part of Self. We can tuck our own Child part back into a Safe Place or utilize our Resource Team. We can be intentional about reflecting upon the client's inner experience, providing a safe, nonjudgmental environment and attune to what the client has experienced in relationships in the past.

Following are brief examples of nonsecure and secure-based responses to clients' vulnerable emotions:

Nonsecure therapist response: "It's not that bad." "I'll tell you what you should do if you'll just listen to me." "If you would just follow my advice, you wouldn't have the problems you do." "Let's change the subject. How was work, today?"

Secure-based therapist response: "It's so good you're able to let your feelings out. I'm right here with you while you experience these emotions." "You can have these emotions and be okay."

Secure-Based Responses to Clients' Trauma Triggers

Clients with an extensive trauma history may be easily triggered, even during the initial intake or history taking or at any moment when a childhood event is recalled. Clients with disorganized attachment regarding traumatic events may experience quick activation of the Child part of Self and become fearful, lose orientation to time, and become highly dissociated. If the therapist has tendencies toward attachment disorganization, the therapist may become overly attuned, experiencing the client's affect state, causing loss of capacity to co-regulate. The therapist with dismissive tendencies may distance, while the therapist with preoccupied tendencies may become anxious and overactive, reducing the capacity for co-regulation either way.

Mindful therapists observe and manage their triggers in order to keep a body posture, face, and voice tone that conveys compassion and calm. The emotionally corrective therapeutic relationship involves recognition of clients' triggers, activated Child parts, and need for attunement, proper pacing, and patient co-regulation from the therapist. The AFTT-A therapist utilizes supervision, peer support, and/or personal therapy to find adaptive resolution with their own unprocessed material to reduce the possibility of triggers.

Following are brief examples of disorganized, nonsecure, and secure-based responses to client triggers:

Disorganized therapist response: Anxiety, confusion, disorientation.

Nonsecure therapist response: "That's all in the past. There's no reason to get all worked up." "Use some self-talk. Take some deep breaths. Try harder." "Let me comfort you. I can provide what you didn't get in the past."

Secure-based therapist response: "I want you to feel free to let me know what helps you feel comfortable and what doesn't help. I'll pace with you. All of your feelings are natural, considering everything you've experienced and the topics we've addressed. You can have these feelings and still be okay."

Secure-Based Therapeutic Responses Regarding Childhood Unmet Needs

The client's Child parts of Self may attempt to get earlier unmet needs met in the present relationship with the therapist. This may be a pattern in many of their adult relationships. For example, when Child parts of Self are activated, the client may ask the therapist for direct messages of affirmation. During interactions in which the client is seeking to get needs met, their voice may sound more child-like or the client's facial expression or posture may show signs of a much younger state.

Statements and actions by clients operating from Child parts of Self who are seeking to get old needs met may include excessive calls, texts, and emails. Statements may include, "You didn't listen to me today, I need you to show me you care, I need more/longer sessions." The attention-seeking client is actually connection seeking. Underlying the connection-seeking behavior is fear of rejection rooted in distressing childhood experiences.

Therapists with dismissive tendencies may be uncomfortable and dismissive toward clients' words and behaviors, while therapists with preoccupied tendencies may give overlong messages of affirmation and attempt to satisfy their clients' demands. Clients who have active Child parts seeking connection remain distressed and unsatisfied in either situation.

When a Child part is seeking attention on the outside, the therapist may *say*... "Perhaps some vulnerable feelings connected to a younger part of you has been activated. How old do you feel right now?" (*Pause for the answer*.) "Before we go any further, let's get Child parts tucked back into Safe Places with their loving and protective figures." Once the Child parts are settled, you can *say*... "Invite that younger part of you to look at your hands and notice how old you are in present time."

Once the client is grounded into the present-day, most adult state, the therapist can *say*... "The kid parts have unmet needs that they're trying to get met through people in your adult life. The problem is that the time for the child to get needs met in the outside world is over. Younger parts of you don't feel safe operating in your adult life, and when they try to get their needs met through your adult relationships, it doesn't work and only escalates their anxiety. The younger parts of you need firm boundaries by directing them back to their Safe Places. They also need your compassion. When they're more settled into Safe Places, we'll be able to safely start reprocessing your traumatic experiences with EMDR therapy and work through the experiences that left kid parts with unmet needs."

Nesting dolls can be used to convey the concept of supporting the Adult part of Self so the Adult can meet the needs of the younger parts of Self (Wesselmann & Potter, 2019). Bring out a set of nesting dolls. Take them apart and reassemble them from biggest to smallest. *Say*... "This bigger doll is me. Here's me, standing behind the next biggest doll that represents you. The little ones around the doll representing your child parts of Self." (Move the little ones around the doll representing the Adult part of the client.) "I'm not directly giving care to those younger parts, but I'm here supporting the Adult part of you so that you can nurture and give care to those younger parts."

Body Postures and Facial Expressions

Ideally, we are mindfully present and attuned to clients in therapy sessions. Being in the emotional and safety "zone" of the ventral vagal part of the parasympathetic part of our autonomic nervous system (ANS) enables us to be calm, at ease, open, and signal safety, security, and approachability with our clients. Sometimes, clients' dysregulation resonates within our own ANS, perhaps activating our sympathetic ANS in which our perceptions narrow and we ready ourselves for danger. As a result, we become anxious, irritable, or even emotionally detached or shut down in response. We signal to clients with the changes in our facial expressions, eye contact, and body postures that we are reacting to a sense of danger, thus decreasing the sense of ease and security in the session and the therapeutic relationship. When we're mindful of our body sensations and facial expressions, we can silently take a few slow, deep breaths, relax any tension, and use our calm body and facial expression to assist our clients with regulation. Radically Open Dialectical Behavioral Therapy (RO DBT; Lynch et al., 2015) suggests that with an overcontrolled client (i.e., dismissive client), it's important not to appear intense or controlling. The therapist might take a sip of coffee, lean back with a relaxed posture, and use the "eyebrow wag." The eyebrow wag is a lift of the eyebrows to exhibit an expression of listening, but with a very relaxed, nonchalant manner.

A common situation involves the dismissive client attempting to avoid emotions and memories by saying something like, "I don't remember much about my childhood, but it was fine, I don't really have anything to talk about today, and I'm not interested in any of that 'new age' woo-woo stuff." The secure-based therapeutic response includes the relaxed body, face, and voice, and the lift to the eyebrows that communicates, "*I hear what you're saying*," while pondering the client's statement for a few moments. The therapist might *say*… "Here's what comes to my mind. I'm wondering if it would be okay with you…" prior to introducing an intervention.

The dismissive individual with a derogatory subtype may use an intimidating manner, perhaps remarking, "I'm here because my partner insisted, not because I want to be here." The secure-based response includes a relaxed facial expression and body posture with an attitude of curiosity. RO DBT (Lynch et al., 2015) calls the therapist's nonverbal communication in this case, the "Big 3 + 1." The therapist takes a deep breath, smiles just enough to crinkle the skin around their eye area but not enough to show their teeth, lifts their eyebrows (affectionately known as the "eyebrow wag"), and leans back in their chair if seated. The therapist might then *say*… "I admire you for coming in, even though your personal feelings are against it."

RO DBT might also be helpful with a client who has a preoccupied attachment tendency and is experiencing intense emotions in therapy. Clients with preoccupied attachment patterns respond best to a posture that shows the therapist is attentive but relaxed, called an "appeasement gesture" (Lynch et al., 2015). The therapist leans forward slightly, rounds their shoulders, and holds their hands out at their waist with their palms up, relaxes their facial expression, and nods a little if it's appropriate to the situation. Because the therapist signals safety to the client, the client can move from their flight/fight/freeze reaction back into the emotional and social safety zone, regulating their emotional intensity and reconnecting them to the therapist.

Providing Insight Into the Client's Effects on Others

With appropriate timing and rapport, we can make observations that may ultimately provide the client with insight into problems experienced in relationships outside of therapy. When a good rapport is already established, we can approach the client with a spirit of collaboration. If we use words like "I'm curious," "maybe," and "I wonder," we're inviting the client to become part of the process, and we're more likely to be perceived as having positive intentions than if we use a direct, more critical approach. We also want to convey a compassionate view of the client's behaviors as trauma based; for example, as a learned way to self-protect during childhood or adolescence.

Consider the client with a dismissive pattern and the derogatory subtype. The therapist finds that the client is frequently sarcastic in session, and the client speaks sarcastically about others in their life as well.

Critical Approach: *Say...* "Your sarcasm makes me feel tense and uncomfortable, and I'm a therapist. If you do that with your friends or family, they must feel even more uncomfortable than I do. This could be one reason your relationships are so unstable."

Collaborative Approach: *Say...* "I've noticed that every so often, your humor has a bit of a sarcastic edge. I wonder, could it have a self-protective purpose? For example, do you think it could be a way you learned to protect yourself when you were younger?" (*Pause for a response.*) "I've also noticed it triggers me a little bit, like I become a little self-protective in response. Do you think this could be happening with anyone else?"

In the first example, the client's defenses are likely to become activated, blocking their capacity to self-reflect. In the second example, the client is more likely to sense the therapist's positive intent, lowering their defenses and allowing them to examine the situation more objectively.

The Unshakable Belief and the Spiritual Core

The client with a difficult childhood history may have a powerful inner critic and a self-concept built around critical messages and damaged by attachment trauma. When we assert the AFTT-A perspective that clients have innate goodness and a Spiritual Essence at the core of their Authentic Self, we are providing clients with a new understanding of their intrinsic value. When we present our unshakable belief that they have everything they need inside of themselves to heal, clients can find hope for healing and wholeness by seeing their potential through our eyes. The therapeutic relationship within the AFTT-A model provides clients with hope and a positive self-view that is new.

As AFTT-A proceeds, we continue to assert our belief in clients' inner potential, giving credit to clients for every small step forward. We consistently call upon clients to look within themselves to find and enhance positive states, qualities, and characteristics during the EMDR preparation phase imagery and resource development work. We use the therapist Self and a secure-based approach to stay firm and grounded in our positive view regarding clients' basic goodness and potential for healing. Ultimately, our belief in clients' capacities and encouragement to look within themselves for what they need ultimately leads clients to reconnect with the Spiritual Essence at their core and reclaim their most Authentic Self.

POINTS TO REMEMBER

- Therapists are human. We may have unprocessed emotions and sensations from earlier experiences that are obstacles to our most therapeutic adult state and secure responses to clients' nonsecure behaviors or words.
- As therapists, we may have some tendencies toward dismissive, preoccupied, or disorganized responses, even when we have a secure or earned secure attachment designation overall.
- As therapists, we have the capacity to operate from our most therapeutic Adult part of Self through mindful self-awareness and the willingness to do our own healing work.

- The therapist's use of Self in the process of therapy provides an emotionally corrective experience for the client, which is a powerful component of the healing process.
- Clients' Child parts of Self may look to the AFTT-A therapist and other relationships in adult life to meet their earlier unmet needs. However, the time for getting needs met on the outside is over. The AFTT-A therapist facilitates healing for Child parts of Self through the adult client and the EMDR resource work.
- The AFTT-A therapist uses Self to provide an emotionally corrective experience for clients by responding to clients' connection-seeking, nonsecure behaviors and words with therapeutic, secure-based words and actions.
- The AFTT-A therapist uses Self and the therapeutic relationship to provide an emotionally corrective experience through their belief in clients' basic goodness and Spiritual Essence at the core as well as the "unshakable belief" that they have everything they need inside to heal.

TROUBLESHOOTING

If you feel you have a positive therapeutic rapport and you're providing secure-based responses to the client's words and behaviors, but the client reminds stuck in negative self-statements or self-defeating behaviors…

- The client may be affected by another Child part of Self that remains blended with the client's Adult part of Self. When the client is stuck in negative self-statements or self-defeating behaviors, *say*… "And how old do you feel right now?" or "Think back to when you were having those behaviors. Ask yourself, how old did you feel right then?" Create a Safe Place for any newly identified Child Part of Self (see Protocol Script 5).
- The Child part of Self may be stuck due to the desire for you, the therapist, to meet the child's old, unmet needs. Facilitate meeting the needs of Child parts through the *Corrective Attachment Experiences Between the Child/Adolescent and True Parent Parts of Self* protocol (see Protocol Script 9).
- Seek an objective perspective on the situation with the help of a peer consultation group, an EMDR consultant, or a supervisor.

PAUSE AND REFLECT FOR THE THERAPIST

BOX 17.1 ANN'S STORY: THERAPIST ATTACHMENT TENDENCY AND IMPACT ON THERAPY

As Deb and I prepared for the presentation on *Attachment Through the Life Span* we gave at the 2019 EMDRIA preconference, I took the opportunity to examine my own attachment pattern and particularly how my attachment tendency manifested in therapy sessions with certain clients and how I modified those responses over the years. To be really honest, I couldn't help but recognize myself in certain descriptions and examples! As I looked back at challenging clients

(continued)

> **BOX 17.1 ANN'S STORY: THERAPIST ATTACHMENT TENDENCY AND IMPACT ON THERAPY** (continued)
>
> over my decades of practice, I could identify with the more dismissive negative cognitions and urges to externalize my own unrecognized anxiety about clients who got "stuck" or didn't make "enough" progress or improve "fast enough." I discouraged in clients what I perceived as "neediness." I got into power struggles with clients who needed to be right (not that I had to be right!).
>
> Then in the mid-1990's, I was trained in Dialectical Behavioral Therapy (DBT) and EMDR therapy, Deb and I became friends and colleagues, and I brought home our sweet baby daughter from China. DBT helped me accept that challenging clients are doing the best that they can and taught me to find balance between and flexibility with approaches that accept clients as they are and those that focus on client change. EMDR gave me effective strategies to help clients resolve traumatic memories and the gift of being present with clients in session. I can't begin to tell you all that Deb teaches me as a friend, but as a colleague, she taught me and continues to teach me that softening how I share something with clients rather than in my usual direct and matter-of-fact way is sometimes more therapeutic (Ha, hard to believe, I know!). And, well, being a mom is really humbling. Sometimes, it's a take-me-to-my-knees questioning of anything I thought I knew or of which I was certain. Doubts that came from a place deep inside me, my own past reminding me it still has a hold, which, thankfully, lead me back to my own personal therapy.
>
> Now I can say I'm humbled by clients' unfathomable courage to face and resolve some of the hardest and most painful experiences we humans live through and I'm honored by their willingness to share those times with me in therapy. I *do* have an unshakable belief that clients really have what they need to heal because I witness over and over their persistence and determination to heal despite years or even decades of internalized messages to the contrary. And now, I also expect that same level of courage from myself as a therapist. I welcome clients who challenge me. I am committed to bringing to light whatever interferes with my being mindful and attuned in therapy sessions. I have colleagues, consultants, consult groups, and my own therapist who are willing and eager to help when I ask. And, luckily, I have learned it's okay to ask.

Since you've been engaging in the "Pause and Self-Reflect" activities, you've developed awareness of your own vulnerable Child parts, and you also have tools to help you operate from your most therapeutic Adult part of Self with competence and sensitivity. Your capacity to self-reflect, self-regulate, attune, and co-regulate your clients will help you navigate situations with clients who have strong nonsecure and/or unresolved/disorganized attachment patterns.

Bring up a picture of a client who is sometimes challenging for you. Notice any internal responses without self-judgment. Approach the discomfort with curiosity. What emotions come up? Anxiety, overwhelm, frustration, hurt, powerlessness? Do you have that urge to try to fix or control that client? Distance or avoid?

Do you feel like the picture in your mind might be activating a Child part of Self? If you had to guess, what age of Self might be activated? What is the associated NC? "I'm not capable"? "I'm not safe"? "I'm powerless"? Consider what you would like to believe about yourself instead. For example, "I'm competent," "I'm safe," or "I can have some impact."

Take a calming breath in and out. Find the body posture associated with your Competent Adult part of Self. Hold your hand over your heart and dialogue with the younger part of you. Remind this younger part that this is present-day adult life. Remind the younger part of you that you are competent and safe, you have resources, and you have supportive others in your life. Encourage the younger part of you to remain in the Safe Place with their Higher Power.

Hold your body in your most competent, confident body position. Next, picture yourself in a future session with your client. Imagine your Resource Team there with you, supporting you. Imagine yourself responding to your client from your most grounded, therapeutic and Competent Adult part of Self. If you notice positive feelings or sensations, add a short, slow butterfly hug by crossing your arms and tapping slowly back-and-forth on shoulders, arms, or chest four or five times to deepen the positive affect.

USEFUL TERMS AND DEFINITIONS

AAI: Adult Attachment Interview

AFTT-A: Attachment-Focused Trauma Therapy for Adults

ANS: autonomic nervous system

DBT: Dialectical Behavioral Therapy

EMDR: Eye Movement Desensitization and Reprocessing

NC: negative cognition

PC: positive cognition

RO DBT: Radically Open Dialectical Behavioral Therapy

REFERENCES

Cohen, D. L. (2005, August). *Exploring the role of secondary attachment relationships in the development of attachment security*. (Publication No. 67292299) [Doctoral dissertation, University of North Texas]. UNT Digital Library. http://digital.library.unt.edu/ark:/67531/metadc4891/

Hesse, E. (1999). The Adult Attachment Interview: Historical and current perspectives. In J. Cassidy & P. R. Shaver (Eds.), *Handbook of attachment: Theory, research and clinical applications* (pp. 395–433). Guilford Press.

Laliotis, D. (2017, November). *The dance of attachment: An EMDR relational approach, a master class for EMDR clinicians*. Presentation, Omaha, Nebraska.

Lynch, T. R., Hempel, R. J., & Dunkley, C. (2015). Radically-open dialectical behavior therapy for disorders of over-control: Signaling matters. *American Journal of Psychotherapy*, 69(2), 141–162. https://doi.org/10.1176/appi.psychotherapy.2015.69.2.141

Saunders, R., Jacobvitz, D., Zaccagnino, M., Beverung, L. M., & Hazen, M. (2011). Pathways to earned-security: The role of alternative support figures. *Attachment & Human Development*, 13(4), 403–420. https://doi.org/10.1080/14616734.2011.584405

Wesselmann, D., & Potter, A. E. (2019, September). *Attachment through the lifespan*. EMDRIA Preconference Presentation, Orange County, California.

CHAPTER 18

Getting Client Permission to Transition From Preparation Phase to Phases 3 to 8 of EMDR Therapy With Attachment-Focused Trauma Therapy for Adults

INTRODUCTION

So far in the Attachment-Focused Trauma Therapy for Adults (AFTT-A) model's Eye Movement Desensitization and Reprocessing (EMDR) preparation phase, therapists helped clients create an internal foundation of safety and nurturing for Adult and Child parts of Self; reconstruct inner parts and relationships among parts; develop Competent Adult and True Parent parts; connect to an inner team of strengths and resources; gain time orientation; and learn skills needed for their adult lives and relationships. The focus of EMDR therapy phases 3 to 8 shifts from accessing and reinforcing strengths and positive affect in the preparation phase to accessing, desensitizing, and reprocessing traumatic memories and associated negative feelings, thoughts, and body sensations. While assessing clients' readiness to transition into phases 3 to 8, therapists need to attune to indications that reflect the potential struggle of clients' internal parts with time orientation and signal that clients don't have consent from their inner parts to move forward.

Time Orientation

Clients who have a history of attachment trauma experience a phenomenon called time disorientation. Parts of Self form around learned behaviors, self-beliefs, and traumatic incidents within the context of childhood attachment relationships. Unprocessed childhood material is stored as alternate configurations of the memory network which AFTT-A calls Child/Adolescent parts of Self or "Kid Brain," separate from the adaptive information processing (AIP) system in "Adult Brain." However, parts of Self contain more than memories of adverse childhood events. Child/Adolescent parts hold past experiences that include relationships, behavior patterns, beliefs, developmental stages, unmet needs, emotions, and coping strategies, thus forming an inner configuration that represents a Child/Adolescent part of Self at a certain age rather than solely a collection of unprocessed traumatic material.

Since the information contained in "Kid Brain" is disconnected from "Adult Brain" or the part of the brain that processes memories in the context of time, Child/Adolescent parts of Self can't tell the difference between "now" in the present moment of a client's adult life and "back then" which, for younger parts, is *still* the present moment. At the beginning of therapy and intermittently throughout therapy, Child/

Adolescent parts as well as the older versions of the Adult and Parent parts of Self get triggered into a time-disoriented state. Parts of Self in a time-disoriented state still believe that danger from the past is present and the coping mechanisms and survival skills they needed to endure the pain and shame during childhood are still critical to survival in adult life.

Child/Adolescent parts in a time-disoriented state also believe that their unmet needs from childhood can still be fulfilled in adult life by using the old, learned coping and survival strategies and by following the old Early Bonding Contract rules from childhood. One of Freud's defense mechanisms is called "repetition compulsion" (1990). He believed that we humans have a need to complete what is incomplete and to finish what is unfinished in our lives. As children, we have access to a limited number of ways to try to get their needs met, largely influenced by our environments. As a result, we repeat the old ways of getting our needs met in our adult lives even though we discover, over and over, that the old ways don't help us meet adulthood needs. For example, children who learn that disregarding their own needs and feelings to take care of an attachment figure might get them a little attention and appreciation, will carry that pattern into their adult life. As adults, they might want to develop a relationship that includes a more balanced give-and-take between them and their partner. However, the client's Competent Adult and Child/Adolescent parts of Self have conflicting motives. The client's Competent Adult part wants a more mutually sharing relationship while, at the same time, an internal Child/Adolescent part finds such a balance threatening. How will they get approval and appreciation if they don't over-function and act as a caretaker in the relationship? The Child part only knows how to use those old patterns and stay true to the old Early Bonding Contract rules and will try, over and over and over again, to get those needs met for approval and appreciation in their present-day life. Unfortunately, we see how those childhood beliefs and patterns not only *can't* help clients get unmet childhood needs met but also sabotage getting their *adulthood* needs met as well.

When clients have parts that are not oriented to the present moment, they are also not ready and able to give permission to move forward in therapy at any step of the AFTT-A process and, in particular, to transition from AFTT-A's enhanced preparation phase to EMDR therapy phases 3 to 8. Clients often demonstrate patterns in their lives and/or therapy that reveal they don't have a consensus from their internal system to move forward; some of these patterns are

- difficulty accessing and experiencing or regulating emotions during/in between sessions;
- lack of follow-through with practice or assignments between sessions, missing or coming late to appointments;
- ongoing crises or relapses in/worsening of symptoms or problem behaviors in present-day life; and
- patterns of fragility, dissociation, withdrawal, willfulness, or argumentativeness in sessions.

Clients who overcontrol emotions may be acting from the overdeveloped Emotion Controller-Regulator aspect of the Adult part of Self. They often have difficulty identifying, connecting to, and experiencing emotions in therapy as well as in their present-day lives. Clients who under-regulate emotions function from the little "a" portion of the Adult part of Self. They tend to have an opposite challenge with emotions as overcontrolled clients: They have intense emotions, unstable moods, and may show intense affect in therapy and in their adult lives. In both cases, the old versions of the Adult part of Self are time disoriented and may resort to old patterns of coping. Additionally, clients need their Competent Adult part in charge of both therapy processes to access and process memories of adverse childhood events and adult-life to make sound decisions.

Sometimes, the Critical Parent part of Self is threatened or gets worried when clients begin to feel better, improve their mood, decrease anxiety and other negative affect, begin to change negative beliefs about themselves, and see positive effects of therapy on the present-day lives. How could the Critical Parent part possibly interpret clients making progress in therapy as dangerous? Remember that the original intent of the Critical Parent part of Self was protection but morphed into an overdeveloped critical voice based on messages given to clients from attachment figures in childhood. Ironically, Critical Parent parts don't really want clients to get hurt in their present-day lives. As a result, they may not want clients to get their hopes up that feeling better and making changes for the better are going to last. *Positive* affect may trigger clients' critical voice to become time disoriented and, despite agreements with the True Parent part of Self and the client's Resource Team, jump in with old protective patterns to remind clients not to feel too optimistic or they will be disappointed.

Clients may show their reluctance to, fear about, or lack of readiness to move forward in therapy as evidenced by their attachment patterns within the therapeutic relationship itself. Clients might present therapists with a sense of fragility ("How could you even expect me to move forward? I can't! You don't understand how hard this is for me!"), disconnection or withdrawal ("I don't know. Nothing. I don't feel anything. Why are we even trying?"), or willfulness and argumentativeness ("Yes, but... You're wrong. You aren't helping me. I don't want to and you can't make me!").

Time orientation is a goal of the protocols in AFTT-A's enhanced preparation phase of EMDR therapy. The *Safe Place and Higher Power for the Adult Part of Self* and *Safe Place and Higher Power for Child/Adolescent Parts of Self* (see Protocol Scripts 4 and 5) protocols act as a foundation for time orientation by assisting clients to begin to differentiate between the past, when there were unmet needs and the danger was real, and the present moment, when the danger has passed and clients have the support and help they need to get their needs met in their adult lives.

Installation of a team of inner resources and integrating old and new versions of Adult and Parent parts of Self as team members foster time orientation by connecting clients to strengths they didn't previously believe they possessed. Accessing and strengthening the Competent Adult and True Parent parts improve time orientation by helping clients develop mature and helpful versions of parts whose growth was stunted in the past. The *Tucking the Child/Adolescent Part of Self Into the Safe Place* protocol (see Protocol Script 11) continues differentiation between the Adult and younger parts of Self with the Competent Adult part empowered to orchestrate the inner system and oversee adult life. Creation of new Bonding Contract rules and the writing of a Therapeutic Story (see Protocol Scripts 12 and

13) assist with time orientation by offering alternative beliefs and perspectives to those engendered in the past.

Overall, time orientation assists clients to reintegrate the whole of their inner system into the present moment. Clients rediscover and reconnect to their Spiritual Essence, their core of strength and goodness. Time orientation also helps clients connect the positive messages and affect from AFTT-A protocols to both their internal personality system and their present-day lives:

- "I'm okay," "I'm lovable," and a sense of calm, safety, and being grounded and centered with their Safe Place and Higher Power; and
- "No matter what, I have what I need" and "I'm not alone anymore" with their Inner Resource Team.

To reorient clients to present time, therapists utilize time orientation techniques to help clients and clients' internal parts discern the difference between present and past (Martin, 2018). Time orientation is incorporated into all AFTT-A's protocols but especially into the *Getting Client's Permission to Transition to EMDR Therapy Phases 3 to 8* protocol. Time orientation procedures can be initiated and repeated at any time in therapy that therapists sense that their clients' internal parts are time disoriented and permission to continue therapy work hasn't been obtained or has been rescinded.

STEPS FOR GETTING CLIENT'S PERMISSION TO TRANSITION FROM THE AFTT-A PREPARATION PHASE TO PHASES 3 TO 8 IN EMDR THERAPY

During the AFTT-A model's preparation phase for EMDR therapy, clients focus on accessing and strengthening positive beliefs and affect as well as reconstructing their internal personality system. In EMDR phases 3 to 8, clients' attention and efforts shift to tapping into painful memories and the associated negative affect. One of the last steps therapists take before moving into phases 3 to 8 is to obtain clients' permission and the permission of all the parts of Self to begin to face and resolve traumatic memories. Getting permission is a pivotal decision point for clients and a final assessment of client readiness for therapists.

Protocol Script 14: *Getting Client's Permission to Transition to EMDR Therapy Phases 3 to 8* builds on protocols aimed at creating a strong sense of Self that is made up of unique parts working together with access to positive qualities, beliefs, and affect whenever needed. Immediately preceding clients' transitioning into trauma desensitization and reprocessing, the protocol offers clients the opportunity to make certain that they have the inner support and protection they need in the form of their Resource Team and that their Competent Adult part of Self will take charge of the subsequent therapy phases. All parts of Self that either have doubts and may be time disoriented or parts that will be helpful to the client's readiness are invited to listen in on the Resource Team meeting and to look through the client's eyes as they get reoriented to the present moment.

Getting permission also reinforces the previously developed methods of communication between clients and the members of their Resource Team and clients and their parts of Self. All parts of Self and Resource Team members take the opportunity to express any doubts, worries, fears, and concerns so that plans for and solutions to potential barriers and problems are explored and put into place. Therapists verify that all parts of the client's Self are oriented to the present moment, knowing that the danger from "back then" has passed. Clients who are ready to give permission to move into subsequent therapy steps feel competent and confident in their capability to complete the upcoming tasks and their related challenges. See the full protocol script at the end of the chapter.

1. Convene the Resource Team Meeting and Explain the Purposes of Meeting

The Resource Team members now include both inner strengths and new versions of the Adult (Competent Adult) and Parent (True Parent) parts of Self. At this point, clients have the internal support and protection they need to shift focus to resolving past traumatic events. Getting permission gives both clients and therapists the chance to bring the client and their Resource Team together to make certain that all parts of Self are oriented to the present moment and make the commitment to help clients with the next phase of therapy. Therapists utilize mindful awareness of and attunement to clients' behaviors in sessions and their reports of situations and occurrences between sessions to assess readiness.

2. Verify That the Child/Adolescent Parts Are in Safe Places With Their Higher Powers. Emphasize to the Resource Team and Higher Powers the Importance of the Child/Adolescent Parts Staying in Their Safe Places

As we've described before, Child/Adolescent parts of Self often "eavesdrop" on clients' adult lives. I remember sitting at the top of the stairs when I was in grade school, listening in when my parents had a party after I was supposed to be tucked into bed and sleeping. Once Child/Adolescent parts overhear what's happening in clients' adult lives, they may feel the need to step in and "help" clients in their child-like ways. As a result, an important component of clients giving permission is to verify that Child/Adolescent parts are in their Safe Places, supervised and protected by their Higher Powers, unconcerned with clients' adult lives, and reassured that their voices will be heard without them needing to leave their places of safety. If needed, therapists help clients revise and install improved aspects of Child/Adolescent parts' Safe Places and/or Higher Powers to ensure they don't feel the need to take charge of the tasks in the next phases of therapy.

3. Introduce Phases 3 to 8 of EMDR Therapy

For clients to give informed consent to move into the next steps of EMDR therapy, they need to understand the purposes, benefits, and potential risks of trauma treatment particularly related to EMDR therapy phases 3 to 8. Therapists explain the tasks involved in the ensuing stages and the differences between the AFTT-A enhanced preparation phase and EMDR therapy phases 3 to 8. Up until this point, clients have accessed and reinforced positive qualities, images, and affect. Bilateral stimulation (BLS) consisted of short sets of slow butterfly tapping or use of tappers. Upcoming EMDR protocols that involve desensitizing and reprocessing present-day triggers and traumatic memories utilize eye movements for BLS rather than tapping and the sets of BLS are longer and much faster.

Therapists may decide that focused reprocessing protocols such as Eye Movement Desensitization (EMD) and restricted/contained reprocessing will be helpful to their clients who still have difficulty with affect regulation and might not be able to tolerate the EMDR standard protocol (Shapiro, 2021a, 2021b, pp. 16–18). Therapists present information about the components of phases 3 to 8 in the standard protocol (selecting target memory, reprocessing memory, linking positive cognition to neutralized memory, and body scan; Leeds, 2016, p. 49; Shapiro, 2018, pp. 85–161). Clients find it helpful for therapists to give them an overview of phases 3 to 8 so they are introduced to the elements of the process and have the time and space to ask questions and voice concerns.

4. Orient All Parts of the Client's Self to the Present Time

Once clients receive a synopsis of the EMDR phases that come next, therapists ask clients to notice if there is any part of them (Child/Adolescent, Critical Parent, Emotion Controller-Regulator, little "a," Competent Adult, or True Parent) that isn't ready to, doesn't want to, doesn't think they can, is scared, or has second thoughts about moving ahead to the next protocols. To paraphrase Kathleen Martin (2018), "Does every part of your being, every cell of your being know that the danger is over?" If the answer is "yes," therapists can skip to Step 5. If the answer is "no," therapists again invite all parts into the session who can be helpful and/or need to hear what will be discussed because they still hold doubts about the danger being over. Parts that are reluctant or afraid are time disoriented to "back then" when danger was real instead of time oriented to "now" when the danger has passed and unmet childhood needs of clients' Child/Adolescent parts can be contacted in previously agreed upon methods of communication in the present moment in their Safe Places with their Higher Powers. Therapists have options for re-orienting clients to time by pointing out how the present moment in the therapist's office is different than the past (Martin, 2018). Therapists may have clients:

- Consider their hands, jewelry, clothes, phone;
- Look at a calendar or phone to see the date and year;
- Scan the therapy office; or
- Discuss the length of relationship with the therapist.

Clients can also be time oriented by being reminded of the results of their work in AFTT-A so far: Creation of Safe Places and Higher Powers for inner Adult and Child/Adolescent parts of Self, their team of internal resources, and new versions of parts of Self; development of corrective attachment relationships among internal parts and improved self-beliefs and self-perceptions; and, most importantly, provision of gifts of safety, protection, caring, and nurturing to all aspects of their inner personality system through their Competent Adult part of Self.

BOX 18.1 CLIENT EXAMPLE: TIME ORIENTATION

Therapist: I'd like you to invite in whatever part or parts of you that don't believe that the danger is past. Let them listen, feel the tones. If they're part of your team, they can stay in your Meeting Place. If they're Kid parts, we want them to stay in their Safe Places and use the Resource Team member assigned to them to communicate with them as needed. Would you check inside to make sure that would be all right?

Client: (Closes her eyes for a moment. Nods her head and opens her eyes.) Yes, it's okay.

(continued)

BOX 18.1 CLIENT EXAMPLE: TIME ORIENTATION (continued)

Therapist: I'd like you to look around my office. How long have you been coming here?

Client: A little less than a year.

Therapist: So, you didn't come to this office when you were young? I didn't know you in the past?

Client: That's right. We didn't know each other.

Therapist: So, we've only known each other this year?

Client: Yes.

Therapist: Not even last year or any time earlier?

Client: No.

Therapist: I'd like you to look at your hands resting on the arms of that chair in my office in this year.

Client: (Nods her head.)

Therapist: What do you notice about your hands?

Client: Well, they're the hands of someone who's older. They have wrinkles and freckles.

Therapist: So, you are older. Your hands have wrinkles and freckles.

Client: (Laughs.) Oh yeah!

Therapist: The ring you have on. When did you get that?

Client: Oh, gosh, about 10 years ago.

Therapist: So, when you were an adult.

Client: Yes.

Therapist: And the bracelet? How long have you had it?

Client: A few years.

Therapist: So, you got it as an adult too?

Client: Yes.

Therapist: How do you feel as you sit here in my office now with your hands on the arms of the chair, seeing your ring and bracelet?

Client: I feel calmer. More solid.

Therapist: Where do you feel the calmer, more solid feelings in your body?

Client: Across my shoulders, in my back and chest.

Therapist: The sensations across your shoulders, in your back and chest?

Client: I feel stronger but relaxed.

Therapist: Hold that in mind and feel the tones.

(Slow short sets of BLS to strengthen and reinforce positive affect.)

5. Discuss With the Resource Team Potential Barriers or Difficulties in the Next Phases of EMDR Therapy and Brainstorm Ways the Resource Team Will Be Helpful: Access and Reinforce the Positive Affect

The AFTT-A model is designed to help clients detect issues and potential problems in their adult lives and bring together all their inner parts and resources to solve those problems and to create lives that are worth both living (Linehan, 1993, 2014) and sharing (Lynch, 2018). AFTT-A also assists clients in identifying and planning ways to overcome barriers to the completion of subsequent phases of EMDR therapy. In the *Getting Client's Permission to Transition to EMDR Therapy Phases 3 to 8* protocol, all parts of Self and Resource Team members have the opportunity to voice their concerns and fears and work together to brainstorm solutions when an issue or problem is identified. Clients apply their newly installed beliefs, the reconfigured inner personality system, and their Resource Team to potentially challenging scenarios in the therapy process.

BOX 18.2 CLIENT EXAMPLE: DISCUSSING RESOURCE TEAM CONCERNS ABOUT MOVING INTO EMDR THERAPY PHASES 3 TO 8

Therapist: Does anyone on your team have doubts or concerns?

Client: Yes, the Guardian-Ad-Litem said the kids are pretty scared. They think they have to go back to the past and be hurt again. I feel kind of anxious, too.

Therapist: What do you think would be helpful for the kids to hear from their Guardian?

Client: Well, it's like we've said before. They don't ever have to go back to past ever again. It's over. They survived and now they have Safe Places and Higher Powers. They can give me information I need but they stay in their Safe Places while I do the work here in your office as my adult self.

Therapist: So, whoever needs to hear that, can feel the tones through your hands.

(Slow, short set to reinforce healthy boundaries among parts.)

Therapist: How do you feel here in my office when you think about that?

Client: Actually, relieved. The kids are taken care of and I can do this.

Therapist: Where do you feel that relief in your body?

Client: In my head. All that movement has slowed down and quieted.

(Slow, short sets to reinforce positive affect.)

---

6. Reinforce the Resource Team's Commitment to Support and Assist the Client During Subsequent Phases

In addition to advice and guidance, a client's Resource Team provides compassion and understanding about their past experiences while, at the same time, providing support and encouragement to move forward with necessary changes. The Resource Team's commitment to help the client no matter what the circumstances is essential for readiness to move into phases 3 to 8.

> **BOX 18.3 CLIENT EXAMPLE: RESOURCE TEAM'S COMMITMENT TO HELP THE CLIENT IN PHASES 3 TO 8**
>
> **Therapist:** What do you need from your team as you move forward in therapy?
>
> **Client:** Well, I really need to know that I'm not doing this by myself. That they will be with me, believing in me and encouraging me.
>
> **Therapist:** Ask them for that and see what you notice.
>
> **Client:** They're all holding out their hands to take mine.
>
> **Therapist:** How does that feel?
>
> **Client:** (Tearful.) Wonderful. I think I can do this.
>
> **Therapist:** Notice that and allow it to strengthen, deepen, expand as much as possible.
>
> (Slow, short sets to reinforce positive affect.)

7. Install the Future Rehearsal of the Client Utilizing the Resource Team's Assistance and Support

Future Rehearsal and future template are EMDR therapy protocols that apply inner resources to challenging present-day situations and link positive affect to clients dealing with tough situations in a competent and confident manner (Shapiro, 2021a, 2021b, pp. 45–60, 145–148). AFTT-A uses Future Rehearsal in the *Getting Client's Permission to Transition to EMDR Therapy Phases 3 to 8* protocol to assist clients in effectively regulating their emotions through the subsequent EMDR stages of therapy by integrating the help of clients' Resource Team and adding the concept of a "Future Self" or the "part of you that already knows" how to effectively access and reprocess traumatic material. The main goals for Future Rehearsal in the AFTT-A protocol of *Getting Client's Permission to Transition to EMDR Therapy Phases 3 to 8* are to recognize potential difficulties for clients in the next steps of therapy, link clients' sense of competence and confidence with working through the identified barriers, and offer clients the opportunity to successfully practice and experience overcoming possible obstacles in their therapy process.

POINTS TO REMEMBER

- Signs clients don't have permission from inner parts of Self to move forward in therapy include difficulty accessing and experiencing or regulating emotions during/in between sessions; lack of follow through with practice or assignments between sessions; missing or coming late to appointments; on-going crises or relapses in/worsening of symptoms or problem behaviors in present-day life; and patterns of fragility, dissociation, withdrawal, willfulness, or argumentativeness in sessions.
- Purposes of time orientation include establishment of re-integration and wholeness in the present moment; rediscovery of and reconnection to inner strength and goodness, Spiritual Essence; reinforcement of the Safe Place and

Higher Power messages of "I'm okay" and "I'm loved" as well as a sense of calm and being grounded and centered; and reinforcement of the Resource Team's messages of "No matter what, I have what I need" and "I'm not alone anymore."

- The time orientation process can be repeated any time the therapist senses that parts of the client's Self are time disoriented or that permission to continue has been rescinded.
- Purposes of Getting Permission protocol are to double check the functionality of the Resource Team so clients have the inner support and protection they need in order to transition to EMDR phases 3 to 8 and have their Competent Adult part of Self in charge of the process; reinforce method(s) so the Child part(s) can communicate with the Resource Team from their Safe Place; give all parts of Self and Resource Team members time and space to express doubts, fears, and concerns as well as a plan for solutions to potential barriers and problems; provide an important opportunity to orient parts of Self to time; and strengthen the client's sense of competence and confidence in moving into the next steps of the EMDR therapy process.

TROUBLESHOOTING

- If the client continues to have difficulty staying time oriented to the present moment, review and revise Safe Places and Higher Powers for Child parts of Self to see if there are still needs for nurturing or protection that are not being met. Review and revise the Resource Team members to ensure that the client has identified needed strengths and team members that can help parts of Self with time orientation.
- If the client has negative affect when practicing overcoming potential obstacles in subsequent therapy phases, use the container from previous protocols to set aside negative affect and refocus on positive cognitions, emotions, and sensations. If negative affect persists, reconvene the Resource Team to explore reasons and brainstorm solutions to include in Future Rehearsal.

PAUSE AND REFLECT FOR THE THERAPIST

As you work with a challenging client who is preparing to move into EMDR phases 3 to 8, notice if all parts of you are ready and able to give permission for you to be mindful, attuned, and present with them from your most authentic Self. What do you observe in your body as you imagine starting into EMDR phase 3 with them? What emotions and cognitions come up for you? Are any parts of you disoriented to time and believe that bringing traumatic memories to light and clients telling the truth about what happened to them is in some way dangerous or taboo? Do you sense an urge to avoid being emotionally involved with clients during the subsequent phases of EMDR therapy? Can you feel an impulse to revert to an old way of emotionally protecting yourself or the client? Meet with your Resource Team member and brainstorm if you need to add another team member that can help you be present in therapy with your client in an open and compassionate way. Talk with your peer consultation group or consultant to get support and to your own therapist if the issues you identify need to be resolved in therapy.

USEFUL TERMS AND DEFINITIONS

"Adult Brain": The parts of the brain that house EMDR's adaptive information processing (AIP) system and include higher cognitive processes such as learning, problem-solving, decision-making, language, understanding of emotions, and narrative memory.

AFTT-A: Attachment-Focused Trauma Therapy for Adults

BLS: bilateral stimulation

DBT: Dialectical Behaviorial Therapy

EMD: Eye Movement Desensitization

EMDR: Eye Movement Desensitization and Reprocessing

"Kid Brain": The neural network clusters in the emotional/social part of the brain that store unprocessed memories of adverse events and are disconnected from a sense of time and from the parts of the brain capable of processing memories and transferring them into narrative memory. AFTT-A views the neural networks as encapsulating more than memories of adverse events and includes the experiences, cognitive development, learning during a particular client age.

PROTOCOL SCRIPT 14. GETTING CLIENT'S PERMISSION TO TRANSITION TO EMDR THERAPY PHASES 3 TO 8

Adapted from Leeds, A. (2016). *A guide to the standard EMDR protocols for clinicians, supervisors, and consultants* (2nd ed.). Springer Publishing Company; Fraser, G. A. (1991). The Dissociative Table Technique: A strategy for working with ego states and dissociative disorders and ego-state therapy. *Dissociation: Progress in the Dissociative Disorders*, 4(4), 205–213; Fraser, G. A. (2003). Fraser's "Dissociative Table Technique" revisited, revised: A strategy for working with ego states in dissociative disorders and ego-state therapy. *Journal of Trauma and Dissociation*, 4(4), 5–28. https://doi.org/10.1300/J229v04n04_02; Potter, A. E. (1994). *Inside out: Rebuilding self and personality through inner child therapy* (therapist manual and client workbook). Taylor and Francis; Shapiro, F. (2018). *Eye movement desensitization and reprocessing (EMDR) therapy: Basic principles, protocols, and procedures* (2nd ed.). Guilford Press; Shapiro, F. (2021a). *Weekend 1 training manual of the two-part EMDR therapy basic training* (revised). EMDR Institute, Inc.; and Shapiro, F. (2021b). *Weekend 2 training manual of the two-part EMDR therapy basic training* (revised). EMDR Institute, Inc.

Prior to starting the protocol, review with the client the AIP system and how the AIP system reprocesses traumatic material. Request that all parts of Self (whether they are parts that have concerns or doubts or parts that can be helpful) that need to be a part of the therapy session listen and look through the client's eyes.

1. **Convene the Resource Team Meeting and Explain the Purposes of Meeting.** *Say...* "Let's get your team together and talk about the next steps in EMDR therapy. In

the AFTT-A enhanced preparation phase, you accessed and strengthened the positive thoughts and emotions by giving yourself a place of respite, tucking Child/Adolescent parts into Safe Places, and creating a Resource Team that now includes the Competent Adult and True Parent parts of Self. We want you to be able to take your new beliefs of 'I'm okay,' 'I have everything I need,' and 'I'm not alone anymore' into the EMDR phases that involve desensitizing present-day triggers and reprocessing traumatic memories. We want to make sure that all parts of you feel safe in the present moment and give permission to move to the next therapy steps." *Ask...* "How does that sound?" *Say...* "Let's get you and your team together." (*Gather Resource Team members together with the client in the Meeting Place. Access and reinforce the positive affect related to reconnecting with team members.*) *Say...* "What would be helpful for your team to know about the purposes of this meeting?"

_____

_____

Ask... "How does your team seem to respond?"

_____

_____

Access and reinforce positive affect with short sets of slow BLS with tappers or butterfly taps. Practice the container for setting aside the negative affect if needed.

2. Verify That the Child/Adolescent Parts Are in Safe Places With Their Higher Powers. Emphasize to the Resource Team and Higher Powers the Importance of the Child/Adolescent Parts Staying in Their Safe Places. *Say...* "The first item on the agenda is to make sure that your Child/Adolescent parts of Self are in their Safe Places with their Higher Powers and that the Child/Adolescent parts' Higher Powers and your Resource Team know how important it is for your Child/Adolescent parts to stay in their Safe Places while you and your team are meeting. We want the Child/Adolescent parts to understand that the team needs to know what they're thinking and feeling about you taking the next steps in therapy but we want to use the new way of communication you agreed on so they stay in their Safe Places while you, the Competent Adult, and the True Parent parts of Self attend the team meeting. Let's have you remind your Child/Adolescent parts and Resource Team members about the new way you all decided to communicate."

3. Introduce Phases 3 to 8 of EMDR Therapy. *Say...* "Let's talk to your team about what the next steps are for therapy. Until now, you've been building positive aspects of yourself and focusing positive emotions and beliefs. So far, we've used very short sets of slow bilateral stimulation (BLS) by using the tappers (or butterfly taps) to strengthen the positive affect related to the protocols. Now, you're going to be accessing, desensitizing, and reprocessing the negative affect related to present-day triggers and memories of adverse events. We'll be using eye movements instead of the tappers for BLS and the sets of eye movements will be longer and much faster."

Ask... "What do you think would be helpful for your team to know about moving onto the next steps of EMDR therapy?"

_____
_____

4. Orient All Parts of the Client's Self to the Present Time. *Ask...* "Is there any part of you that doesn't think it's time to move forward in therapy? Does every part of you know that it's 'now' and not 'back then' and the danger is past?"

_____
_____

If parts are oriented to time, go to Step 5. If not, invite any parts who have doubts about the danger being past to listen in on the discussion and all parts and Resource Team members who can be helpful to join in the discussion. Ask the client to look at their hands. Note the age of their hands. Think about when they bought or received any jewelry they're wearing. Ask the client to look around the office and remember how long they have been coming to therapy, that they didn't know the therapist as a child. Prompt the client to keep in mind the Safe Places and Higher Powers they've given to the Adult and Child/Adolescent parts of Self. They gifted safety, protection, caring, and nurturing to their inner parts in the present moment. Ask... "What do you notice?"

_____
_____

Access and reinforce the positive affect.

5. Discuss With the Resource Team Potential Barriers or Difficulties in the Next Phases of EMDR Therapy and Brainstorm Ways the Resource Team Will Be Helpful. *Encourage Resource Team members to express any doubts or worries.* Say... "Let's open up the meeting so your Resource Team members can raise concerns or worries; so they can talk about possible difficulties in or barriers to the next steps in therapy." *Ask...* "What do you notice? How can your team help?"

_____
_____

Access and reinforce the positive affect.
   Say... "Is there anything else you feel like you'll need from your Resource Team as you take the next steps in therapy?"

_____
_____

Ask... "How will your team help you?"

_____

_____

Access and reinforce the positive affect.

6. Reinforce the Resource Team's Commitment to Support and Assist the Client During Subsequent Phases. *Say...* "Take a few moments to let yourself notice how it feels to have your Resource Team committed to helping you with whatever you need and however you need their help." (*Access and reinforce the positive affect.*)

7. Install the Future Rehearsal of the Client Utilizing the Resource Team's Assistance and Support. *Say...* "I'd like you to think about a time in therapy when (***name one of the challenges brought up in discussion***) might happen. Notice how your Resource Team helps by (***mention ways the Resource Team has agreed to help***)." *Ask...* "What do you notice?"

_____

_____

Access and reinforce the positive affect.

REFERENCES

Leeds, A. (2016). *A guide to the standard EMDR protocols for clinicians, supervisors, and consultants* (2nd ed.). Springer Publishing Company.

Linehan, M. (1993). *Cognitive-behavioral treatment of borderline personality disorder*. Guilford Press.

Linehan, M. (2014). *DBT skills training manual* (2nd ed.). Guilford Press.

Lynch, T. (2018). *The skills training manual for radically open dialectical behavior therapy: A clinician's guide for treating disorders of overcontrol*. Context Press.

Martin, K. (2018, April). *Mastering the treatment of complex trauma: Transforming theory into practice*. Presentation, Omaha, Nebraska.

Shapiro, F. (2018). *Eye movement desensitization and reprocessing (EMDR) therapy: Basic principles, protocols, and procedures* (2nd ed.). Guilford Press.

Shapiro, F. (2021a). *Weekend 1 training manual of the two-part EMDR therapy basic training* (revised). EMDR Institute, Inc.

Shapiro, F. (2021b). *Weekend 2 training manual of the two-part EMDR therapy basic training* (revised). EMDR Institute, Inc.

CHAPTER 19

Client Transition From Enhanced Preparation Phase in Attachment-Focused Trauma Therapy for Adults to EMDR Phases 3 to 8

INTRODUCTION

A history of ongoing abuse and neglect within clients' primary attachment relationships during childhood complicates posttraumatic symptomology and requires a multi-modal approach to trauma therapy. Attachment-Focused Trauma Therapy for Adults (AFTT-A) utilizes Eye Movement Desensitization and Reprocessing (EMDR) therapy's preparation phase and integrates theory and practice from a variety of therapy approaches to address the complexities of attachment trauma. The AFTT-A model regards its application of EMDR therapy preparation phase as a stand-alone treatment for resolving the impact of attachment trauma on clients' personality structures and both internal and present-day attachments *in addition to* providing the essential emotional groundwork for phases 3 to 8 of EMDR therapy.

Like the Kintsugi process of creating unique works of art from shattered pottery pieces by celebrating and accentuating the scars of brokenness, AFTT-A protocols aren't intended to restore clients to an original state or to whom they were at an earlier time, but rather to move clients into a new state of strength and resilience (Kitty, 2020; Santini, 2019). Thus, the main outcomes of the AFTT-A preparation phase are

- transformation of clients' sense of Self with a core of spiritual goodness;
- reconstruction of their internal systems with integration of healthier, more helpful versions of personality parts;
- restoration of healthy boundaries, attachments, communication, and teamwork among inner parts;
- development of strong positive self-beliefs;
- reconnection to inner resources and a Spiritual Essence;
- orientation to time in the present moment;
- formation of balanced and fulfilling present-day relationships; and
- emotional readiness to move into the subsequent desensitization and trauma reprocessing phases of EMDR therapy.

Up to this point in AFTT-A therapy, clients developed a strong inner foundation and support system and became ready to integrate and apply all their resources, skills, and experiences to the next steps in their therapy process. One of the most positive outcomes of the AFTT-A preparation phase is a marked improvement in clients' affect regulation during desensitization and reprocessing protocols. Clients who tend to under-control emotions are less likely to get triggered into flashbacks or abreactions. Clients who demonstrate more emotion overcontrol can more easily access, experience, and process emotions. Clients are less likely to get "stuck" or loop during processing and, if they have difficulty, they move through challenges and barriers more quickly and with emotional balance because they have already learned positive self-beliefs, connected with the inner guidance and support, and experienced time orientation.

Therapists begin by reviewing the process they utilized to gain permission from all parts of clients' Self and members of their Resource Team to move forward in the therapy process. They remind clients about the tasks involved in the ensuing therapy stages and, if needed, give clients more time and space to ask questions and voice concerns. Therapists also reiterate the differences between the AFTT-A preparation phase they recently completed and EMDR therapy phases 3 to 8 into which they will transition. For example, clients focus primarily on positive aspects of themselves and their lives and access and reinforce positive qualities, images, and affect in the preparation phase while upcoming protocols in phases 3 to 8 concentrate on desensitizing and reprocessing present-day triggers and traumatic memories with associated negative thoughts, emotions, and body sensations.

Therapists may decide to utilize focused reprocessing protocols such as Eye Movement Desensitization (EMD) and restricted/contained reprocessing with clients who may still have difficulty regulating affect (Shapiro, 2018, pp. 220–222; Shapiro, 2021a, 2021b, pp. 16–18) instead of or prior to the full reprocessing standard EMDR protocol (Leeds, 2016, p. 49; Shapiro, 2018, pp. 85–161). Another difference between the preparation phase and subsequent phases is in the use of bilateral stimulation (BLS). In the preparation phase, BLS consisted of short sets of slow butterfly taps or use of tappers. In phases 4 to 8, BLS is achieved through eye movements rather than tapping and the sets of BLS are longer and much faster.

In AFTT-A's preparation phase, clients identified overall goals for therapy and their associated positive characteristics and Resource Team representatives. Clients now narrow down their overall therapy goals into what they want to achieve in therapy related to phases 3 to 8. Clients can even set goals for a particular protocol or with a specific memory. What do they want to accomplish in trauma resolution phases of EMDR therapy? What place do they want their past to have in their life or what kind of influence do they want their past to have on their life? How do they want to feel about themselves? What differences do they want to see in themselves? In their relationships?

Prior to starting the *Transition From the AFTT-A Preparation Phase to EMDR Phases 3 to 8* protocol, therapists and clients review initial therapy goals, strengths, current Resource Team members, and Meeting Place. Child/Adolescent parts of Self get tucked into Safe Places with their Higher Powers and reassured that the job of the Competent Adult part of Self is to take charge of the emotional work involved in the next therapy steps with the support and protection of their own Higher Power and their Resource Team members. Therapists help clients get reconnected to the belief of "I'm okay" and the positive affect linked to their Adult Safe Place and Higher

Power. They also assist clients to reinforce the positive affect they have related to their Resource Team that now includes the Competent Adult and True Parent parts of Self, the beliefs of "No matter what, I have what I need" and "I am not alone anymore," their Meeting Place for Resource Team meetings with the transitional object they brought from their Adult Safe Place, their new Bonding Contract rules, and their Therapeutic Story.

STEPS FOR TRANSITIONING FROM THE AFTT-A ENHANCED PREPARATION PHASE TO EMDR PHASES 3 TO 8 PROTOCOL

In the *Transition From the AFTT-A Preparation Phase to EMDR Phases 3 to 8* protocol (see Protocol Script 15 at the end of this chapter), clients gather their Resource Team members for a meeting or a series of meetings to identify goals for the upcoming phases of EMDR therapy, the strengths clients will need to access to meet their goals, and representatives of those strengths on their Resource Team. The plan created with the client's Resource Team focuses on how the current configuration of their Resource Team might help them meet their goals for EMDR phases 3 to 8 and whether the client's strengths and team members need to be reworked.

At times, the clients' Resource Teams can apply the strengths they already identified and use the current configuration of Resource Team members to accomplish their goals for transitioning to subsequent therapy phases. Sometimes, clients don't need all the of the strengths and team members they originally determined and comprise a "subcommittee" of team members to address clients' needs as they move forward in therapy. At other times, clients need to add strengths and supplement their current Resource Team with new members. Although the formal Resource Team meeting doesn't convene until Step 4 of the *Transition From the AFTT-A Preparation Phase to EMDR Phases 3 to 8* protocol, therapists encourage clients to engage their existing Resource Team any time during the protocol to assist with difficulties or barriers in Steps 1 to 3.

1. Identify the Goals Specific to EMDR Therapy Trauma Protocols
Therapists remind clients that they will integrate and apply all the changes they made in their internal personality system, skills they learned, and inner resources they developed during the AFTT-A preparation phase to the next phases of therapy, specifically to the EMDR therapy desensitization and reprocessing protocols. They start by reviewing with clients their overall goals set early in the therapy process during the preparation phase and reworking their initial goals to concentrate on what clients want to accomplish during the later steps of EMDR therapy. If clients have difficulty brainstorming new goals or modifying existing goals, they can open the discussion up with their current Resource Team.

Clients create goals related to overcome potential impediments to their therapy process; for example:

- I access and process my feelings easily during EMDR sessions.
- I use my Resource Team to balance my emotions while I reprocess memories.
- I let my therapist know when I feel overwhelmed.
- When I place my hand on my chest, I connect to my Higher Power and my Resource Team to remind me that I'm okay, I can do this, and I have the support I need.

- I ask my therapist for help when I can't get connected to my feelings.
- I use that feeling of anxiety to alert me that a Child/Adolescent part might be out of their Safe Place and needs to be tucked in.

2. Brainstorm the Needed Strengths/Positive Characteristics/Inner Resources to Meet Goals

Next, therapists and clients re-examine the strengths they decided would help them reach their original goals and determine whether those positive characteristics will benefit them as they move into the next stages of therapy. Again, if clients have difficulty brainstorming strengths/positive characteristics/inner resources, they can open the discussion to their present Resource Team.

Clients have the options of including all their original strengths, choose one or two of their current strengths, add strengths, or completely generate new strengths to aid them in meeting their goals for the trauma resolution protocols. For example, one of my clients initially identified self-compassion, faith in their convictions, persistence, and determination for positive characteristics. When we started the *Transition From the AFTT-A Preparation Phase to EMDR Phases 3 to 8* protocol, they created a goal for getting emotional support and help throughout the rest of the therapy process during and between sessions, so they added willingness to ask for help as a resource.

3. Decide Whether Existing Resource Team Members Can Act as Representatives of Needed Strengths

By this point in therapy, clients are very familiar with their Resource Team members, have utilized them to assist with both the emotional tasks of the AFTT-A preparation phase and challenges of their adult lives and relationships, and linked a sense of competence and confidence to collaborating with them. I find that as clients progress through the preparation phase, they develop an intuitive knowing or wisdom about ways their team can be helpful to them in a variety of situations and circumstances and an automatic connection to them when needed. As with the goals and inner strengths or resources, therapists clarify with clients whether the present makeup of the Resource Team will represent the positive characteristics they chose to assist in transitioning to the next steps in therapy. Clients can open the discussion with current Resource Team members if they have difficulty assigning new roles to current members or brainstorming new team representatives.

Again, clients may move forward with the Resource Team intact, add team members, select a "subcommittee" of members, or start over with a new Resource Team membership. When I (A.P.) was doing the *Transition From the AFTT-A Preparation Phase to EMDR Phases 3 to 8* protocol with one of my clients, they got stuck when assessing the ability of their existing Resource Team to benefit them as they moved forward in therapy. When the client discussed the difficulty with their team, the client realized that the initial Resource Team was more focused on protecting and meeting the needs of the Child/Adolescent parts of Self than on assisting the Competent Adult part to navigate the client's adult life and relationships. As a result, the client thanked the first Resource Team for their service thus far and reassured them that they had ensured the safety of inner Child/Adolescent parts. Since the client now had a Competent Adult part in the leadership role, the client offered the first Resource Team early retirement with full benefits, chose new strengths, and designed a new Resource Team with representatives for the positive characteristics needed to take the next steps in therapy.

BOX 19.1 CLIENT EXAMPLE: GOALS, STRENGTHS, AND RESOURCE TEAM MEMBERS

Therapist: Last time we talked about your goals for the next steps in EMDR when you'll be reprocessing memories of adverse events. You said that you had three goals: First, to face the past with courage and take back beliefs about yourself and your own feelings from your abusers; second, to experience feelings needed for healing; and third, to regain your sense of being a free spirit without getting out of control. How do those goals sound to you today?

Client: They're still true.

Therapist: You also added a willingness to ask for help to your inner strengths of courage and self-compassion. Does that quality still seem to fit?

Client: Yes. I thought about my team since then and I think the team members I already have can help me with willingness.

Therapist: How so?

Client: Well, my True Parent part can remind me that it's okay to trust safe people like you. That you and the team will be there for me no matter what. And even when it's painful or when I'm scared, it's okay to ask for what I need.

---

4. Access and Install a Revised Resource Team

If clients are confident that their original Resource Team will meet their needs while transitioning to the next phases of EMDR therapy, therapists ask clients to reconvene with their team in their Meeting Place and take them back into the sensory experience of the Meeting Place and the way in which they gather their team members. Therapists invite clients to access and strengthen the positive affect linked to client re-engaging with their Resource Team, using butterfly taps or tappers for short sets of slow BLS. If clients struggle with setting aside any negative affect, therapists remind them to practice the use of a container as needed. If clients revised their Resource Team membership, therapists invite them to gather the new team in their Meeting Place, focusing on the sensory experience of their Meeting Place and the way in which they want to gather their newly configured team. Therapists coach clients to access and strengthen the positive affect linked to meeting with their new Resource Team, using butterfly taps or tappers for short sets of slow BLS. If clients struggle with setting aside any negative affect, therapists help them practice the use of a container as needed.

5. Discuss Potential Barriers or Difficulties in Phases 3 to 8 and Ways the Resource Team Will Assist the Client to Resolve the Identified Issues

As previously stated in this chapter's introduction, clients who complete the AFTT-A enhanced version of EMDR therapy's preparation phase tend to move through protocols involving triggering events, traumatic memories, and negative affect quickly; are less likely to get "stuck" or loop; and use positive self-beliefs and new skills to work efficiently through barriers and challenges. They developed trusting inner attachments with personality parts and resources, within the personality system itself, and between parts and internal resources. The healthy inner attachment relationships serve as a foundation for time orientation, emotion regulation, guidance, and support essential to the trauma resolution process.

The AFTT-A model helps clients create and strengthen an Authentic Self consisting of an inner system based in trust; firm and flexible boundaries; healthy communication; regulated emotions; and an internalized sense of nurturance, safety, competence, and confidence. The *Transition From the AFTT-A Preparation Phase to EMDR Phases 3 to 8* protocol gives clients the opportunity to gather, organize, and activate all the resources, parts of Self, and skills they need to face and resolve attachment trauma in the upcoming therapy phases. The protocol enables clients to evaluate their needs for moving forward in therapy, predict potential obstacles, and plan how they will maximize their approach to future challenges, *using tools they have already developed and strengthened.*

> ### BOX 19.2 CLIENT EXAMPLE: BRAINSTORMING THE RESOURCE TEAM'S WAYS TO HELP FOR EMDR PHASES 3 TO 8
>
> **Therapist:** Okay, you're back in the mountains on the flat rock around the campfire with your team. The Secret Service agents are standing guard at the top of the path. You can hear the sound of the stream from your Safe Place. What do you notice?
>
> **Client:** I feel safe and cared about. I can tell by the faces of my team that they're there for me no matter what. So, I feel strong too. Like, "I can do this."
>
> **Therapist:** Let's talk to your team about any fears, doubts, or worries you have about moving into the next steps of EMDR. Is that okay with you?
>
> **Client:** Yes.
>
> **Therapist:** What do you think is important for your team to know?
>
> **Client:** That I'm scared to have my feelings. That I'm not sure I can handle revisiting those bad times.
>
> **Therapist:** How does your team seem to react as you say that?
>
> **Client:** They're nodding their heads like they understand. My New Parent puts her hand on my back and the Competent Adult takes my hand.
>
> **Therapist:** How will the team know that you need them?
>
> **Client:** Well, the fairies will be able to tell if the Kid parts are starting to feel like they need to come out and take over. My Competent Adult can act as a barometer of my emotions.
>
> **Therapist:** How can your team help when they can tell that you need them?
>
> *(continued)*

> **BOX 19.2 CLIENT EXAMPLE: BRAINSTORMING THE RESOURCE TEAM'S WAYS TO HELP FOR EMDR PHASES 3 TO 8 (continued)**
>
> **Client:** My True Parent part can remind me that it's okay to trust safe people like you. That you and the team will be there for me no matter what. And even when it's painful, I won't be alone. My Competent Adult part will help with my feelings by telling me that I am in your office as an adult and am doing EMDR. The fairy will tuck Kid parts in their Safe Places and sprinkle fairy dust around them so they know they don't have to go through what happened in the past again but can be in their Safe Places and give me the information I need to heal the past. And I have my Higher Power, my whole team, and you to help.
>
> **Therapist:** What do you notice as you sit around the campfire, hearing your team members talk about how they'll help you?
>
> **Client:** Warm, relaxed, confident.

6. Install Future Rehearsal to Resolve the Identified Issue in Phases 3 to 8

Clients with a history of attachment trauma bring their negative self-beliefs and emotional distress into therapy. They view their ability to successfully complete therapy through the lens of "I can't do it," "There's something defective about me," "I don't have what it takes to...," or "What's the point in trying?" Anxiety, fear, self-doubt, insecurity, frustration, helplessness, and/or hopelessness accompany such negative self-beliefs. Clients who complete AFTT-A's enhanced and expanded preparation phase transform harmful internalized messages into affirming beliefs, under- and overdeveloped parts of Self into a balanced and functional inner personality system, and a disbelief in their abilities and strengths into an internal team of strengths and resources.

EMDR Future Rehearsal and future template protocols assist clients to link *positive* affect such as confidence, competence, safety, security, and hope with challenging situations that are already linked to negative beliefs and affect (Shapiro, 2021a, 2021b). The *Transition From the AFTT-A Preparation Phase to EMDR Phases 3 to 8* protocol utilizes Future Rehearsal to link client's strengths, positive beliefs and affect, and skills to potentially difficult and distressing tasks in EMDR phases 3 to 8. In particular, therapists help clients apply their newly installed beliefs of "I'm okay," "No matter what, I have everything I need," and "I am not alone anymore" to the components of EMDR trauma protocols that clients identify as possible emotional challenges. The protocol affords clients the experience of navigating difficult therapy tasks while feeling safe, supported, competent, and confident. Any time clients have difficulty during the protocol, they can access and use whatever resources they need to overcome the immediate obstacle.

Therapists employ the *Transition From the AFTT-A Preparation Phase to EMDR Phases 3 to 8* protocol to link clients to their Future Self, "the part that already knows," or the version of themselves at a point in the future after which they have worked through whatever needs to be resolved so they can effectively and fully participate in EMDR trauma protocols. Clients have the option to add their Future Self to their team of internal resources to support and guide them through the EMDR therapy process and navigate their present-day lives and relationships.

POINTS TO REMEMBER

- Use the *Transition From the AFTT-A Preparation Phase to EMDR Phases 3 to 8* protocol between AFTT-A's enhanced EMDR preparation phase and phases 3 to 8 regardless of prong or prong sequence.
- Maintain the unshakable belief that clients have the wisdom and resources they need to resolve attachment trauma in their Authentic Self, connected to all parts, Spiritual Essence, and inner resources.
- Use the Future Rehearsal to strengthen the sense of competence and confidence in preparing for and mastering potential challenges with EMDR phases 3 to 8.
- Link the client in the present moment to their Future Self, the "part of them that already knows" how to overcome obstacles in their therapy process and present-day lives.
- In addition to installing Future Rehearsal, use EMD or contained/restricted reprocessing (short sets of rapid BLS focusing on disturbing emotions/sensations) to decrease anticipatory anxiety related to trauma work.

TROUBLESHOOTING

- If the client has difficulty brainstorming goals, strengths, and/or Resource Team members for use in EMDR phases 3 to 8, convene a meeting with the current Resource Team to identify reasons for and solutions to the barrier.
- If the client has problems accessing and reinforcing a positive affect related to reconnecting with their Resource Team and/or installation of Future Rehearsal, use the container generated and utilized in earlier protocols, check that Child/Adolescent parts are tucked into their Safe Places with their Higher Powers, and verify that Adult and Parent parts of Self are time-oriented.

PAUSE AND REFLECT FOR THE THERAPIST

We invite you to imagine helping your challenging client work through EMDR phases 3 to 8. As before, notice what emotions, cognitions, body sensations come up for you. Is there a particular aspect or step that brings up negative affect? Imagine watching yourself on a movie or television screen at a time in the future when you have worked through whatever you've needed to resolve so that you are at ease and confident in a session with the client related to the identified step or aspect of therapy. Picture the "Future You," the part of you that "already knows how" to handle the situation effectively and with self-assurance. What do you notice about your posture, your voice, your facial expressions? How can you tell by watching yourself that you feel at ease? If needed, ask your Resource Team for help. Make sure any Child/Adolescent parts of Self are tucking into their Safe Places. If you want, reinforce your positive affect with short sets of slow butterfly taps. When you're ready, step into the scene and give yourself a few moments to get used to the different perspective, to experience what it feels like in your body at this time in the future when you are at ease and self-assured about handling the identified step or aspect in session with the client. Again, if you want, reinforce your positive affect with short sets of slow butterfly taps. As you come back to the present moment, bring back a gift from your Future Self that you can use to remind yourself that you are capable and you have the inner strengths and support you need in order to be present with the client in the future sessions. You can choose an object, a word or phrase, a picture or photo, a song, or an anchor on your body. Imagine using the gift from your Future Self when needed and reinforce your positive affect with short sets of slow butterfly taps.

USEFUL TERMS AND DEFINITIONS

AFTT-A: Attachment-Focused Trauma Therapy for Adults

BLS: bilateral stimulation

EMD: Eye Movement Desensitization

EMDR: Eye Movement Desensitization and Reprocessing

PROTOCOL SCRIPT 15. TRANSITION FROM THE AFTT-A PREPARATION PHASE TO EMDR PHASES 3 TO 8

Adapted from Leeds, A. (2016). *A guide to the standard EMDR protocols for clinicians, supervisors, and consultants* (2nd ed.). Springer Publishing Company; Fraser, G. A. (1991). The Dissociative Table Technique: A strategy for working with ego states and dissociative disorders and ego-state therapy. *Dissociation: Progress in the Dissociative Disorders*, 4(4), 205–213; Fraser, G. A. (2003). Fraser's "Dissociative Table Technique" revisited, revised: A strategy for working with ego states in dissociative disorders and ego-state therapy. *Journal of Trauma and Dissociation*, 4(4), 5–28. https://doi.org/10.1300/J229v04n04_02; Potter, A. E. (1994). *Inside out: Rebuilding self and personality through inner child therapy* (therapist manual and client workbook). Taylor and Francis; Shapiro, F. (2018). *Eye movement desensitization and reprocessing (EMDR) therapy: Basic principles, protocols, and procedures* (2nd ed.). Guilford Press; Shapiro, F. (2021a). *Weekend 1 training manual of the two-part EMDR therapy basic training* (revised). EMDR Institute, Inc.; and Shapiro, F. (2021b). *Weekend 2 training manual of the two-part EMDR therapy basic training* (revised). EMDR Institute, Inc.

Prior to the protocol, review initial goals, strengths, Resource Team members, and Meeting Place. Check to see if any Child/Adolescent parts need to be tucked into Safe Places with their Higher Powers and reassured that the Competent Adult part of Self will be completing the next therapy steps (EMDR phases 3 to 8) with the support and protection of their own Higher Power, their Resource Team, their therapist, and the safe people in their life. Reconnect the client to the positive affect and beliefs from their Adult Safe Place and Higher Power, the transitional object they brought from their Safe Place to their Meeting Place, and their Resource Team in the Meeting Place. Access and reinforce positive affect with shorts sets of slow bilateral stimulation (BLS) with tappers or butterfly tapping.

1. Identify the Goals Specific to EMDR Therapy Trauma Protocols. *Say…* "One of the purposes of the *Transition* protocol is to help you set goals and connect all of your resources and strengths you developed and strengthened in the preparation phase to the next phases of therapy. As we just discussed, when you first started EMDR therapy, you created Safe Places and Higher Powers for both your Adult and Child/Adolescent parts of Self. You set goals for therapy, picked positive characteristics to help you meet those goals, and developed an Inner Resource Team with members who represent those strengths for you. You and your team work together to protect and nurture your Child/Adolescent parts and strengthen the Competent Adult and the True Parent parts of you. Now, we want to bring your sense of being okay, having everything you need to meet your goals, and being connected to an inner team of resources to reprocessing traumatic memories or in your adult life. *Ask...* "Making sense? Any questions?" *Say...* "Let's look at your goals and decide which ones you want to keep for the next therapy steps and if there are any goals you want to add or change."

_____

_____

2. Brainstorm the Needed Strengths/Positive Characteristics/Inner Resources to Meet Goals. *Say...* "Let's look at the inner strengths you accessed and used so far in therapy and let's brainstorm which ones you want to keep on your team and whether you want to add any other positive characteristics to help you meet your goals for the next phases of therapy (*repeat client's new goals*)."

_____

_____

3. Decide Whether Existing Resource Team Members Can Act as Representatives of Needed Strengths. *Say...* "Now let's look at your Resource Team. First, I invite you to think about who on your team will be helpful to you as you move forward in therapy. Which ones will represent (*repeat strengths*) for you now? Do you need to change or add any team members?"

_____

_____

4. Access and Install a Revised Resource Team. **If the client retains the same members as the original Resource Team, access and reinforce the positive affect and beliefs related to client re-engaging with their team, using short sets of slow BLS with tappers or butterfly tapping. Practice the container for setting aside the negative affect if needed. Skip to Step 5.*

*If the client revised their Resource Team, say... "Your Resource Team now includes (*repeat members with strengths they represent*). Let's get you all together in your Meeting Space. Let me know when you're in (*name Meeting Place*) with your new team." *Ask...* "What do you notice?"

Access and reinforce a positive affect with BLS.

5. Discuss Potential Barriers or Difficulties in Phases 3 to 8 and Ways the Resource Team Will Assist the Client to Resolve the Identified Issue. *Say...* "Let's brainstorm parts of trauma reprocessing that might be hard for you or times you think you might get stuck."

Ask... "How do you think your team can help?" or "How would you like your team to help?"

Access and reinforce a positive affect with short sets of slow BLS.

6. Install Future Rehearsal to Resolve the Identified Issue in Phases 3 to 8. *Say...* "I'd like you to imagine yourself at a future moment when you are at the point in therapy when (*repeat situation from Step 5*). First, picture yourself on a movie screen at a time in the future when you can handle (*repeat situation from Step 5*) in the way you identified in your goals. Notice everything about the future you, that part of you that already knows how to deal with the situation with a feeling of competence and confidence. How you look, act, how your body moves, how you seem to be feeling." *Ask...* "What do you notice?"

If client has difficulty creating a positive movie, say... "That's okay, imagine fast forwarding in the movie to a time farther in the future when whatever you needed to work through and resolve has been worked through and resolved and you automatically know how to handle the situation." *Access and reinforce a positive affect with short sets of slow BLS. Say...* "Now, I'd like you to step into the movie. Give yourself a few moments to get used to this different perspective." *Ask...* "What do you notice?"

Use fast forward again if the client has trouble creating a positive image and affect. Access and reinforce a positive affect with short sets of slow BLS. Say... "I invite you to bring back a gift from the future you, something you can bring back to the present moment so that when you see it or hear it or hold it in your hand, you'll remember,

'Oh, that's right. I have that part of me that already knows how to do this, that can help me and be with me through this.'" **Ask…** "What do you notice?"

_____

_____

Access and reinforce a positive affect with short sets of slow BLS. **Ask…** "Is there anything else that is needed to complete the scene?"

_____

_____

Access and reinforce positive affect with short sets of slow BLS.

Repeat the protocol with other potential obstacles for phases 3 to 8.

REFERENCES

Kitty, A. (2020). *The art of Kintsugi: Learning the Japanese craft of beautiful repair.* Schiffer Publishing.

Leeds, A. (2016). *A guide to the standard EMDR protocols for clinicians, supervisors, and consultants* (2nd ed.). Springer Publishing Company.

Santini, C. (2019). *Kinstsugi: Finding strength in imperfection.* Andrews McMeel Publishing.

Shapiro, F. (2018). *Eye movement desensitization and reprocessing (EMDR) therapy: Basic principles, protocols, and procedures* (2nd ed.). Guilford Press.

Shapiro, F. (2021a). *Weekend 1 training manual of the two-part EMDR therapy basic training* (revised). EMDR Institute, Inc.

Shapiro, F. (2021b). *Weekend 2 training manual of the two-part EMDR therapy basic training* (revised). EMDR Institute, Inc.

CHAPTER 20

Adaptations for EMDR Reprocessing and Desensitization in Attachment-Focused Trauma Therapy for Adults

INTRODUCTION

Clients with a history of attachment trauma often present with complex symptoms, problems, memories, and triggers. This chapter describes the process of collaborating with the client to identify the present-day problem area and associated memory network with which to begin the work. It outlines considerations for choosing a sequence and initial target for clients with a history of attachment trauma. It provides tools therapists can use to assist clients with safe and effective desensitization and reprocessing, including restricted reprocessing and interweaves that access the healthy aspects of the client's inner system and the client's connection with the therapist.

IDENTIFYING REMAINING PRESENT-DAY PROBLEMS

Clients who experienced serious attachment trauma typically present for therapy with multiple issues, symptoms, and problems. Through the Attachment-Focused Trauma Therapy for Adults (AFTT-A) preparation phase work involving creation of a healthy internal system and reclaiming and strengthening of the Authentic Adult part of Self (see checklist for AFTT-A steps, Exhibit 22.1 in Chapter 22, or access the form online through Springer Publishing Connect: Use the code on the opening page of this book to access the digital product and select Chapter 22), some initial symptoms, issues, and problems may be already resolved or partially resolved. Following the preparation phase, the AFTT-A therapist should re-evaluate the client's functioning by revisiting the initial assessment and collaborating to identify which presenting issues, symptoms, or problem areas remain problematic. Some new areas that were previously unreported may come to light, as clients develop greater self-awareness and insight during the preparation phase work as well as increased trust and capacity for sharing sensitive and distressing information.

While taking stock of remaining issues, the therapist should stay mindful of the possibility of stored, unprocessed traumatic memories related to clients' social and cultural identity that they may not have felt comfortable sharing previously. As therapeutic trust grows, some clients become more comfortable describing experiences of marginalization or discrimination. The therapist should demonstrate humility regarding the client's cultural and social identity and experiences of marginalization or discrimination and an openness to learning more (Nickerson, 2017).

In some cases, the therapist may notice signs that their client holds prejudice toward specific groups of people and perhaps is hurtful toward a social or cultural group. The adaptive information processing (AIP) model explains that such prejudice is associated with early events involving misinformation and strong emotional impact (Nickerson, 2017). With a therapeutic alliance, the therapist may be able to inquire about the client's negative cognitions (NCs). From there, the Eye Movement Desensitization and Reprocessing (EMDR) therapist can suggest that the client think back to their earliest experiences to learn more about the sources of their negative thoughts and feelings.

IDENTIFYING RELEVANT MEMORIES FOR REPROCESSING

Once a priority problem area has been identified, the therapist asks, "What is the earliest memory you have related to this issue?" If the client has no response to this direct line of questioning, the therapist can ask the client to access the emotions, sensations, and/or thoughts associated with the present issue and then *say*... "Let your mind float back, as far back as you can go. What comes up for you? Any memories? A certain age? Certain people who were in your life?" Next, ask about other similar situations or events (Shapiro, 2018).

Another method of identifying a past memory for reprocessing is to begin with an "early bonding rule" that remains problematic (see Table 15.1). *Say*... "Hold that early bonding rule in mind and let your mind float back to when you were a child. What comes to mind?" Identify an "earliest" and a "worst" memory related to the "early bonding rule," if possible.

Leeds (2016) suggests identifying the emotions, sensations, and perceptions experienced during a recent triggering situation that is typical for the client. Next, invite the client to bring up the trigger and the emotions, sensations, and perceptions. Once accessed, ask them to float back to childhood and see what comes up. Using a present-day trigger to begin a float back is a way to identify relevant memories for reprocessing.

An additional method for identifying relevant memories for reprocessing is to bring out the Therapeutic Story (Lovett, 2007, 2015; Wesselmann et al., 2014; see Protocol Script 13). Even if the story has been read more than once with bilateral stimulation (BLS) and there is an overall increase in comfort level for the story, some specific events in the story may still hold disturbance. *Say*... "I'm going to start reading the story from the beginning. Raise your hand to let me know when I get to a part that still holds an emotional charge for you." Even a preverbal event from the story may bring up disturbing emotions. Even though the event is not consciously remembered, the client may have an imagined picture or sound, smell, or sensation that can be used as a target to begin the EMDR reprocessing phases. Once one event from the story is identified and reprocessed with EMDR therapy, the therapist can re-read the story to identify the next memory that still holds disturbance. Continue until the entire story can be read without disturbance.

BOX 20.1 CLIENT EXAMPLE: FLOATING BACK TO THE MOST RELEVANT TRAUMA TARGET

During the initial intake, history-taking and treatment planning, this client identified their priority issue was reactivity. They told me (D.W.) that they would frequently lash out at others with angry or sarcastic words. Both their marriage

(continued)

> **BOX 20.1 CLIENT EXAMPLE: FLOATING BACK TO THE MOST RELEVANT TRAUMA TARGET (continued)**
>
> and their job were at stake. The client stated that they were triggered by interactions in which they felt their partner or their boss wasn't listening or when they sensed they were being ignored. However, by the end of the preparation phase, these behaviors were nearly eliminated.
>
> Before commencing the EMDR reprocessing phases, I invited the client to collaborate with me and revisit the history-taking and treatment planning procedures to identify the remaining issues, problems, or symptoms from which we would identify targets for EMDR reprocessing. The client identified that their social anxiety was still a major issue. They described their fear of looking foolish to others and a distressing feeling of being an outsider, both of which were triggered when they were in groups of people. I asked the client to focus on a recent time when they were triggered by being in a group. They identified the associated NCs "I'm shameful" and "I don't belong." They identified emotions of shame and sadness as well as disturbing sensations in their stomach. I asked the client to momentarily stay with the NCs, emotions, and body sensations and to let their mind float back as far as they could go. The client said they were heavy as a child and recalled incidents they had not previously mentioned involving harsh criticism from their father as well as bullying from classmates in grade school due to their weight. The client also recalled traumatic incidents in middle school in which they were shamed by a teacher in front of the other boys in physical education class. Together, we decided to begin with the earliest incident first, followed by the worst, which was the shaming from the teacher. EMDR reprocessing was facilitated through the client's most Competent Adult part of Self. After the memories were brought to adaptive resolution, the client reprocessed the present-day triggers and developed future templates in which they imagined themself using adaptive interpersonal skills and operating from their most Competent Adult part of Self. By the end of therapy, the client felt confident they could manage previously triggering situations without distress.

CONSIDERATIONS REGARDING PAST-PRESENT-FUTURE SEQUENCE

The EMDR standard sequence suggests reprocessing the touchstone (earliest) memory related to the problem or issue first, followed by the worst memory, and finally any related ancillary memories that remain disturbing, unless the client prefers a different order. The past memory work is followed by reprocessing of remaining present-day triggers. Finally, the therapist and client identify anticipated future challenges. They collaborate to develop and reprocess a future template (positive picture), imagining effective future behaviors using EMDR standard future template procedures.

The past-present-future sequence can be changed to adapt to the needs of the client with serious attachment trauma. Sometimes a present-day behavior or emotional reaction causes such serious misery or consequences in present-day life that addressing the present-day trigger feels urgent. For example, a client who becomes angry at a partner due to triggered fears of abandonment may be creating instability in the relationship. Or a client who is triggered by a supervisor may be so immobilized that they could lose their job. Targeting present-day triggers first may provide timely relief to problematic situations.

The past-present-future sequence can also be changed for clients who may still have difficulty tolerating the stored, unprocessed affect associated with highly disturbing traumatic memories (Shapiro, 2018). For this situation, beginning with present triggers is a way to provide a successful experience with EMDR reprocessing of a target that is less intense, allowing the client to develop more confidence with EMDR reprocessing before addressing the earlier traumatic events.

Reverse Protocol and Inverted Protocol

Adler-Tapia (2012) suggests a Reverse Protocol for complex clients. The clinician helps the client identify a future feared situation and then reprocesses the feared situation with standard EMDR reprocessing procedures. Reprocessing the imagined future eliminates the disturbance and changes the NC, such as *I'll fail*, to a positive cognition (PC), such as *I'll do fine*. Prior to reprocessing, the clinician helps the client develop positive imagery of adaptive behaviors or skills to use to cope with the future situation.

Hofmann's Inverted Protocol (2009) for complex clients also starts with the future prong prior to addressing the present and then the past. To address the future, the clinician and client identify resources needed to meet challenges in the next few days. For each needed resource, the clinician and client collaborate to identify a memory in which the client demonstrated the resource. The body sensations associated with the resourced state are strengthened with BLS in a simplified version of Resource Development and Installation (RDI; Korn & Leeds, 2002). The client is then guided to bring all of the strengthened resources and associated body sensations together, followed by deepening of the resourced positive state with a slow set of BLS.

The next step of the Inverted Protocol involves orienting the client to present time and deepening the present time orientation with slow BLS as described by Knipe (2015). When the client shows success with present-day coping, EMDR reprocessing of past traumas is initiated.

The AFTT-A therapist may begin the past-present-future sequence by bringing a developed resource or skill into a Future Rehearsal. The traditional RDI procedure as developed by Korn and Leeds concludes with a Future Rehearsal, utilizing the strengthened, chosen resource. Any newly developed or strengthened resource or skill can be accessed and utilized with an imaginal Future Rehearsal. The AFTT-A therapist can suggest clients access their newly developed resources and skills to bring to the imaginal situation. For example, clients can access the Higher Powers, Resource Team members, the strengthened Competent Adult part of Self or True Parent part of Self to assist with Future Rehearsals (see Protocol Scripts 4, 6, 7, 8, and 9).

Next, reprocess the present-day trigger with EMDR phases 3 to 8. This can be repeated for various challenging situations until clients feel ready to reprocess traumatic memories.

STEPS FOR CONDUCTING AN EMDR FUTURE REHEARSAL USING RESOURCES FROM THE HEALTHY INNER SYSTEM

1. In collaboration with the client, identify a challenging situation the client expects to face in the future and identify exactly how the client would like to respond.

2. Ask the client to access their Competent Adult part of Self through the previously learned methods.
3. Ask the client to check and make sure all Child parts of Self are settled into Safe Places.
4. Collaborate with the client to identify any appropriate PC that would be helpful in the situation. When the Future Rehearsal involves a relationship, the PC may be pulled from their Bonding Contract list of preferred new rules.
5. Suggest the client invite any member of their Resource Team or a Higher Power they believe could be helpful to accompany them into the Future Rehearsal.
6. Suggest the client match their body position with the Competent Adult state and visualize a "mental movie" of managing the future situation with Resource Team members or a Higher Power at their side. Check in regarding the client's experience. If the client reports positive affect, the clinician asks the client to "run the movie again" while adding a short set of slow BLS to deepen the positive affect.

If the client reports any difficulty, reassure the client that they have what they need inside to accomplish this task. Suggest the client re-access the Competent Adult part of Self through the Competent Adult body position and then visualize stepping into the Meeting Place to meet with the whole Resource Team. Suggest the client ask the team for advice or help, taking time to access the needed adaptive information. If the client reports helpful information or affect, deepen the positive shift with a short set of slow BLS and then repeat the Future Rehearsal. (Note: Future Rehearsal utilizing resources should be implemented with slow, shorter sets of BLS to avoid associations to unprocessed material.) After developing and reinforcing one or more Future Rehearsals, the therapist can choose to address past memories or present-day triggers next.

BOX 20.2 CLIENT EXAMPLE: FUTURE REHEARSAL WITH ASSISTANCE FROM A TEAM MEMBER

This client wanted to change the way they reacted to their boss at work. Instead of feeling panicky and shut down, they wanted to respond with confidence and assertiveness. The client identified that anytime their boss asked them a question about their work, the client froze up, certain that their boss didn't trust them to do the job. The client accessed their most Competent Adult part of Self through their posture and cue word. Then the client visualized a quick meeting with their Resource Team and invited their imaginal assertiveness coach to assist them with developing a confident and assertive demeanor. The client imagined their boss questioning their handling of a situation and visualized a movie of a confident and assertive response, with the assertiveness coach at their side. After checking that the client had a positive response to the future movie, the therapist asked the client to run the movie again and added a slow, short set of tactile BLS. Next, the therapist asked the client to step into the movie and experience the feelings in their body and their body posture as the client imagined responding from their most Competent Adult part of Self with the assertiveness coach at their side. The therapist applied another slow, short set of tactile BLS.

ACCESSING THE COMPETENT ADULT AND RESOURCE TEAM FOR THE EMDR REPROCESSING PHASES

Ensure the client is in their most Competent Adult part of Self for starting reprocessing by suggesting recall of their Competent Adult memory and/or cue word and shifting their posture to match (see Protocol Script 8). Check in with the client as to whether there are any Child parts of Self activated, and if so, direct the client to invite the Child part of Self back to their Safe Place and remind the Child part that the Adult part will be working on the memory. Suggest reminding the Child part that the memory is all over, even though the Adult might have thoughts and feelings about the memory.

Additionally, if needed, suggest the client choose any Resource Team members who might be helpful to stay by their side and assist as needed throughout the memory work (see Protocol Scripts 6 and 7). Remind the client that they have everything they need inside to heal. Remind the client that they won't be searching for new memories. They can trust that they will remember what they *need* to remember to heal.

PHASE 3: TARGET ASSESSMENT

If the therapist and client make a decision to focus on a present-day trigger, the "worst image" related to the situation that triggered their distress is the initial EMDR target. If the therapist and client make a decision to focus on the past prong, the "worst image" associated with the memory is the initial target. If the client reports they are not visual or don't seem to have access to an image, a sound, smell, or sensation can be identified as the target.

The client is asked to identify the worst image, the NC and preferred PC, the Validity of Cognition (VOC), the emotion, the Subjective Units of Disturbance (SUD), and the body sensations. The purpose of this phase is to get baseline readings, but even more importantly, to access the visual, perceptual, emotional, and sensory channels for reprocessing. Research has found that activation of emotions may be particularly important for effective EMDR reprocessing (Littel, 2017).

PHASE 4: DESENSITIZATION AND REPROCESSING OF TRIGGERS OR MEMORIES

Once the client has accessed emotions, perceptions, and sensations of the memory or present-day trigger through the phase 3 target assessment procedures and the client is still grounded in the Competent Adult part of Self, phase 4 desensitization and reprocessing is implemented (Shapiro, 2018). Sets of eye movements are applied, moving the client's eyes at a pace that is as rapid as the client can comfortably tolerate. Alternatively, tactile BLS may can be used if the client prefers. In between sets, the clinician checks in with the client only briefly by asking "What's there now?" After the client responds, the clinician says, "Go with that" or "Notice that" and proceeds with another set of rapid BLS.

Although the goal is to activate the client's own natural information processing system, it's common for clients with a history of attachment trauma to occasionally get stuck and require assistance. This isn't surprising, as attachment trauma can negatively impact social, emotional, and cognitive development, and clients may hold misperceptions or have other holes in their store of adaptive information.

Restricted/Contained Reprocessing of Present-Day Triggers or Memories

The EMDR therapist allows the client to freely reprocess without restrictions if the client is well-resourced and able to tolerate their emotions. However, the clinician may choose to restrict/contain the reprocessing to keep the client's focus on the memory or present-day trigger if: (a) the therapist is concerned about dissociation; (b) the therapist observes that reprocessing activates multiple triggering situations or memories, leading to intense emotions beyond what the client can tolerate or reprocess safely; or (c) the client reports a high level of anxiety about reprocessing the particular trigger or memory before beginning phase 4. In these situations, restricting/containing clients' focus to the original memory or trigger increases clients' sense of control, safety, and tolerance for the EMDR desensitization and reprocessing phases.

To prepare the client for restricted reprocessing, the therapist can *say...* "At least for today, I'd like to help you restrict your reprocessing to this one memory/present-day trigger and avoid accessing other events or situations. I'd like you to picture your container (developed during the preparation phase) and imagine sweeping everything into your container except for the one thing we chose to work on."

Restricted/contained reprocessing is on a continuum from very restricted to slightly restricted Eye Movement Desensitization (EMD). EMD desensitizes without allowing associations by using shorter sets of fast BLS (10 to 20 passes) and returning to the memory and taking a SUD with each set (Shapiro, 2018). More flexible restricted reprocessing allows some associations without accessing too many memories or intense emotions. Sets of BLS are somewhat shorter, the therapist returns the client to the memory more frequently but not every time, and the SUD may be taken more frequently but not every time.

If a client seems stuck and needs to access other information to gain insight or perspective, the therapist can lengthen the sets and/or return to the memory less frequently, or even return to EMDR standard reprocessing procedures.

Cognitive Interweaves During Reprocessing of Present-Day Triggers or Memories

Sometimes clients loop during the EMDR reprocessing phases because they lose access to their present-day adaptive perspective and become overwhelmed by their stored negative childhood perceptions and affect. For example, a client may be stuck in the perception that was present during some type of childhood abuse, repeating after each set, "I'm trapped, I'm trapped." Or a client who is triggered by a present-day situation in which they experience criticism and rejection from a boss may loop on the thought, "I'm not good enough; I'm never going to be good enough."

Sometimes clients have no movement during the EMDR reprocessing phases because the fear of experiencing their emotions causes them to keep a defensive wall around them. Instead of over-accessing their emotions, they're under-accessing.

Cognitive interweaves are quick statements or questions to help clients access a present-day perspective, overcome a fear or block, or create a sense of connection or safety in the session that helps them bring down their defenses (Shapiro, 2018). In AFTT-A, the cognitive interweave may suggest that the client access an internal resource by accessing a Resource Team figure or Higher Power figure or may call the client's attention to the therapeutic relationship for grounding and support. Once the internal shift is made through the cognitive interweave, EMDR reprocessing is allowed to continue naturally.

In the case of reprocessing with present-day triggers, cognitive interweaves can be used to help clients separate the present from the past. Examples include: "And how is this present-day situation different from situations in childhood?" "How high can you reach now, and how high could you reach then?"

If the SUD is not moving toward zero well into the reprocessing, a standard interweave question is, "What keeps it from being a zero?" Some clients with attachment trauma resist the idea of achieving a SUD of 0, believing that it invalidates the seriousness of the emotional pain that was experienced at the time of the trauma. It can be helpful to follow with a clarifying interweave: "Remember that the number you give me has nothing to do with the seriousness of what happened or how harmful the event was. The number tells me how much actual disturbance is inside of you now or in your physical being right this minute when you go to the memory." If the client still feels a 0 would be invalidating or the remaining SUD of 1 or 2 is related to other memories that are yet unprocessed, the number should be accepted as ecological.

Cognitive interweaves are usually nondirective and open-ended, although sometimes small pieces of information are provided directly. The therapist tries not to interrupt the client's internal reprocessing by use of minimal words and resuming BLS as soon as possible. The BLS can be applied right after the cognitive interweave statement, right after the client has answered a cognitive interweave question, or right after the cognitive interweave question is posed.

Table 20.1 provides common interweaves used during EMDR reprocessing within AFTT-A.

PHASES 5 THROUGH 7 WITH PRESENT-DAY TRIGGERS OR MEMORIES

During phase 5, installation of the PC is implemented. If the client has numerous memories associated with the same PC, it may not be reasonable to expect a VOC of 7. Sometimes, the PC can be changed to a "process PC," meaning a PC that acknowledges the client is moving toward a more definitive belief. For example, the PC "I am lovable" may be changed to a "process PC": "I am learning that I am lovable."

During phase 6, the client focuses on any remaining body sensations with BLS. The BLS remains fast, as the body sensation could be associated with an unprocessed channel or another associated memory. Rather than activate new material at the end of a session, the therapist should close the session as incomplete before beginning phase 6 and resume phase 6 at the beginning of the follow-up session.

Phase 7 involves closing the session as an incomplete session or as a complete session (with a SUD of 0 or a number that is ecological to the situation and a VOC

Table 20.1 Therapist Cognitive Interweaves in Attachment-Focused Trauma Therapy for Adults

Type of Cognitive Interweave	Examples of Cognitive Interweaves
Integrating Reorganized Internal Attachments/ Personality Structure	How can your team help you? Ask your team for help with … Notice how it feels to have my support and the support of your team right now. Remember how it feels to know you're not alone anymore. What do you/your Child part need from the True Parent part of you? What do you think your team would say to you about …? Remember how it feels, knowing you have everything you need. Connect to that sense of being okay from your Safe Place while you … Remember the (object) you took from your Safe Place and … What does your Higher Power say when … Stay with that and connect to that sense of your Higher Self/ Spiritual Essence.
Corrective Attachment Relationship With Therapist	I will pace with you. We can go as slowly as you need. You are here in the office with me, right now, today. I am here to support Adult you so that you can care for the younger parts of you. I will be right here next to Adult you, so that Adult you can step into that memory and stand next to the Younger you. Here in this office, with me, there are no judgments.
Reducing Affect Avoidance	During this set, notice your emotions and remind yourself that your feelings won't hurt you, feelings come and then feelings go. I am with you right here in this office as you feel whatever you feel. By feeling your feelings, you can heal your feelings.
Accessing Competent Adult Part of Self	Can you look at this memory from your Authentic Adult Self right now? Access both the Competent Adult and True Parent parts of you. Imagine that the True Parent part of you could go back in time and be there with the Child you. Just think of that. What does the New Parent part of you want to say to your Child Self about this? If Adult you could speak to _____ today, what would Adult you say?
Time Orientation	Use of Post-It Note: The memory is an old photo on this wall. It's black and white and it's faded with time. Use of Little Shoes: You could have worn these shoes back then. Compare them to your shoes now. Take a look at your hands and remember the age you are now. Take a look at this calendar and see what day and year it is now. Does every part of you understand that you are here in this office with me now?

Source: Data from Laliotis, D. (2017, November). *The dance of attachment: An EMDR relational approach,* a master class for EMDR clinicians. Presentation, Omaha, Nebraska; Shapiro, F. (2018). *Eye movement desensitization and reprocessing (EMDR) therapy: Basic principles, protocols, and procedures* (3rd ed.). Guilford Press; and Wesselmann, D., & Potter, A. E. (2019, September). *Attachment through the lifespan.* EMDRIA Preconference Presentation, Orange County, California.

of 7 or a number that is ecological to the situation). An incomplete session can be closed safely by asking for a positive idea that was discovered during the session and by asking for assistance from the Resource Team or Higher Power figure to help. Furthermore, the therapist may ask the client to ensure they are operating from their most Competent Adult part of Self by adjusting their body position and recalling a competency memory.

Phase 8 involves re-evaluation of the client's affect and recent functioning at the follow-up session and the present SUD associated with the memory. If the prior session was incomplete, resume reprocessing in phases 4, 5, or 6, depending on the point at which the session was previously closed.

Follow Reprocessing of Triggers With Future Templates

A future template follows any reprocessing of a present-day trigger (Shapiro, 2018). A future template involves targeting an image of positive functioning related to the triggering situation in the future. The therapist implements fast BLS during the imagery to deepen the associated positive affect but also to allow associations to be made that may be important and relevant to resolution of their problems or issues.

POINTS TO REMEMBER

- After the AFTT-A preparation phase, assess to determine remaining present-day problems/issues/symptoms.
- Starting with the present-day priority problem/issue/symptom, ask for the earliest and worst related memory or suggest the client focus on the present-day disturbance and then let their mind "float back" as far as it can go to see what comes up.
- The present-day problem may be identified as a troublesome "Early Bonding Contract rule" (see Table 15.1 for list of common Early Bonding Contract rules) or a present-day situation or event that has been triggering for the client.
- Another method for identifying relevant EMDR targets involves re-reading the Therapeutic Story to identify events in the story that still hold disturbance (see Protocol Script 13).
- The Resource Team developed during the AFTT-A preparation phase (see Protocol Scripts 6 and 7) can be accessed to help with a Future Rehearsal prior to addressing the past or present. Following the Future Rehearsal, reprocess the present-day trigger. Repeat with other present-day challenges until the client is comfortable addressing the past.
- The Resource Team developed during the AFTT-A preparation phase (see Protocol Scripts 6 and 7) can be accessed prior to beginning EMDR reprocessing.
- If EMDR standard reprocessing opens up too many memories or more emotions than can be tolerated, restrict the number of passes and bring the client back to target more frequently.

- EMDR cognitive interweaves can help access resources from the healthy internal system to assist with stuck points during EMDR reprocessing of present-day triggers and memories.

TROUBLESHOOTING

If the client with a history of attachment trauma struggles with co-occurring conditions such as obsessive-compulsive disorder, schizophrenia, addictions, or intermittent explosive disorder that impair day-to-day functioning, seek additional information and/or training regarding the condition and specific EMDR information or specialized EMDRIA-approved trainings, found through EMDRIA (www.emdria.org/publications-resources) and the EMDR Institute (www.emdr.com).

PAUSE AND REFLECT FOR THE THERAPIST

As you have implemented the AFTT-A protocols with clients and/or EMDR reprocessing with traumatic memories and triggers, do you feel unsure or have an urge to avoid any specific aspects of the therapy? For example, do you get anxious implementing the protocol for creating attachment experiences between the True Parent and Child parts? Or do you feel nervous about conducting EMDR reprocessing with abuse memories? Jot down any parts of the therapy that create anxiety. What Resource Team/Higher Power figure(s) might you bring in to assist you the next time you approach this part of the protocol?

Conduct a Future Rehearsal. Step into your most Competent Adult part of Self (see Protocol Script 8) and invite the Resource Team member(s) (see Protocol Script 7) to assist while you imaginally implement that piece of the therapy and apply slow BLS with butterfly tapping (crossing your arms and tapping bilaterally on either shoulder or arm). Notice how that feels. Further strengthen any positive shift in affect with another short, slow set of BLS.

USEFUL TERMS AND DEFINITIONS

AFTT-A: Attachment-Focused Trauma Therapy for Adults

AIP: adaptive information processing

BLS: bilateral stimulation

EMD: Eye Movement Desensitization

EMDR: Eye Movement Desensitization and Reprocessing

NC: negative cognition

PC: positive cognition

RDI: Resource Development and Installation

SUD: Subjective Units of Disturbance

VOC: Validity of Cognition

REFERENCES

Adler-Tapia, R. (2012). *Child psychotherapy: Integrating developmental theory into clinical practice.* Springer Publishing Company.

Hofmann, A. (2009). The inverted EMDR standard protocol for unstable complex posttraumatic stress disorder. In M. Luber (Ed.), *EMDR scripted protocols. Special populations* (pp. 313–328). Springer Publishing Company.

Knipe, J. (2015). *EMDR toolbox: Theory and treatment of complex PTSD and dissociation.* Springer Publishing Company.

Korn, D. L., & Leeds, A. M. (2002). Preliminary evidence of efficacy for EMDR resource development and installation in the stabilization phase of treatment of complex posttraumatic stress disorder. *Journal of Clinical Psychology, 58*(12), 1465–1487. https://doi.org/10.1002/jclp.10099

Leeds, A. (2016). *A guide to the standard EMDR protocols for clinicians, supervisors, and consultants* (2nd ed.). Springer Publishing Company.

Littel, M., Kenemans, J. L., Baas, J. M., Logemann, H. A., Rijken, N., Remijn, M., Hassink, R. J., Engelhard, I. M., Van den Hout, M. A. (2017). The effects of β-adrenergic blockade on the degrading effects of eye movements on negative autobiographical memories. *Biological Psychiatry, 82*(8), 587–593. https://doi.org/10.1016/j.biopsych.2017.03.012

Lovett, J. (2007). *Small wonders: Healing childhood trauma with EMDR.* Free Press/Simon & Schuster.

Lovett, J. (2015). *Trauma-attachment tangle: Modifying EMDR to help children resolve trauma and develop loving relationships.* Routledge/Taylor & Francis Group.

Nickerson, M. (Ed.). (2017). *Cultural competence and healing culturally based trauma with EMDR therapy: Innovative strategies and protocols.* Springer Publishing Company.

Shapiro, F. (2018). *Eye movement desensitization and reprocessing (EMDR) therapy: Basic principles, protocols, and procedures* (3rd ed.). Guilford Press.

Wesselmann, D., Schweitzer, C., & Armstrong, S. (2014). *Integrative team treatment for attachment trauma in children: Family therapy and EMDR.* W. W. Norton & Company.

CHAPTER 21

Applications of Attachment-Focused Trauma Therapy for Adults With a Dissociative Identity Disorder Diagnosis

INTRODUCTION

Clients who have a diagnosis of dissociative identity disorder (DID) are on the severe end of the dissociative continuum. The internal system of the client with DID is usually complex and may include more than one Adult part as well as multiple Child/Adolescent parts. At least some parts may operate with autonomy and with dissociative barriers between themselves and other parts resulting in lack of co-consciousness and creating significant complications in adult life. Clients who live with severe dissociation experience fragmentation of both time and sense of Self.

Attachment-Focused Trauma Therapy for Adults (AFTT-A) is not designed to be a comprehensive treatment for the DID client; however, with adaptations and consideration for the increased complexity of the internal personality system, the protocols of the AFTT-A model can help create stabilization through work with the internal personality system and an emotionally corrective therapeutic relationship in the preparation phase of Eye Movement Desensitization and Reprocessing (EMDR).

The following assessments are helpful in diagnosing a dissociative disorder and determining level of severity of dissociation:

- Dissociative Experiences Scale (DES-II; Carlson & Putman, 1993)
- Multiscale Dissociation Inventory (MDI; Briere et al., 2005)
- Multidimensional Inventory of Dissociation (MID; Dell, 2006)

See Chapter 6 for more information on assessment, treatment planning, and EMDR readiness in AFTT-A.

Clients who live with a dissociative disorder experience fragmentation of both time and sense of Self (Boon et al., 2011; Bryant, Kessler, & Shirar, 1992; Dell, 2006; Fraser, 2003; Holmes & Holmes, 2007; International Society for the Study of Trauma and Dissociation [ISST-D], 2011; Ross, 2013; van der Hart et al., 2006). Clients with DID may enter therapy fully aware of their diagnosis and familiar with their system or they may have little to no awareness of their parts, little memory for their traumatic past, and memory gaps in their present-day lives. As a result, the therapist may learn very little about the client's system in the early weeks of therapy sessions. Gaining a thorough understanding of the internal system is a process that often requires careful listening and observation. However, as the client's internal system gains trust in the therapist, more of the system becomes willing to make itself known and cooperate with therapy.

Any therapist treating clients with dissociative disorders should complete training and consultation specific to the disorder. EMDR therapy is appropriate for addressing traumatic memories with DID clients with appropriate stabilization and preparation phase work which may be lengthy and include a multimodal approach that includes skills training as well as restructuring work with the internal system (Carvalho, 2012; Fisher, 2017; Forgash, 2008; Gonzales & Mosquera, 2012; Knipe, 2015; Lanius & Paulsen, 2014; Martin, 2012; Parnell, 1999; Paulsen, 2009; Phillips, 2008; Schmidt, 2020). When the client meets the criteria for readiness to begin reprocessing, the therapist should be prepared to choose less disturbing EMDR targets to begin and apply restricted reprocessing and other modifications designed to increase safe and effective EMDR application with dissociative disorders. With flexibility and consideration for the increased complexity of the internal personality system, the protocols of the AFTT-A model can help provide stabilization and readiness through the preparation phase of EMDR therapy as well as safe and effective application of the reprocessing phases.

AFTT-A, Structural Dissociation Model, and Adaptive Information Processing Model

The Structural Dissociation model (van der Hart et al., 2006) is consistent with our theoretical view of dissociation. AFTT-A views clients with DID as having Adult and Child/Adolescent parts of Self that may play numerous roles and tend toward disconnected internal relationships rather than the more common enmeshed or partially disconnected internal relationships seen in clients with posttraumatic stress disorder (PTSD), complex PTSD (C-PTSD), and dissociative disorder not otherwise specified (DDNOS). For example, the Competent Adult part of Self in the AFTT-A model is termed the apparently normal part (ANP) within the framework of structural dissociation. In the case of DID, there may exist more than one functional ANP (Adult part of Self). In the Structural Dissociation model, the AFTT-A model's Child/Adolescent parts of Self are labeled emotional parts (EPs; van der Hart et al., 2006). EPs are viewed as holding the intolerable emotions and sensations that were present during traumatic events. Similarly, AFTT-A regards the Child/Adolescent parts as the aspects of Self that hold disturbing memories and associated affect.

Shapiro's adaptive information processing (AIP) model explains that everyday experiences are processed and either discarded from memory as unimportant or stored along with appropriate adaptive information. The AIP model is consistent with the Structural Dissociation model in its view that traumatic memories can overwhelm the AIP and become stored in memory networks in an unprocessed form, along with emotions, sensations, and perceptions separate from adaptive information in the brain. This stored material constitutes the EP in structural dissociation terms and the Child/Adolescent part of Self in AFTT-A. When attachment figures are the source of trauma for children, the hurt, betrayal, anger, fear, need, and associated perceptions and sensations are easily triggered by present-day attachments. In the case of DID, the triggered affect is so strong that the state of consciousness shifts completely to the remembered child state, thus moving executive control to the Child/Adolescent part of Self (EP) from the Adult part of Self (ANP) and leaving the adult client with amnesia for specific periods of time.

The Structural Dissociation model explains primary structural dissociation as involving a single EP that holds emotions related to a single incident trauma or more than one traumatic event with at the most, mild symptoms of dissociation related to EP activation. Secondary structural dissociation involves more than one EP, and the EPs may be more complex and more autonomous in their functioning, with dissociative symptoms about mid-range on the dissociation continuum. DID is considered tertiary structural dissociation, often involving more than one ANP and multiple and autonomous EPs with various roles. The EPs take executive control of the personality and leave the ANPs with little or no memory for those periods of time.

Interrupting the Dissociative Patterns

Adults at the most severe end of the dissociative continuum developed the capacity for dissociation as young children. Attachment disorganization in young children is associated with high risk for dissociative disorders by adolescence. Young children with the disorganized designation are observed to be caught in the classic double-bind struggle with their parents: The parent to whom the child wants to run for comfort is simultaneously the source of their fear (Main et al., 1985). Ross (2013) points out that the struggle between the desire for closeness and the fear of closeness leads to dissociation between the attachment system and the defensive system. The ANP who depends upon closeness with parents for survival is able to maintain attachment to the frightening parent by creating an EP that holds the fear.

The capacity for dissociation that starts in early childhood persists into adulthood. Just as learning to speak a second language at a very young age allows us to become adept at learning additional languages later in our lives, the capacity to create parts at a very young age becomes an established pattern for making new parts into adulthood.

The Structural Dissociation model posits that the pattern of dissociation becomes further entrenched due to the phobias of the ANP (van der Hart et al., 2006) for their memories, emotions, for the EPs, and for attachment relationships. The phobias trigger activation of the EPs.

By working with the ANPs to reduce the phobias, the need for protection provided by dissociative barriers is lessened over time. AFTT-A is not designed to be a comprehensive treatment for DID clients. However, with adaptations and consideration for the increased complexity of the personality system, the protocols of the AFTT-A model reduce phobias and help provide DID clients with

- an understanding of the Spiritual Essence that still exists at the core;
- development of skills and resources for improved functioning of Adult part(s);
- internal safety, nurturing, time orientation, and appropriate boundaries for younger parts of Self;
- decreased need to get childhood needs met through outside relationships in adult life;
- greater access to internal positive resources and qualities;
- understanding of the self-protective intentions underlying the behaviors of various parts of themselves;

- improved internal communication, cooperation, and new roles among parts;
- adoption of new Bonding Contract rules for improved relationships;
- an emotionally corrective therapeutic relationship; and
- an organized, coherent story.

ADAPTING AFTT-A STEPS WITH THE DISSOCIATIVE IDENTITY DISORDER DIAGNOSIS

Informed Consent for Clients With a Dissociative Identity Disorder Diagnosis

It is beneficial for clients with a DID diagnosis to know what to expect and what is expected of them up front. Through informed consent, the therapist is more likely to have agreement and cooperation from all parts.

The therapist *says...* "Science tells us that trauma underlies the development of dissociation and dissociated parts of Self. All parts of you are doing the best they can right now, and it's important that you understand that there are no bad parts of you at all. However, my overall goal is to work with you and your internal system of parts of Self so that your system is healthier. We'll work to help your 'Adult Brain' become stronger and more skilled and to help younger parts of you find safety, security, and nurturing on the inside. We'll work together to help access your internal resources and to help you re-connect with the Spiritual Essence with which you were born. You and I will help all parts of you work together in a more helpful way so you can replace unhealthy coping behaviors with healthy coping behaviors. When you're ready, we can utilize EMDR therapy to help heal your traumatic memories. Overall, does this model fit the goals you have for yourself? ... Do you have any questions?"

The *Guidelines for Treating Dissociative Identity Disorder in Adults, Third Revision* (ISST-D, 2011), suggest stopping the creation of additional parts by leaving unnamed parts with no name and avoiding creation of additional alternate identities. We directly ask clients with DID up front to agree to avoid making any new parts. The therapist *says...* "Before we get started with treatment, I'd like to go over therapy expectations that will help ensure that therapy is helpful for you. Is that okay with you? ... First, I'd like to request that no part of you creates any new parts. Creation of new parts will set us back, as we're working to create awareness, cooperation, and communication among your present parts of Self. Are all parts of you in agreement with this?

"Another agreement I'd like to make is that we have a shared goal for the parts on the inside to develop better communication between one another, and for the younger parts inside of you, over time, to learn to communicate things they want me to know by going through the Adult part(s) of you. This doesn't mean that I think any parts aren't important or that their message isn't important. It's just that the world of adult life is not a place where younger parts can feel comfortable or safe, and younger parts shouldn't have to take care of problems without assistance from an older part of Self. Does this goal seem reasonable? Do you sense a willingness from all parts to work on this? ...

"Another important expectation is for regular attendance. Consistency is important for developing our therapeutic relationship and for developing healthy relationships between all parts of you on the inside. Can we agree on keeping our work consistent? ...

"Another important expectation is regarding self-harming. I'd like you to contact me if you think you're going to harm yourself, with the expectation that the phone call will focus on identifying the coping skills you'll need to use until our next appointment and with a goal that you'll feel better by the end of the call. And, again, if younger parts are struggling, I'd like to help them learn to ask for help through the Adult part(s) of you. Does this seem reasonable to you and all parts on the inside (Linehan, 1993)?" ...

If you know that you'll be asking the client to attend a skills training class, it will be important to describe the class and the expectations of class participation. Sometimes it's helpful to explain the differences between a skills training class and a therapy group. It's also important to go over the cost of sessions and insurance coverage and to explain how payments are made. Additionally, go over your Consent for Treatment and under what conditions confidentiality is broken. Have any permissions to exchange information with other providers signed at this time.

If the client reports that some parts of Self are hesitant to participate in therapy, ask what the client thinks is getting in the way. If the client is unsure, *say*..."I have an unshakable belief that within your internal system, you have what you need to heal and that some parts of you will have ideas and solutions for any problems that come up. If parts are listening in that have anything that may be helpful right now, I hope those parts will communicate through an Adult part of you so that we can work together and find solutions. Of course, the final decision to participate in therapy is yours."

Bilateral Stimulation During Preparation Phase AFTT-A Protocols

Bilateral stimulation (BLS) should be applied with care during the AFTT-A preparation phase protocols for restructuring the internal system. BLS during EMDR resource work helps deepen and integrate the positive shifts but should be applied very carefully for DID clients. For clients with mild to moderate dissociation, very slow tactile BLS with only four to six passes may be safely applied. In the case of DID, slow BLS may need to be shortened to two to three passes. Offer the option of imaging with eyes open to assist with staying grounded or holding onto an item that is grounding such as a rock from the therapist's office or a meaningful object brought from home. The therapist can offer some options for BLS that might provide more grounding, such beating on a drum with bilateral movements, shaking maracas back and forth, or tapping the floor back and forth with their feet. If any form of BLS seems activating, the imagery should be conducted without the BLS until the client develops more stability.

Explaining the Parent-Adult-Child Model With Adaptations for Dissociative Identity Disorder

When explaining the Parent-Adult-Child (P-A-C) model (see Protocol Scripts 1, 2, and 3) in the case of a client with DID, special emphasis should be given to the AFTT-A tenet that every human being is born connected to a Spiritual Essence that is still present and unharmed by adverse events or attachment relationships during childhood, and that the purpose of AFTT-A is for clients to reconnect to their Spiritual Essence to which they were bonded at birth. The AFTT-A therapist also emphasizes with DID clients their "unshakable belief" that clients have everything they need inside of themselves to heal. It's the therapist's job to help them access their own internal qualities for healing and help them create a healthy internal personality system in which parts of Self communicate and work together for more effective functioning.

When explaining the P-A-C model to a client with DID, the complexity and multiplicity of parts is explained through the trauma lens. The therapist may *say*... "In the case of severe trauma, young children protect themselves by cutting off the parts of themselves holding intolerable feelings or memories. Once a young child learns how to create dissociated parts, it becomes easy to continue making parts, especially when there is anxiety about a situation or a task. There are no bad parts, and even though some parts may have behaviors that cause some problems, those behaviors are meant to be self-protective in some way. We'll work as a team to figure that out and find new ways to self-protect that don't create problems.

"Another difficulty is that parts of Self may sometimes confuse the past with the present. There is even more confusion when there is a lot of shifting of consciousness back-and-forth from one part of Self to another part of Self, causing all parts to have gaps in awareness and memory for present-day life. The good news is that we can work together as a team to improve the way things are working."

The Creation of a Safe Place and Higher Power for Adult Part(s) of Self

A Safe Place provides the Adult part(s) of Self with a place of respite created in the mind's eye that is clearly from imagination, not in any way connected to any difficult memories, and provides a sense of comfort, safety, and protection. If the word "safety" triggers thoughts related to "lack of safety," use words like calm and respite to describe the imaginal place. By imagining a fantasy figure that represents their Higher Power there in their place of respite, clients are reminded of the Spiritual Essence that remains at their core (see Protocol Script 4). If clients with DID have multiple Adult parts, they can decide with their therapist whether Adult parts have separate Safe Places and Higher Powers or have their own space within a shared Safe Place.

Creation of a Safe Place and Higher Power for the Child/Adolescent Part(s)

The client with DID may view some Child/Adolescent parts of Self with derision due to difficulties caused by challenging, self-protective behaviors. The therapist *says*... "Children and adolescents don't have the skills to operate effectively in adult life or cope well with difficult emotions. They need adults to set boundaries and take care of them. When younger parts are operating in adult life, they don't feel safe. If it's okay with you, I can guide you (*speaking to Adult part*) in creating a Safe Place and providing a Higher Power figure to care for your younger parts. In this way, you can provide them with the structure, safety, and care all youngsters need" (see Protocol Script 5).

The therapist works through the Adult part to create a Safe Place and fantasy figure representing a Higher Power for Child/Adolescent parts of Self as well (see

Protocol Script 5). The therapist encourages communication from the Adult part(s) of Self to the Child/Adolescent parts and from the Child/Adolescent parts to the Adult part(s) to avoid activating a transference response from the Child/Adolescent parts toward the therapist. Child/Adolescent parts will likely take executive control during sessions at times, but with great kindness and respect, the therapist communicates the message that Adult life is not a place that will ever feel completely safe for younger parts. Therefore, younger parts should stay safely tucked into Safe Places as much as possible and communicate "to" and "through" the Adult parts.

Some younger parts of Self will actively seek direct nurturing from the therapist. If the therapist were to attempt to provide nurturing messages directly to younger parts, any sense of satisfaction in the younger part would be temporary and lead to intense appeals for more. The therapist's boundaries need to be very clear and firm for the welfare of the Child/Adolescent parts.

Adapting the Resource Team Protocol

Although the Resource Team procedures are not intended to create new parts of Self, they are modified for clients with DID to ensure that new parts are not unintentionally created. The client should be reminded that the agreement for making no more parts remains in effect.

DID clients often have existing parts that already have helpful roles or potentially helpful talents or skills. The therapist helps the internal system work together by delineating the roles of existing parts. For example, the therapist may point out that one part brings strength and assertiveness to the personality system, while another part brings wisdom and problem-solving skills. The therapist can invite Adult parts to become a cooperative team. Resources can be deepened by accessing the associated posture or physical sensations and adding a slow, short set of BLS.

Alternatively, clients may be invited to visualize an imagined team member—a resource figure that cannot be mistaken for a part of Self—for the purpose of developing a specific needed resource. For example, the client may visualize a guardian angel or Yoda to access inner wisdom and peace.

Strengthening the Competent Adult Part of Self Protocol

A basic tenet of both the Structural Dissociation model and the AFTT-A model is the importance of improving skills and functioning of Adult part(s) of Self for adult life. The AFTT-A therapist emphasizes that Child/Adolescent parts of Self should not carry out the tasks of adult life. Child/Adolescent parts that are operating in adult life experience high anxiety and have inadequate skills for adult jobs.

However, when there is a DID diagnosis, Adult part(s) may have a significant deficit in interpersonal skills and emotion coping skills due to the negative impact of chronic trauma on social and emotional development. Therefore, we recommend Dialectical Behavioral Therapy (DBT; Linehan, 2014) for clients who demonstrate under-controlled affect and behavior or Radically Open Dialectical Behavioral Therapy (RO DBT; Lynch, 2018) for clients who are emotionally and behaviorally overcontrolled.

In addition to skills training, The AFTT-A therapist asks about and listens for stories about moments in which an Adult part of Self handled a situation with competence or a helpful skill. The therapist enhances the associated positive affect and body state with the *Strengthening the Competent Adult Part of Self* protocol (see Protocol Script 8). The protocol is not meant to be a one-time activity, but a procedure that can be repeated both in sessions and at home to enhance competence and confidence related to the use of skills in various present-day situations and tasks.

Creation of Emotionally Corrective Experiences Between Adult and Child/Adolescent Parts of Self

Although the time for meeting childhood needs on the outside is past and simply won't be helpful, the good news is that the Adult part(s) can provide corrective emotional experiences through affirming and reassuring messages for the younger part(s) of Self along with clear boundaries, safety, and structure (see Protocol Script 9). If the Adult part(s) is unable or unwilling to directly nurture the younger part(s), it may be more doable to visualize the Higher Power/Caregiver figure providing the nurturing care. Nurturing imagery for the Child/Adolescent part(s) can improve feelings of trust, safety, and worthiness for younger part(s) and lessen the drive to find others in outside adult life to meet their needs.

The Adult part(s) of Self may be resistant to the activity due to judgments about the behaviors of the Child/Adolescent part(s). It can be helpful to provide psychoeducation about the behaviors common to children who have experienced extensive trauma. Conducting guided imagery in which the Adult part experiences nurturing care from their own Higher Power figure within their own Safe Place may increase their willingness to provide nurturing messages or imagery for the younger part(s).

Parts' Work: Negotiating Roles

Parts' work is basically family therapy conducted through a Meeting Place with a team of Adult parts of Self learning to work cooperatively. The meeting is conducted with the most functional Adult part (or Adult parts with co-consciousness) present in the therapy office. The therapist guides the Adult part in the use of imagery to establish the Meeting Place and invite attendees.

The AFTT-A therapist makes suggestions to the Adult part who reports to the therapist any comments, complaints, demands, questions, or suggestions from all parts involved in the meeting. The therapist gives assistance as needed by providing suggestions to the Adult part regarding possible questions or solutions, which are then brought for discussion into the Meeting Place. The therapist strongly insists that every Adult part speaks respectfully with all other parts and that all behaviors have positive intentions and were developed to be self-protective in some way.

Meetings help negotiate new roles when there is a part functioning as an Emotion Protector-Controller or a part operating as a Critical Parent (see Protocol Script 10). Meetings can be called to ask one of the Adult parts to replace a harmful behavior with a new skill or set of new skills. For example, a part acting out aggressively to avoid vulnerability is thanked for participating and asked whether they might consider alternate means of avoiding vulnerability. Parts' work often involves discussions and agreements about opening communication or bringing down walls between parts of Self for greater teamwork.

One of the tenets of AFTT-A is that adults, not children, are responsible for adulthood tasks and that adults are responsible for keeping children safe and protected. Therefore, our view is that creation of a healthy internal system that is in the best interest of the whole person and that Adult parts of Self should be encouraged to keep younger parts of Self settled into Safe Places during meetings with Adult parts, emphasizing, "Meetings are grown-up business and not something kids need to be concerned about." If a Child/Adolescent part is acting out in some way, the Adult part(s) visits the younger part in the Safe Place or talks through an open door or window or through a creative method such as an intercom system. Behaviors of Child/Adolescent parts should be addressed with both compassion, boundary-setting, and reassurance of present-day safety. The therapist can guide the Adult parts in relieving Child/Adolescent parts from adulthood roles, reminding the younger part that it's time to relax and "just be a kid," while Adult part(s) step up to manage adult life.

Sometimes a part of Self believed to be an Adult turns out to be a Child/Adolescent part of Self behaving as a "pseudo-adult." While growing up, the child may have been parentified due to a neglectful or abusive environment. It can be reassuring to the pseudo-adult Child/Adolescent part to be relieved of adult roles and provided a Safe Place and Higher Power appropriate for a youngster.

> **BOX 21.1 CLIENT EXAMPLE: PATIENT WITH DISSOCIATIVE IDENTITY DISORDER**
>
> A thirty-year old client with a long history of self-harming was diagnosed with DID. Through parts' work it was discovered that an Adolescent part of Self had started cutting during a traumatic time in adolescence to numb emotional pain. The Adult part was encouraged to create a Safe Place protected by an angel for the Adolescent part. The Adult part gave affirming and nurturing messages to the Adolescent part as an emotionally corrective experience. Later, after another experience of self-harming, the Adult part agreed to encourage the younger part to stay in their Safe Place with the Higher Power and then offered additional comforts there for the younger part. They visualized a soft quilt, a rocking chair, a cat, and a picture window overlooking a forest. The angel became a team of angels. The Adult part agreed to reassure the younger part that the trauma was all over and that the Adult part was practicing new skills for managing triggered emotions and memories.

The Emotionally Corrective Therapeutic Relationship

In addition to the unresolved/disorganized status of DID clients related to trauma and loss, they may have dismissive or preoccupied attachment patterns within their significant relationships. Different parts of Self may operate with different patterns, so depending upon what part of Self is operating, interpersonal behaviors and defenses may vary. As a result, the therapist can be caught off-guard, as the client's behaviors and words can be unexpected at times. Thus, it's even more important for the AFTT-A therapist to attune to clients, providing secure-based responses to dismissive, preoccupied, or disorganized behaviors or words. (See Chapter 17, The Emotionally Corrective Therapeutic Relationship.) The AFTT-A therapist also stays mindful of personal emotions and self-regulates as needed to provide secure-based responses, staying attuned and respectful, validating emotions, looking for self-protective intentions in the behaviors, and providing time orientation as needed.

New Rules for the Early Bonding Contract

The client with DID can benefit from the protocol for *Revising the Early Bonding Contract Rules* (see Protocol Script 12). Stay aware that different functioning Adult parts of Self may be operating with different rules and therefore need to work through the *Revising the Early Bonding Contract Rules* protocol individually, or they may work together as a team to gain consensus on and set priorities for new rules. Also, in the case of DID, Child/Adolescent parts may need extra reassurance regarding present-day time and present-day safety for considering changes in the Early Bonding Contract rules.

Therapeutic Story

Clients with a DID diagnosis have unresolved/disorganized attachment patterns with respect to recall of traumatic memories (Liotti, 2004). Their narrative is confused and confusing related to sequence of events and who did what and who was responsible. They become dissociated and disoriented during a recounting of any part of their story. The tendency for confusion and disorientation can interfere with effective EMDR reprocessing of individual traumatic events. Creating a simple Therapeutic Story can be an effective way to help DID clients create internal organization, begin desensitization for discussion of their story, and begin integration of adaptive information (see Protocol Script 13).

The difficulty with writing a Therapeutic Story for clients with DID is the amount of material and the speed with which the Adult part(s) may become overwhelmed. For the client with extensive traumatic material, it helps to break the story down; for example, into chapters for infancy and toddlerhood, preschool years, elementary school years, middle school years, and high school years. Create a separate timeline for each chapter and complete the writing of the chapter following the storytelling outline (see Exhibit 22.13 in Chapter 22 or access the form online through Springer Publishing Connect: Use the code on the opening page of this book to access the digital product and select Chapter 22) before moving onto the next timeline. Keep identification of traumatic events or situations very brief. Give extra emphasis in the story to the positive beliefs/adaptive information related to each event/situation.

BLS is traditionally added throughout the reading of the Therapeutic Story. The therapist may wish to offer the option of adding BLS only during the parts that describe positive, preferred beliefs to deepen the positive shifts. Allow the client to choose the speed and modality of the BLS. Offer the options for BLS that might be more grounding to the client, such as beating a drum, shaking maracas, or tapping the feet. Optionally, the story can be read without BLS if the client prefers.

Getting Permission to Do Emotional Work and Time Orientation

Before moving into the EMDR reprocessing phases of therapy, it's important to get permission to do the trauma work from all parts of the client and make sure all parts are time oriented. No parts should feel pressured or coerced. Address any concerns, doubts, and worries from any parts of Self with sensitivity and attunement (see Protocol Script 14).

Transitioning From AFTT-A Preparation to EMDR Phases 3 to 8

The *Transition From the AFTT-A Preparation Phase to EMDR Phases 3 to 8* protocol ensures the DID client is fully prepared to move into the reprocessing phases, working the phases in a grounded, adult state, with Child/Adolescent parts of Self tucked into Safe Places (see Protocol Script 15). Adult parts of Self should have achieved at least some co-consciousness and agreement to share the eyes in viewing the memory during EMDR reprocessing.

EMDR Reprocessing Phases

When clients with DID have a strengthened capacity to operate from an Adult part of Self with present-day time orientation and manage emotions through appropriate coping skills, they may meet readiness criteria for beginning the reprocessing phases of EMDR standard protocol. However, when beginning EMDR trauma reprocessing with clients with DID, the work may made be safer and more manageable by keeping the focus on just one memory at a time and placing all other memories in a container—whether something concrete in the office such as a box or drawer or an imaginary container. To avoid unwanted associations, the therapist should use shorter sets of BLS and return to the memory more frequently. The therapist should also be prepared to use cognitive interweaves as often as necessary to help clients re-access the adult, present-day perspective and reduce dissociation. (See Chapter 20 for more AFTT-A recommendations regarding the reprocessing phases.)

Integration

Integration is not a solitary "step" in the AFTT-A model. All protocols within the AFTT-A model are naturally integrative over time. As the Adult part(s) of Self are strengthened through skills and resourcing of adaptive behaviors, they become more adept at communicating with one another, managing emotions, and providing needed safety and nurturing for younger parts, all of which are integrative for the system. The work reduces fears of danger and orients all parts of Self to present time and present-day perspective, reducing the phobias for memories. EMDR trauma reprocessing integrates the past with the present-day perspective and creates a sense of continuity of consciousness: "This happened to me in the past, and now that is over and I am here in this place and time."

Through the preparation and reprocessing phases of EMDR therapy and the AFTT-A model overall, the brain learns to access the different parts of the brain simultaneously. As connections are made between the various parts of the brain that hold different information, perspectives, emotions, and memories, the client experiences an emerging continuity of consciousness and sense of Authentic Self.

POINTS TO REMEMBER

- The client with DID is on the severe end of the dissociative continuum.
- The internal system of the client with DID is usually complex and may have more than one functioning Adult part as well as multiple Child/Adolescent parts of Self.
- The Structural Dissociation model describes parts of Self as EPs holding intolerable emotions and memories. It describes the functioning Adult parts of Self as the ANPs. The model promotes parts' work through the ANP(s) as integrative.
- The Structural Dissociation model posits that the ANP has phobias for emotions, memories, parts of Self, and attachments.
- The AFTT-A protocols, with appropriate adaptations for DID, reduce phobias by developing resources for managing emotions, strengthening the Adult parts of Self, giving protection and safety to Child/Adolescent parts, and creating new attachment rules and an organized trauma story.
- Child/Adolescent parts may be persistent in their attempts to get childhood needs met through relationships on the outside. Adult part(s) should be guided in meeting the needs of Child/Adolescent parts on the inside. Attempts of the therapist to directly meet the needs of Child/Adolescent parts will intensify the transference and fail to provide satisfaction.
- The therapist should minimize direct work with Child/Adolescent parts or other parts and facilitate the majority of therapeutic work through the Adult part(s) of Self.
- Behaviors that create difficulties are self-protective in some way. The AFTT-A therapist works with the system to find new ways to meet needs of the various parts of Self and communicates the consistent message that the system has everything it needs inside to heal.
- Younger parts that are activated within the therapy session should be listened to and treated with respect, but the therapist should consistently communicate to younger parts that adult life is not a place where they will feel safe. Guided imagery can create internal safety for younger parts.
- AFTT-A and EMDR therapy are naturally integrative, as the work strengthens the Adult parts, orients parts of Self to present-day time, reduces fears of emotions, memories, other parts, and attachment relationships, and internal cooperation, communication, and co-consciousness.

TROUBLESHOOTING

- **Clients may have mixed feelings about increasing conscious awareness and reducing or eliminating dissociation.**

Dissociation allows the Adult part to mentally leave during stressful situations, emotions, or triggered memories. However, there are consequences to dissociation as well. *Say...* "You may have mixed feelings about staying present to more of your adult life, which is understandable, because change is hard. But remember, we can go as slowly as you need, and ultimately, the decision to stay present will always be yours. I want to help you be more conscious of your choices and more skillful with present-day situations. Remember, the younger parts of you feel better when there's an adult managing adulthood tasks. Kids just don't feel safe operating in adult life because they don't have the skills."

- **Child/Adolescent parts may continue to seek nurturing and affection directly from the therapist.**

It's critical that the therapist avoid the temptation to satisfy younger parts seeking affection, nurturing, and reassurance through affectionate words or any type of physical touch. Attempts by the therapist to "fix" the early wounds of the Child/Adolescent part of Self don't lead to a sense of satisfaction for the Child/Adolescent part and can intensify problematic transference. *Say...* "The time for younger parts to get needs met from others on the outside is over." Validate and attune to feelings of sadness, grief, loss, and anger. Avoid caregiving in response.

Say... "However, I can assist the Adult part of you (or Adult parts of you working together as a team) with providing love and care to the younger parts of you on the inside." Bring out a set of nesting dolls and explain, "The two biggest dolls here represent the Adult part of you and the therapist—me." Place the therapist doll behind the doll representing the client. The smaller dolls are grouped in front of the Adult. *Say...* "The dolls illustrate how I will be here to support and guide the Adult part of you, while the Adult part provides a Safe Place and meets the needs of the younger parts of you."

PAUSE AND REFLECT FOR THE THERAPIST

Providing secure responses to nonsecure words and behaviors of clients' parts is critical to creation of an emotionally corrective therapeutic relationship. However, work with complicated systems of clients with DID can be overwhelming at times, and therapists' emotions can get in the way of staying intentional and even-keel in the therapy office. Mindful awareness is the key. Write down answers to the following questions in your journal.

1. What situations in working with the DID client trigger anxiety? What are your negative cognitions (NCs)? What positive cognitions (PCs) help you when you get anxious?
2. What situations trigger frustration? What are your NCs? What do you need to remind yourself (PCs) when you get frustrated?
3. What situations trigger an urge to caretake? What are your NCs? What do you need to remind yourself (PCs) when you want to caretake?
4. What situations trigger anger? What are your NCs? What do you need to remind yourself (PCs) when you feel angry?

5. What situations trigger feelings of inadequacy? What are your NCs? What do you need to remind yourself (PCs) when you feel inadequate?

USEFUL TERMS AND DEFINITIONS

AFTT-A: Attachment-Focused Trauma Therapy for Adults

AIP: adaptive information processing

ANP: apparently normal part

BLS: bilateral stimulation

DBT: Dialectical Behavioral Therapy

DDNOS: dissociative disorder not otherwise specified

DES-II: Dissociative Experiences Scale

DID: dissociative identity disorder

EMDR: Eye Movement Desensitization and Reprocessing

EP: emotional part

ISST-D: International Society for the Study of Trauma and Dissociation

MDI: Multiscale Dissociation Inventory

MID: Multidimensional Inventory of Dissociation

NC: negative cognition

P-A-C: Parent-Adult-Child

PC: positive cognition

PTSD: posttraumatic stress disorder

RO DBT: Radically Open Dialectical Behavioral Therapy

REFERENCES

Boon, S., Steele, K., & van der Hart, O. (2011). *Coping with trauma-related dissociation.* W. W. Norton & Company.

Briere, J., Weathers, F. W., & Runtz, M. (2005). Is dissociation a multidimensional construct? Data from the Multiscale Dissociation Inventory. *Journal of Traumatic Stress, 8*(3), 221–231. https://doi.org/10.1002/jts.20024

Bryant, D., Kessler, J., & Shirar, L. (1992). *The family inside: Working with the multiple.* W. W. Norton & Company.

Carlson, E. B., & Putnam, F. W. (1993). An update on the Dissociative Experience Scale. *Dissociation: Progress in the Dissociative Disorders, 6*(1), 16–27.

Carvalho, E. R. (2012). *Healing the folks who live inside: How EMDR can heal our inner gallery of roles.* EMDR Treinamento e Consultoria Ltda.

Dell, P. F. (2006). A new model of dissociative identity disorder. *Psychiatric Clinics of North America, 29*(1), 1–26. https://doi.org/10.1016/j.psc.2005.10.013

Fisher, J. (2017). *Healing the fragmented selves of trauma survivors: Overcoming internal self-alienation*. Routledge.

Forgash, C. (2008). Integrating EMDR and ego state treatment for clients with trauma disorders. In C. Forgash & M. Copeley (Eds.), *Healing the heart of trauma and dissociation with EMDR and ego state therapy* (pp. 1–60). Springer Publishing Company.

Fraser, G. A. (2003). Fraser's "Dissociative Table Technique" revisited, revised: A strategy for working with ego states in dissociative disorders and ego-state therapy. *Journal of Trauma and Dissociation*, 4(4), 5–28. https://doi.org/10.1300/J229v04n04_02

Gonzales, A., & Mosquera, D. (2012). *EMDR and dissociation: The progressive approach* (1st ed., revised). Self-Published.

Holmes, T., & Holmes, L. (2007). *Parts work: An illustrated guide to your inner life*. Winged Heart Press.

International Society for the Study of Trauma and Dissociation. (2011). Guidelines for treating dissociative identity disorder in adults, third revision. *Journal of Trauma & Dissociation*, 12(2), 115–187. http://dx.doi.org/10.1080/15299732.2011.537247

Knipe, J. (2015). *EMDR toolbox: Theory and treatment of complex PTSD and dissociation*. Springer Publishing Company.

Lanius, U., & Paulsen, S. (2014). *Neurobiology and treatment of traumatic dissociation: Towards an embodied self*. Springer Publishing Company.

Linehan, M. (1993). *Cognitive-behavioral treatment of borderline personality disorder*. Guilford Press.

Linehan, M. (2014). *DBT skills training manual* (2nd ed.). The Guilford Press.

Liotti, G. (2004). Trauma, dissociation, and disorganized attachment: Three strands of a single braid. *Psychotherapy: Theory, Research, Practice, Training*, 41(4), 472–486. https://doi.org/10.1037/0033-3204.41.4.472

Lynch, T. (2018). *The skills training manual for Radically Open Dialectical Behavior Therapy: A clinician's guide for treating disorders of overcontrol*. Context Press.

Main, M., Kaplan, N., & Cassidy, J. (1985). Security in infancy, childhood, and adulthood: A move to the level of representation. *Monographs of the Society for Research in Child Development*, 50(1/2), 66–104. http://dx.doi.org/10.2307/3333827

Martin, K. M. (2012). How to use Fraser's Dissociative Table Technique to access and work with emotional parts of the personality. *Journal of EMDR Practice and Research*, 6(4), 179–186. https://doi.org/10.1891/1933-3196.6.4.179

Parnell, L. (1999). *EMDR in the treatment of adults abused as children*. W. W. Norton & Company.

Paulsen, S. (2009). *Looking through the eyes of trauma and dissociation*. The Bainbridge Institute for Integrative Psychology.

Phillips, M. (2008). Combining hypnosis with EMDR and ego state therapy for ego strengthening. In C. Forgash & M. Copeley (Eds.), *Healing the heart of trauma and dissociation with EMDR and ego state therapy* (pp. 91–120). Springer Publishing Company.

Ross, C. (2013). *Structural dissociation: A proposed modification of the theory*. Manitou Communications, Inc.

Schmidt, S. L. (2020). *Ego state therapy interventions to prepare attachment-wounded adults for EMDR*. DNMS Institute LLC.

van der Hart, O., Nijenhuis, E. R. S., & Steele, K. (2006). *The haunted self: Structural dissocaition and the treatment of chronic traumatization*. W. W. Norton & Company.

CHAPTER 22

Supplemental Materials for Use With Clients in Attachment-Focused Trauma Therapy for Adults

> **EXHIBIT 22.1 CHECKLIST: STEPS FOR ATTACHMENT-FOCUSED TRAUMA THERAPY FOR ADULTS (AFTT-A)**
>
> Note: This checklist is original to the authors. The initial outline was created by Lisa Ripperton, LCSW, LCAS; North Carolina Department of Health and Human Services.
>
> ☐ **Introduce Parent-Adult-Child (P-A-C) Model**
>   ☐ Identify parts of Self, impact of childhood experiences on internal system, patterns, and unmet childhood needs
>   ☐ Complete diagram/sand tray picture/drawing of current P-A-C diagram
>   ☐ Complete diagram/sand tray picture/drawing of future/ideal P-A-C diagram
> ☐ **Develop Safe Place and Higher Power for Adult Self**
>   ☐ Nurturing and protective
>
> | Safe Place | Higher Power |
> |---|---|
> | _____ | _____ |
> | _____ | _____ |
> | _____ | _____ |
> | _____ | _____ |
> | _____ | _____ |
>
> ☐ **Deepen associated positive affect with slow bilateral stimulation (BLS)**
>
> *(continued)*

Access digital versions of these forms online through Springer Publishing Connect: Use the code on the opening page of this book to access the digital product and select Chapter 22.

EXHIBIT 22.1 CHECKLIST: STEPS FOR ATTACHMENT-FOCUSED TRAUMA THERAPY FOR ADULTS (AFTT-A) (continued)

☐ **Develop Safe Place and Higher Power for Child Parts**
  ☐ Nurturing, protective, and age-appropriate

Child Part's Age	Unmet Needs	Safe Place	Higher Power

☐ **Deepen positive affect with slow BLS**

☐ **Resource Team**
Identify:
  ☐ Client goals
  ☐ Strengths and characteristics needed to accomplish goals
  ☐ Team members who represent those characteristics
  ☐ Meeting Place (not adult Safe Place)—nurturing and protective
  ☐ Transitional object to carry from Safe Place to Meeting Place: _____

Goals	Characteristics	Team Member	Meeting Place

(continued)

EXHIBIT 22.1 CHECKLIST: STEPS FOR ATTACHMENT-FOCUSED TRAUMA THERAPY FOR ADULTS (AFTT-A) (*continued*)

- [ ] Invite team to gather—strengthen and reinforce positive affect
- [ ] Discuss ways Resource Team can assist in meeting goals—strengthen and reinforce
- [ ] Add visual/tactile/auditory links to sense of competence/confidence—strengthen with slow BLS
- [ ] Future Rehearsal with use of Resource Team

- [ ] **Strengthen the Competent Adult Part of Self**
  - [ ] Identify positive memories of operating from Competent Adult part of Self
  - [ ] Use Popky's "video and step into" process to deepen the positive memory and associated body position, facial expression, and voice tone
  - [ ] Install cue word
  - [ ] Identify preferred method(s) for accessing Competent Adult part of Self (body, face, voice, cue word)
  - [ ] Competent Adult Future Rehearsal with present-day challenge

Memory	Imagery	Body Position/Posture	Cue Word	Future Rehearsal
_____	_____	_____	_____	_____
_____	_____	_____	_____	_____
_____	_____	_____	_____	_____

- [ ] **Create Corrective Attachment Experience Between Child/Adolescent and True Parent Parts of Self**
  - [ ] Ground client in Competent Adult part of Self to begin
  - [ ] Invite Adult part to place hand on heart to access nurturing aspects and peek or step into Safe Place of Child part
  - [ ] Invite True Parent to reach out in some way, with assistance from Higher Power or Resource Team to help if needed
  - [ ] Dialogue messages of reassurance, time orientation, worthiness, belonging with slow BLS
  - [ ] Check in regarding response of True Parent and Child parts
  - [ ] Magical Cord of Love. Deepen with slow BLS
  - [ ] "Enfold" Child part of Self inside Safe Place in client's heart

- [ ] **Parts' Work: Negotiating Roles for Critical Parent (CP) and Emotion Controller-Regulator (ECR)**
  - [ ] [ ] Convene meeting with Resource Team—strengthen and reinforce positive affect

(*continued*)

EXHIBIT 22.1 CHECKLIST: STEPS FOR ATTACHMENT-FOCUSED TRAUMA THERAPY FOR ADULTS (AFTT-A) (*continued*)

- ☐☐ Decide which part (CP or ECR) to bring into meeting
  Describe what part looks like
- ☐☐ Bring part into meeting to discuss:
  Past roles of part in client's life, including positive and negative effects
  Thank part for helping client survive in the past
  Explain need to change to continue to help part and become a Resource Team member
  Gain commitment to change/consider the possibility of change
  Brainstorm new roles
  Open Resource Team for comments, concerns, including from Child parts (tucked into Safe Places)
- ☐☐ Strengthen and reinforce positive affect with slow BLS
- ☐☐ Time orientation
  Repeat process with other part

☐ **Parts' Work: Tucking in Child Parts**
  - ☐ Identify enmeshment between "Adult Brain" and "Kid Brain"
  - ☐ Find location of Child part is NOW
  - ☐ Invite Adult Self to talk to Child part about:
    Why child snuck out of Safe Place—link to past roles, beliefs, and so on
    Thank part for helping client survive in the past
    Time orientation
    Reinforce education about unmet childhood needs, now for Adult/New Parent to meet
    Reinforce time orientation
    Set firm boundaries about child staying in Safe Place. Make sure Higher Power is aware/able to maintain these boundaries
    Make sure there is a communication path between child Safe Place and Resource Team

☐ **Revise Early Bonding Contract Rules**
  - ☐ Orient to Competent Adult part of Self
  - ☐ Explain Early Bonding Contract as unspoken relationship rules developed in early childhood
  - ☐ Brainstorm the Early Bonding Contract old rules together
  - ☐ Make list of opposing, healthy new rules for present-day relationships

(*continued*)

EXHIBIT 22.1 CHECKLIST: STEPS FOR ATTACHMENT-FOCUSED TRAUMA THERAPY FOR ADULTS (AFTT-A) (*continued*)

- ☐ Dialogue with Child part of Self:
  "Picture Child part of you in Safe Place. Dialogue: It's OK to change rules because the child is safe no matter what." Repeat with other young parts as needed. Add slow BLS throughout to strengthen.
- ☐ Future Rehearsal with person with whom you have a difficult relationship:
  Read new rules while client views themselves in room with person at some point in the future
  Read new rules while client "steps into" room with person at some point in the future
  (Add constant, slow BLS throughout each visualization to deepen)

Old Rules	New Rules

(*continued*)

EXHIBIT 22.1 CHECKLIST: STEPS FOR ATTACHMENT-FOCUSED TRAUMA THERAPY FOR ADULTS (AFTT-A) (*continued*)

- ☐ **Therapeutic Story**
  - ☐ Orient to Competent Adult part of Self
  - ☐ Introduce idea of story to create coherent narrative of past
  - ☐ Draw a timeline with client including preverbal events (by family stories, etc.). Note negative cognitions, positive cognitions
  - ☐ Write the story beginning in the following format:
    An adult with many positive qualities, such as . . ., enjoys . . . and lives . . .
    Like most people they had both positive and difficult things happen in life.
    The adult has inside and outside resources such as . . .
  - ☐ Continue the story as follows:
    A positive event was . . .
    A difficult event was . . .
    The youngster felt . . . and began to believe . . . (NCs)
    The Competent Adult wants the younger part to know . . . (PCs)
    A positive event/wonderful thing was . . .
    Repeat italicized section until story is complete
  - ☐ Close the story:
    Today the adult sometimes struggles with believing . . .
    But with the help of inside and outside resources and supports, they are continuing to heal and learn . . .

- ☐ **Permission to Do the Work and Time Orientation**
  Permission to Do the Work:
  - ☐ Convene Resource Team meeting. Encourage Resource Team to communicate with Child parts, as needed. Invite all parts who would be helpful or who do not believe the danger is past, including child parts in their Safe Places, to observe the meeting
  - ☐ Brainstorm with Resource Team barriers to trauma processing and how Resource Team can help
  - ☐ Use Future Rehearsal protocol to practice using Resource Team in trauma processing

  Time Orientation:
  - ☐ Invite all parts that are disoriented to time, including Child parts, to listen in during the session
  - ☐ Time orientation: Note hands, jewelry, clothes, office space, relationship with therapist
    Does every part of you and every cell in your body know that the danger is past and it's "now," not "back then"?

(*continued*)

EXHIBIT 22.1 CHECKLIST: STEPS FOR ATTACHMENT-FOCUSED TRAUMA THERAPY FOR ADULTS (AFTT-A) (*continued*)

- ☐ **Transition From Preparation to Phases 3 to 8**
    - ☐ Develop client goals specific to EMDR protocol
    - ☐ Brainstorm needed strengths, characteristics and resources, Resource Team members
    - ☐ Discuss how Resource Team can help
    - ☐ Brainstorm potential "stuck points" in protocols and use Future Rehearsal to strengthen sense of competence and confidence to master challenges
    - ☐ Review and revise Safe Place(s), Meeting Place, Resource Team members until client feels ready to proceed

Goals	Characteristics	Team Members	Possible "Stuck" Points	Ways Resource Team Can Help
_____	_____	_____	_____	_____
_____	_____	_____	_____	_____
_____	_____	_____	_____	_____
_____	_____	_____	_____	_____
_____	_____	_____	_____	_____
_____	_____	_____	_____	_____
_____	_____	_____	_____	_____
_____	_____	_____	_____	_____
_____	_____	_____	_____	_____
_____	_____	_____	_____	_____

- ☐ Prior to EMDR phase 3, identify targets relevant to client goals using:
    Present-day triggers
    First/worst memory associated with trigger
    Timeline events

EXHIBIT 22.2 THERAPIST DISCLOSURE STATEMENT

(Therapist's Name and Contact Information)

EDUCATION, LICENSURE, AND CERTIFICATION

TREATMENT
(Include therapist approaches to therapy, what to expect from therapy, and risks and benefits of therapy.)

THE NATURE OF OUR RELATIONSHIP
(Clarify professional relationship and specify confidentiality and limits to confidentiality, professional boundaries, therapist's individual boundaries, and process for reporting boundary violations.)

EMERGENCIES
(Define and specify contact with therapist for both emergencies and non-emergency matters.)

FEES FOR SERVICES
(Include fees for initial session, differing lengths of individual sessions, and group therapy if relevant; policy about cancellation with late cancellation and no-show charges; and expectations about payment of client portion of fee.)

TERMINATION OF THERAPY
(Include process and expectations for termination when client has completed goals for therapy and when client and/or therapist decides that therapy is not effective or not being used effectively, client's needs are beyond therapist's scope of practice, and state licensure statutes related to ethical termination of therapy.)

DATED STATEMENT OF UNDERSTANDING AND AGREEMENT WITH CLIENT AND THERAPIST SIGNATURES

EXHIBIT 22.3 INITIAL ASSESSMENT

Client Name _____ Date _____

Age _____ Date of Birth _____ Last 4 Digits of SSN _____

Presenting Problem
_____
_____

Highest Level of Education _____

or Grade in School _____

Name of School _____

Employment History _____

Religious Preference _____

Interests _____

Friends _____

Current Relationship Status _____

Children _____

Relationship History _____

Family History

Parents
_____
_____

Siblings
_____
_____

Family History of Mental Illness/Substance Abuse
_____
_____

(*continued*)

EXHIBIT 22.3 INITIAL ASSESSMENT (continued)

History of Abuse/Neglect

Neglect _____

_____

_____

Abuse (including emotional, verbal, physical, witnessing violence, bullying, sexual, date or acquaintance rape, socially based adversity/trauma)

_____

_____

Strengths, Skills, and Internal and External Resources

_____

_____

EXHIBIT 22.4 MENTAL STATUS EXAMINATION

Note: Adapted from Aas, I.H. M. (2011). Guidelines for rating Global Assessment of Functioning (GAF). *Annals of General Psychiatry*, 10, Article No. 2. https://doi.org/10.1186/1744-859X-10-2; American Psychiatric Association. (2013). *Diagnostic and statistical manual of mental disorders* (5th ed., pp. 265–290). American Psychiatric Publishing; and Martin, D. C. (1990). The mental status examination. In H. K. Walker, W. D. Hall, & J. W. Hurst (Eds.). *Clinical methods: The history, physical, and laboratory examinations* (3rd ed; Chapter 207). Butterworth Publishers.

Client _____ Date _____

Last 4 Digits of SSN _____ Age _____ Date of Birth _____

Presenting Problem _____

_____

_____

Relevant History

Grade in School _____

Employment History _____

Family History

Mental Illness/Alcoholism _____

Current Status

Legal _____

Ethanol/Drug Use/Abuse _____

Previous Treatment _____

Physical Problems _____

Medications _____

Current Symptoms
- ☐ Depressed Mood
- ☐ Short Attention Span/Poor Concentration
- ☐ Memory Impairment
- ☐ Appetite Loss/Gain
- ☐ Significant Weight Loss/Gain
- ☐ Overeating/Binge Eating

(continued)

EXHIBIT 22.4 MENTAL STATUS EXAMINATION (continued)

- ☐ Feelings of Worthlessness
- ☐ Hypersomnia
- ☐ Insomnia (onset)
- ☐ Early Morning Awakening
- ☐ Nightmares/Night Terrors
- ☐ Anhedonia
- ☐ Fatigue
- ☐ Anxiety
- ☐ Panic Attacks
- ☐ Indecisiveness
- ☐ Marked Mood Swings
- ☐ Racing Thoughts
- ☐ Mania/Hypomania
- ☐ Irritability
- ☐ Purging/Self-Induced Vomiting
- ☐ Persistent Anger
- ☐ Outbursts of Anger
- ☐ Outbursts of Aggression
- ☐ Antisocial Behavior
- ☐ Self-Mutilating Behavior
- ☐ Suicide Attempt
- ☐ Suicidal Ideation
- ☐ Dissociative Episodes
- ☐ Impairment in Job/School/Home Functioning
- ☐ Flashbacks/Disturbing Recollections
- ☐
- ☐

Recent Changes (Last 6 Months)

Mood/Affect _____

Weight _____

Eating Habits _____

Sleeping Habits _____

Appearance

Age __ Gender __ Cau. __ Black __ Hisp. __ Asian __ Native Amer. __ Other __

Apparent Age: Greater __ As stated __ Younger __

Build: Malnourished __ Thin __ Medium __ Heavy __ Obese __

Hygiene: Clean __ Disheveled __ Odorosis __

Dress: Neat __ Untidy __ Peculiar __

Behavioral/Facial Expressions

Normal __ Immobile __ Sad __ Worried __ Angry __ Happy __

Eye Contact: Good __ Avoided __ Stared Into Space __

Attention Span: Poor __ Satisfactory __ Distractable __

Motor: Normal __ Hypoactive __ Stupor __ Hyperactive __

Posture: Normal __ Slumped __ Rigid __ Other __

Mannerisms: Normal __ Posturing __ Echopraxia __ Stereotyic __ Pacing __ Tics __ Handwriting __ Involuntary Movements __

(continued)

EXHIBIT 22.4 MENTAL STATUS EXAMINATION (continued)

Demeanor: Normal __ Tearful __ Crying __ Blushing __ Sweating __ Tremorous __ Other __

Involuntary Movements: Tremor __ Chorea __ Myoclonius __ Athetosis __

Speech
Rate: Normal __ Slow __ Rapid __ Pressured __
Word-Finding Ability: Normal __ Impaired __ Aphasia __
Rhythm: Normal __ Abnormal __
Other: Defect/Slur __ Stutter __ Echolalia __

Level of Consciousness
Alert __ Drowsy __ Somnolent __ Confused __ Comatose __

Affect
Appropriate: Yes __ No __
Lability: Yes __ No __
Range: Constricted __ Full __
Intensity: Mild __ Moderate __ Severe __

Thought Processes
Confabulation __ Tangential __ Circumstantial __
Blocking __ Non-Sequitor __ Looseness of Assoc. __ Flight of Ideas __ Other __

Thought Productivity
Normal __ Slow __ Accel. __

Thought Content
Suicidal Ideation: Y __ N __ Plan __ Means ____ Intent ____ (0–10)
Homicidal Ideation: Y __ N __ Plan __ Means ____ Intent ____ (0–10)
Persecutory Delusions: Y __ N __
Grandiose Delusions: Y __ N __
Violence to Others: Y __ N __ Preoccupation __
Ideas of Reference __ Ideas of Control __ Thought Broadcasting __

Perception
Hallucinations: Visual __ Auditory __ Tactile __ Olfactory __ Gustatory __
Describe _____

Mental Status
Orientation: Person __ Place __ Time __
Concentration: Serial 7s _____ Serial 3s _____

(continued)

EXHIBIT 22.4 MENTAL STATUS EXAMINATION (*continued*)

16	32
795	648
2671	5394
81327	62859
472851	196583

Digit Span #FRD ___ #BKWD ___ Not Tested ___

Memory: Remote ___ Not Tested ___

        Recent ___ Not tested ___

Recall: Verbal Recall (Immed.) # _____ /3

        Verbal Recall (at 5 Minutes) _____ Not Tested ___

Multiplication: _____ Not Tested _____

Presidents: ___ ___ ___ Not Tested ___

Gen. Info/Assessed IQ: Avg. ___ Below Avg. ___ Above Avg. ___

                         Unable to Access ___

Similarities:

Apple and Banana _____

Table and Chair _____

Fly and Tree _____

Poem and Statue _____

Idiom: "Cold Shoulder" _____

Proverbs: Not Tested _____

        Spilled Milk _____

        Glass House _____

Reasoning Level: Concrete ___ Mostly Concrete ___ Mostly Abstract ___ Abstract ___

Judgment: Mail _____

               Fire _____

               Test Judgment Intact _____ Impaired _____ Unable to Assess _____

               Social Judgment Intact _____ Impaired _____ Unable to Assess _____

Diagnoses   Axis I: _____

                Axis II: _____

                Axis III: _____

                Axis IV: (Stressors) Absent ___ Mild ___ Moderate ___ Severe ___

                          Catastrophic ___

                Axis V: (GAF) Current _____ Highest Past Year _____

Goals for Therapy

_____

_____

Signature _____   **Date** _____

EXHIBIT 22.5 CLIENT MEDICAL HISTORY

NAME: _____ DATE: _____

CURRENT PRIMARY MEDICAL CARE PROVIDERS (PRIMARY CARE PHYSICIAN, SPECIALIST, PSYCHIATRIATRIC MEDICATION MANAGER)

Name: _____ Title: _____

Phone: _____ Address: _____

Name: _____ Title: _____

Phone: _____ Address: _____

Name: _____ Title: _____

Phone: _____ Address: _____

How would you rate your overall health: ☐ Excellent ☐ Good ☐ Fair ☐ Poor

What, if any, concerns do you have about your health: _____
_____

When was your last complete physical examination: _____

Please list any medication/substance/food/environmental allergies:
_____
_____

Please list any medication/food/environmental sensitivities or intolerances:
_____
_____

Health Risk History

☐ YES ☐ NO Do you smoke? If yes, how long, how many cigarettes per day: _____

☐ YES ☐ NO Have you smoked in the past? If so, how long? _____ How long ago did you quit? _____

☐ YES ☐ NO Do you use alcohol? If yes, how often, how much: _____

☐ YES ☐ NO Do you use drugs? If yes, how often, how much: _____

☐ YES ☐ NO Have you or your partner(s) ever injected drugs and when: _____

☐ YES ☐ NO Have you ever had a problem with alcohol, drugs, other addiction?

☐ YES ☐ NO Do you think you should cut down on your drinking or drug use?

(continued)

EXHIBIT 22.5 CLIENT MEDICAL HISTORY (continued)

☐ YES ☐ NO   Have you been annoyed when others question your drug or alcohol use?

☐ YES ☐ NO   Have you ever felt guilty about how much you drink or use drugs?

☐ YES ☐ NO   Have you ever had a drink/used drugs to get going, to treat a hangover, or to prevent withdrawal symptoms?

☐ YES ☐ NO   Has anyone ever been concerned or complained about your drinking/using?

☐ YES ☐ NO   Have you ever gotten into trouble when drinking/using?

With family members _____   With friends _____   Others _____

☐ YES ☐ NO   With the law

No. of DUI(s): _____   What year(s): _____ / _____ / _____ / _____ / _____

No. of MIP(s): _____   What year(s): _____ / _____ / _____ / _____ / _____

Other: _____   What year(s): _____ / _____ / _____ / _____ / _____

☐ YES ☐ NO   Have you ever had a sexually transmitted disease? If so, specify: _____

☐ YES ☐ NO   Have you ever been tested for HIV? If yes, what were the results? _____

Do you now have, or have you ever had, conditions involving the following? Please check all that apply and describe your symptoms or diagnoses.

☐ Skin: _____

☐ Eyes: (Changes in vision, glaucoma, cataracts, etc.) _____
_____

☐ Ears: (Changes in hearing, hearing loss, problems with ears, etc.)
_____
_____

☐ Teeth and Mouth: (Dentures/missing teeth, mouth pain, etc.)
_____
_____

(continued)

EXHIBIT 22.5 CLIENT MEDICAL HISTORY (continued)

☐ Lungs: (Asthma, persistent cough, shortness of breath, COPD) _____
_____

☐ Urinary: (Chronic bladder or kidney infections, difficulty urinating, etc.)
_____
_____

☐ Muscles/Joints (arthritis, fibromyalgia, joint pain/inflammation, muscle weakness/pain, etc.)
_____
_____
_____

☐ Neurological: (Head injury, seizures, dizziness, problems with balance, falls, severe/persistent/chronic headaches, loss of consciousness, numbness/tingling/weakness in extremities, speech problems, clumsiness, etc.)
_____
_____
_____

☐ Gastrointestinal: (Diabetes, gastric reflux, irritable bowel syndrome, hepatitis, stomach/abdominal pain, nausea/vomiting, difficulty swallowing, vocal problems, etc.) _____
_____
_____

☐ Reproduction/Sexual: (Menstrual or menopausal difficulties, breast disease, pain/cysts/drainage from breasts, prostate problems, erectile difficulties, difficulty with orgasm, other sexual difficulties, etc.)
_____
_____

☐ Endocrinological: (Diabetes, adrenal fatigue, hypo- or hyperthyroidism, etc.)
_____
_____

☐ Heart or Blood: (High/low blood pressure, high cholesterol or triglycerides, heart attack, stroke, congestive heart failure, anemia, abnormal heartbeat, bruising easily, etc.)
_____
_____
_____

(continued)

EXHIBIT 22.5 CLIENT MEDICAL HISTORY (continued)

☐ Other: (immune disorders, sore/swollen neck/glands, etc.)
_____
_____

☐ Past Injuries/Surgeries: _____
_____

Referred for Physical Exam: ☐ YES ☐ NO

To Whom: _____ Client Accepting Referrals: ☐ YES ☐ NO

Referred for Psychiatric Evaluation: ☐ YES ☐ NO

To Whom: _____ Client Accepting Referrals: ☐ YES ☐ NO

_____   _____
Client Signature   **Date**

_____   _____
Therapist Signature   **Date**

EXHIBIT 22.6 CURRENT AND PAST MEDICATION LIST

Please feel free to request a copy from your pharmacy; they will print a current list including the below information.

CLIENT NAME: _____ DOB: _____ DATE: _____

Please list all your current medications:

➣ Medication: _____ Dose: _____

Diagnosis/Purpose: _____ How Long on Rx: _____

Side Effects: _____ Cautions: _____

Prescribing Physician: _____ Phone No.: _____

Pharmacy: _____ Phone No.: _____

➣ Medication: _____ Dose: _____

Diagnosis/Purpose: _____ How Long on Rx: _____

Side Effects: _____ Cautions: _____

Prescribing Physician: _____ Phone No.: _____

Pharmacy: _____ Phone No.: _____

➣ Medication: _____ Dose: _____

Diagnosis/Purpose: _____ How Long on Rx: _____

Side Effects: _____ Cautions: _____

Prescribing Physician: _____ Phone No.: _____

Pharmacy: _____ Phone No.: _____

Please list any medications you have tried and have discontinued in the past 2 years/24 months below:

Medication	Length of Time Taken	Reason for Discontinuing Medication
_____	_____	_____
_____	_____	_____

(continued)

EXHIBIT 22.6 CURRENT AND PAST MEDICATION LIST (*continued*)

Medication	Length of Time Taken	Reason for Discontinuing Medication
_____	_____	_____
Medication	Length of Time Taken	Reason for Discontinuing Medication
_____	_____	_____
Medication	Length of Time Taken	Reason for Discontinuing Medication
_____	_____	_____
Medication	Length of Time Taken	Reason for Discontinuing Medication
_____	_____	_____
Medication	Length of Time Taken	Reason for Discontinuing Medication
_____	_____	_____
Medication	Length of Time Taken	Reason for Discontinuing Medication
_____	_____	_____
Medication	Length of Time Taken	Reason for Discontinuing Medication
_____	_____	_____

EXHIBIT 22.7 ADVERSE CHILDHOOD EXPERIENCES QUESTIONNAIRE FOR ADULTS

Note: Questionnaire is from the Centers for Disease Control and Prevention, https://www.cdc.gov/violenceprevention/aces/index.html

Our relationships and experiences—even those in childhood—can affect our health and well-being. Difficult childhood experiences are very common. Please tell us whether you have had any of the experiences listed in the following, as they may be affecting your health today or may affect your health in the future. This information will help you and your provider better understand how to work together to support your health and well-being.

Instructions: Following is a list of 10 categories of Adverse Childhood Experiences (ACEs). From the list, please place a checkmark next to each ACE category that you experienced prior to your 18th birthday. Then, please add up the number of categories of ACEs you experienced and put the total number at the bottom.	
Did you feel that you didn't have enough to eat, had to wear dirty clothes, or had no one to protect or take care of you?	
Did you lose a parent through divorce, abandonment, death, or other reason?	
Did you live with anyone who was depressed, mentally ill, or attempted suicide?	
Did you live with anyone who had a problem with drinking or using drugs, including prescription drugs?	
Did your parents or adults in your home ever hit, punch, beat or threaten to harm each other?	
Did you live with anyone who went to jail or prison?	
Did a parent or adult in your home ever swear at you, insult you, or out you down?	
Did a parent or adult in your home ever hit, beat, kick, or physically hurt you in anyway?	
Did you feel that no one in your family loved you or thought you were special?	
Did you experience unwanted sexual contact (such as fondling and/or oral/vaginal intercourse/penetration)?	
Your ACE score is the total number of checked responses	

EXHIBIT 22.8 EMDR READINESS QUESTIONNAIRE (ERQ)

Note: Sine, L., Vogelmann-Sine, S., Wade, T. C., & Wade, D. K. (1997). *EMDR Readiness Questionnaire*. Reprinted with permission by EMDR Institute.

Name: _____   Date: _____

Please circle which of the following items apply to you:

BN

1. I have a permanent place to live.	Not at All ☐	Rarely ☐	Sometimes ☐	Often ☐	Always ☐
2. My basic needs (food, clothing) are met.	Not at All ☐	Rarely ☐	Sometimes ☐	Often ☐	Always ☐
3. I have enough money to pay for basic needs.	Not at All ☐	Rarely ☐	Sometimes ☐	Often ☐	Always ☐
4. I live in a safe environment.	Not at All ☐	Rarely ☐	Sometimes ☐	Often ☐	Always ☐

SS

1. I have a spouse or partner I confide in.	Not at All ☐	Rarely ☐	Sometimes ☐	Often ☐	Always ☐
2. I have a family to talk to.	Not at All ☐	Rarely ☐	Sometimes ☐	Often ☐	Always ☐
3. I have close friends or coworkers I confide in.	Not at All ☐	Rarely ☐	Sometimes ☐	Often ☐	Always ☐
4. I am involved in community organizations.	Not at All ☐	Rarely ☐	Sometimes ☐	Often ☐	Always ☐
5. I am involved in support groups.	Not at All ☐	Rarely ☐	Sometimes ☐	Often ☐	Always ☐
6. I make friends easily.	Not at All ☐	Rarely ☐	Sometimes ☐	Often ☐	Always ☐

F

1. I am able to identify my feelings.	Not at All ☐	Rarely ☐	Sometimes ☐	Often ☐	Always ☐
2. I know why I feel the way I do.	Not at All ☐	Rarely ☐	Sometimes ☐	Often ☐	Always ☐
3. I recognize how the past affects my feelings now.	Not at All ☐	Rarely ☐	Sometimes ☐	Often ☐	Always ☐
4. When I grew up, it was safe to express my feelings.	Not at All ☐	Rarely ☐	Sometimes ☐	Often ☐	Always ☐
5. My parents or caretakers overreacted emotionally (angry outbursts, depression, anxiety).	Not at All ☐	Rarely ☐	Sometimes ☐	Often ☐	Always ☐
6. I am able to express my feelings appropriately to the people I trust.	Not at All ☐	Rarely ☐	Sometimes ☐	Often ☐	Always ☐

(continued)

EXHIBIT 22.8 EMDR READINESS QUESTIONNAIRE (ERQ) (*continued*)

		Not at All	Rarely	Sometimes	Often	Always
7.	When appropriate, I am able to show my feelings.	☐	☐	☐	☐	☐
8.	I am able to accept and tolerate intense feelings (fear, anger, sadness, hurt) in myself/others.	☐	☐	☐	☐	☐

EL

		Not at All	Rarely	Sometimes	Often	Always
1.	If I show feelings, I am afraid that others will not like me.	☐	☐	☐	☐	☐
2.	I alternate feeling love and hate for the same person.	☐	☐	☐	☐	☐
3.	My feelings change rapidly and unexpectedly.	☐	☐	☐	☐	☐
4.	I overreact to people and situations.	☐	☐	☐	☐	☐
5.	I have a short fuse.	☐	☐	☐	☐	☐
6.	I feel empty.	☐	☐	☐	☐	☐
7.	Presently, I get so depressed I feel suicidal.	☐	☐	☐	☐	☐
8.	As I look over my life, I have gotten so depressed that I have felt suicidal.	☐	☐	☐	☐	☐
9.	Presently, I get so angry I feel like hurting others or destroying things.	☐	☐	☐	☐	☐
10.	As I look over my life, I have gotten so angry that I have like hurting others or destroying things.	☐	☐	☐	☐	☐
11.	When I feel bad, I act impulsively in ways that can be harmful to myself (spending, sex, eating, alcohol/drugs, gambling).	☐	☐	☐	☐	☐
12.	When I feel bad, I do things to hurt my body (cutting, burning).	☐	☐	☐	☐	☐
13.	When I feel bad, I do things to hurt others or destroy things.	☐	☐	☐	☐	☐

(*continued*)

EXHIBIT 22.8 EMDR READINESS QUESTIONNAIRE (ERQ) (continued)

R

	Not at All	Rarely	Sometimes	Often	Always
1. I need to be in control and want things to be done my way.	☐	☐	☐	☐	☐
2. I tolerate changes well.	☐	☐	☐	☐	☐
3. I am flexible.	☐	☐	☐	☐	☐

ES

	Not at All	Rarely	Sometimes	Often	Always
1. I like myself.	☐	☐	☐	☐	☐
2. I am confident.	☐	☐	☐	☐	☐
3. I trust myself.	☐	☐	☐	☐	☐
4. I feel people are out to get me.	☐	☐	☐	☐	☐
5. I hear or see things others may not be hearing or seeing.	☐	☐	☐	☐	☐

O

	Not at All	Rarely	Sometimes	Often	Always
1. I share my innermost thoughts and feelings with others when appropriate.	☐	☐	☐	☐	☐
2. I get defensive when questioned about my past.	☐	☐	☐	☐	☐

D

	Not at All	Rarely	Sometimes	Often	Always
1. I have lapses in my memory for the present/past.	☐	☐	☐	☐	☐
2. I have bodily symptoms that physicians cannot explain.	☐	☐	☐	☐	☐
3. I view the world as strange and unreal.	☐	☐	☐	☐	☐
4. I feel like I am an observer of my thoughts and body.	☐	☐	☐	☐	☐
5. I feel like I am in a dream.	☐	☐	☐	☐	☐
6. I hear voices inside my head.	☐	☐	☐	☐	☐
7. I have feelings that come out of the blue without any way to explain them.	☐	☐	☐	☐	☐

(continued)

EXHIBIT 22.8 EMDR READINESS QUESTIONNAIRE (ERQ) (*continued*)

8. I cope with feelings by going away inside.	Not at All ☐	Rarely ☐	Sometimes ☐	Often ☐	Always ☐
9. I cope with feelings by pushing them down.	Not at All ☐	Rarely ☐	Sometimes ☐	Often ☐	Always ☐

A/D

1. Presently, I use alcohol/drugs to cope.	Not at All ☐	Rarely ☐	Sometimes ☐	Often ☐	Always ☐
2. Alcohol/drugs have negative effects on my life now.	Not at All ☐	Rarely ☐	Sometimes ☐	Often ☐	Always ☐
3. I have used alcohol/drugs to cope in the past.	Not at All ☐	Rarely ☐	Sometimes ☐	Often ☐	Always ☐
4. Alcohol/drugs have caused negative effects on my life in the past.	Not at All ☐	Rarely ☐	Sometimes ☐	Often ☐	Always ☐

For the following, please circle Yes or No.   If Yes, please explain.

SMI

1. I use medication for depression, anxiety, or hearing voices.	Yes	No	
2. In the past, I have used medication for depression, anxiety, or hearing voices.	Yes	No	
3. I have been in the hospital for emotional/psychiatric reasons.	Yes	No	
4. I have received treatment for alcohol/drug abuse.	Yes	No	
5. I have attempted suicide.	Yes	No	

M

1. I have heart problems.	Yes	No	
2. I have high blood pressure.	Yes	No	
3. I have eye problems.	Yes	No	
4. I have respiratory problems.	Yes	No	
5. I have neurological problems.	Yes	No	
6. I have a seizure disorder.	Yes	No	
7. I am pregnant.	Yes	No	
8. Other medical conditions.	Yes	No	

(*continued*)

EXHIBIT 22.8 EMDR READINESS QUESTIONNAIRE (ERQ) (*continued*)

4. I have been in a physical fight in the past year.	Yes	No	
5. I have attempted/committed homicide.	Yes	No	
6. I often have to fight to defend my rights.	Yes	No	
7. I often have to lie to get by.	Yes	No	

If needed, use this space for continuing explanations of YES responses in the preceding.

EXHIBIT 22.9 NEGATIVE COGNITIONS QUESTIONNAIRE – INITIAL FORM (NCQ-IF)

Note: Sine, L., & Vogelmann-Sine, S. (1997). *Negative Cognitions Questionnaire – Initial Form*. Reprinted with permission by EMDR Institute.

NAME: _____ DATE: _____

Please circle the number in the following to indicate how true each of the following statements feels about you at a gut level. The scale goes from 1 being "Untrue" to 7 being "Totally True."

NOTE: If you begin to experience very distressing/unpleasant feelings or sensations while completing this questionnaire, discontinue immediately and discuss this situation with your therapist at the next session.

	Untrue						Totally True
1. I don't deserve love	1	2	3	4	5	6	7
2. I am a bad person	1	2	3	4	5	6	7
3. I am terrible	1	2	3	4	5	6	7
4. I am worthless (inadequate)	1	2	3	4	5	6	7
5. I am shameful	1	2	3	4	5	6	7
6. I am not loveable	1	2	3	4	5	6	7
7. I am not good enough	1	2	3	4	5	6	7
8. I deserve only bad things	1	2	3	4	5	6	7
9. I cannot be trusted	1	2	3	4	5	6	7
10. I cannot trust myself	1	2	3	4	5	6	7
11. I cannot trust my judgment	1	2	3	4	5	6	7
12. I cannot succeed	1	2	3	4	5	6	7
13. I am not in control	1	2	3	4	5	6	7
14. I am powerless (helpless)	1	2	3	4	5	6	7
15. I am weak	1	2	3	4	5	6	7
16. I cannot protect myself	1	2	3	4	5	6	7
17. I am stupid (not smart enough)	1	2	3	4	5	6	7
18. I am insignificant (unimportant)	1	2	3	4	5	6	7
19. I am a disappointment	1	2	3	4	5	6	7
20. I deserve to die	1	2	3	4	5	6	7
21. I deserve to be miserable	1	2	3	4	5	6	7
22. I cannot get what I want	1	2	3	4	5	6	7
23. I am a failure (will fail)	1	2	3	4	5	6	7

(continued)

EXHIBIT 22.9 NEGATIVE COGNITIONS QUESTIONNAIRE – INITIAL FORM (NCQ-IF) (continued)

	1	2	3	4	5	6	7
24. I have to be perfect (please everyone)	☐	☐	☐	☐	☐	☐	☐
25. I am permanently damaged	☐	☐	☐	☐	☐	☐	☐
26. I am ugly (my body is hateful)	☐	☐	☐	☐	☐	☐	☐
27. I should have done something	☐	☐	☐	☐	☐	☐	☐
28. I did something wrong	☐	☐	☐	☐	☐	☐	☐
29. I am in danger	☐	☐	☐	☐	☐	☐	☐
30. I cannot stand it	☐	☐	☐	☐	☐	☐	☐
31. I cannot trust anyone	☐	☐	☐	☐	☐	☐	☐
32. I cannot let it out	☐	☐	☐	☐	☐	☐	☐
33. I do not deserve	☐	☐	☐	☐	☐	☐	☐
34. It's not okay to feel (show my emotions)	☐	☐	☐	☐	☐	☐	☐
35. I cannot stand up for myself	☐	☐	☐	☐	☐	☐	☐
36. I am different (don't belong)	☐	☐	☐	☐	☐	☐	☐
37. I should have known better	☐	☐	☐	☐	☐	☐	☐
38. I am inadequate	☐	☐	☐	☐	☐	☐	☐

Please insert in the following any negative statements about yourself not covered in the preceding. Then rate them in the same manner.

	Untrue						Totally True
	1 ☐	2 ☐	3 ☐	4 ☐	5 ☐	6 ☐	7 ☐
	1 ☐	2 ☐	3 ☐	4 ☐	5 ☐	6 ☐	7 ☐
	1 ☐	2 ☐	3 ☐	4 ☐	5 ☐	6 ☐	7 ☐
	1 ☐	2 ☐	3 ☐	4 ☐	5 ☐	6 ☐	7 ☐

EXHIBIT 22.10 TREATMENT GOALS AND CONCERNS

Note: Leeds, A. (2016). *A guide to the standard EMDR protocols for clinicians, supervisors, and consultants* (2nd ed., p. 365). Springer Publishing Company. Reprinted with permission by Springer Publishing Company.

Name: _____   Date: _____

BEHAVIORAL: WANTS MORE	WANTS LESS	CONCERNS

AFFECTIVE: WANTS MORE	WANTS LESS	CONCERNS

COGNITIVE: WANTS MORE	WANTS LESS	CONCERNS

SOMATIC: WANTS MORE	WANTS LESS	CONCERNS

EXHIBIT 22.11 TREATMENT PLAN TEMPLATE

Client Name _____   Date _____

PROBLEM/ISSUE/DIAGNOSIS:
_____

Long-Term Goal:	Estimated Time Frame	Achieved
_____	_____	_____

Short-Term Goals:	Progress	Date
1. _____	_____	_____
2. _____	_____	_____
3. _____	_____	_____

Therapist Interventions:

1. _____
   _____ Initiated _____ Reviewed _____
2. _____
   _____ Initiated _____ Reviewed _____
3. _____
   _____ Initiated _____ Reviewed _____

PROBLEM/ISSUE/DIAGNOSIS:
_____

Long-Term Goal:	Estimated Time Frame	Achieved
_____	_____	_____

Short-Term Goals:	Progress	Date
1. _____	_____	_____
2. _____	_____	_____
3. _____	_____	_____

Therapist Interventions:

1. _____
   _____ Initiated _____ Reviewed _____

(continued)

EXHIBIT 22.11 TREATMENT PLAN TEMPLATE (continued)

2. _____

_____ Initiated _____ Reviewed _____

3. _____

_____ Initiated _____ Reviewed _____

PROBLEM/ISSUE/DIAGNOSIS:

_____

Long-Term Goal:	Estimated Time Frame	Achieved
_____	_____	_____

Short-Term Goals:	Progress	Date
1. _____	_____	_____
2. _____	_____	_____
3. _____	_____	_____

Therapist Interventions:

1. _____

_____ Initiated _____ Reviewed _____

2. _____

_____ Initiated _____ Reviewed _____

3. _____

_____ Initiated _____ Reviewed _____

Strengths and Limitations Affecting Goal Achievements:

_____

_____

_____

Discharge Plan/Termination/Relapse Prevention Plan:

_____

_____

_____

(continued)

EXHIBIT 22.11 TREATMENT PLAN TEMPLATE (continued)

_____   _____
Client Signature   Date

_____   _____
Therapist Signature   Date

EXHIBIT 22.12 STYLES OF COPING WORD-PAIRS

Note: Lynch. (2018). *The skills training manual for Radically Open Dialectical Behavior Therapy: A clinicians' guide for treating disorders of overcontrol.* New Harbinger Publications. Reprinted with permission by New Harbinger Publications.

Read each word-pair in each row and place a check-mark next to the word that best describes you. Make sure you pick only ONE word or phrase in each row. If you are unsure which word best describes you, imagine what your friends or family members might say about you. If neither of the words describe you, pick the one that is the closest to how you would describe yourself. Make sure you pick one word from each row.

A		B	
Impulsive		Deliberate	
Impractical		Practical	
Naïve		Worldly	
Vulnerable		Aloof	
Risky		Prudent	
Talkative		Quiet	
Disobedient		Dutiful	
Fanciful		Realistic	
Fickle		Constant	
Act without thinking		Think before acting	
Changeable mood		Stable mood	
Haphazard		Orderly	
Wasteful		Frugal	
Affable		Reserved	
Impressionable		Not easily impressed	
Erratic		Predictable	
Complaining		Uncomplaining	
Reactive		Unreactive	
Careless		Fastidious	
Playful		Earnest	
Intoxicated		Clear-headed	
Self-indulgent		Self-controlled	
Laid-back		Hard-working	
Unconventional		Conventional	
Dramatic		Modest	
Brash		Unobtrusive	
Obvious		Discreet	

(continued)

EXHIBIT 22.12 STYLES OF COPING WORD-PAIRS (continued)

Column A		Column B	
Vacillating		Determined	
Unrealistic		Sensible	
Gullible		Shrewd	
Unpredictable		Dependable	
Dependent		Independent	
Improper		Proper	
Chaotic		Organized	
Susceptible		Impervious	
Unstable		Steadfast	
Volatile		Undemonstrative	
Excitable		Stoical	
Lax		Precise	
Unsystematic		Structured	
Thoughtless		Thoughtful	
Inattentive		Attentive	
Short-lived		Enduring	
Perky		Despondent	
Passionate		Indifferent	
Immediate gratification		Delay gratification	

Styles of Coping Word-Pairing Scoring Instructions

Tally up the number of checks in each column. The column with the greatest number represents your overall personality style.

If you have a higher score for column A, this indicates you tend to be more under-controlled.

If you have a higher score for column B, this indicates you tend to be more overcontrolled.

Note: This scale measures overall personality styles. A high score on either subscale does not necessarily indicate maladaptive overcontrolled or maladaptive under-controlled coping. For assessing maladaptive overcontrolled coping, refer to a Radically Open Dialectical Behavioral Therapy (RO DBT) trained therapist.

EXHIBIT 22.13 THERAPEUTIC STORYTELLING OUTLINE

Note: Adapted from Lovett, J. (1999, 2007). *Small wonders: Healing childhood trauma with EMDR*. Free Press/Simon & Schuster; Lovett, J. (2015). *Trauma-attachment tangle: Modifying EMDR to help children resolve trauma and develop loving relationships*. Routledge/Taylor & Francis Group; and Wesselmann, D., Schweitzer, C., & Armstrong, S. (2014). *Integrative team treatment for attachment trauma in children: Family therapy and EMDR*. W. W. Norton & Company.

An adult with positive qualities, such as _____,

enjoys _____ and

lives _____. The adult has inside and outside

resources, such as _____.

Like everyone else in the world, this adult experienced both positive and difficult events/situations in life.

A positive event/situation was _____.

A difficult event/situation was _____.

The youngster began to believe _____.

The (Competent Adult part of them/the therapist/caring others) wants the younger part(s) of them to know that _____.

Another positive event/situation was _____.

Another difficult event/situation was _____.

The youngster began to believe _____.

The (Competent Adult part of them/the therapist/caring others) wants the younger part(s) of them to know that _____.

Another positive event/situation was _____.

A difficult event/situation was _____.

The youngster began to believe _____.

The (Competent Adult part of them/the therapist/caring others) wants the younger part(s) of them to know that _____.

Another positive event/situation was _____.

Today, the adult sometimes struggles with _____
_____.

But with the help of inside and outside resources and supports, they are continuing to heal and learn _____
_____.

Index

AAI. *See* Adult Attachment Interview. *See also* assessments
AAP. *See* Adult Attachment Projective. *See also* assessments
abuse/neglect, 6
ACEs. *See* Adverse Childhood Experiences
adaptive information processing (AIP), 20, 27, 28, 45, 141, 153, 266, 278
Adult Attachment Interview (AAI), 19, 32, 61, 217
Adult Attachment Projective (AAP), 32, 61
Adult part of Self. *See* Self
Adverse Childhood Experiences (ACEs), 41, 54, 69
  Adverse Childhood Experiences (ACE) Questionnaire for Adults, 59, 313. *See also* assessments
affect regulation, 60, 116, 122
  affect dysregulation, 11, 62, 63
AFTT-A model. *See* Attachment-Focused Trauma Therapy for Adults model
Ainsworth, Mary, 19, 26. *See also* Bowlby
AIP. *See* adaptive information processing
alcoholism, 2
  Alcoholics Anonymous, 95
ANS. *See* autonomic nervous system
appeasement gesture, 234
assessments, 44, 53
  Adult Attachment Interview (AAI), 19, 32, 61, 217
  Adult Attachment Projective (AAP), 32, 61
  Adverse Childhood Experiences (ACE) Questionnaire for Adults, 59, 313
  Behavior and Symptom Identification Scale (BASIS-32), 58
  client readiness for EMDR, 53, 60
  Detailed Assessment of Posttraumatic Stress (DAPS), 61
  Depression Checklist and Anxiety Inventory, 58
  Dissociative Experiences Scale (DES-II), 61
  EMDR Readiness Questionnaire (ERQ), 60, 314
  Experiences in Close Relationships (ECR) scale, 61
  initial assessment/interview, 44, 53, 56, 301
  Inventory of Altered Self-Concept (IASC), 61
  Mental Status Examination (MSE), 57, 303
  Multidimensional Inventory of Dissociation (MID), 61
  Multiscale Dissociation Inventory, 61
  Negative Cognitions Questionnaire–Initial Form (NCQ-IF), 61, 319
  Personality Assessment Inventory (PAI), 58
  Psychotherapy Assessment Checklist (PAC), 58
  screenings, 58
  Strange Situation, 19, 26, 31, 206
  Styles of Coping Word-Pairs checklist, 63, 325
  Substance Abuse Subtle Screening Inventory 3 (SASSI-3), 59
  Therapeutic Storytelling Outline, 327
  Trauma Systems Inventory–2 (TSI-2), 61
attachment
  adult attachment
    categories/patterns, 27, 32
      disorganized/unresolved, 28
      earned secure, 21, 218
      nonsecure/dismissive, 28, 32, 154, 207
        derogatory subtype, 28
        idealizing subtype, 29
      nonsecure/preoccupied, 28, 29, 32, 154, 207, 227
      secure, 20, 22–23, 28, 32, 229
      unresolved/disorganized, 2, 26, 28, 30, 32, 218, 227
    mothers, 32
  childhood attachment, 26, 28
    categories/patterns, 28
      disorganized, 26, 28
      in therapy, 33
      nonsecure/ambivalent/resistant, 26, 28, 206
      nonsecure/avoidant, 26, 28, 206
      secure, 20, 26, 28, 206
    qualities, 26
  continuum of, 21, 31, 34

attachment (*cont.*)
  experiences
    corrective attachment experiences, 43, 53, 154
    early attachment experiences, 1, 27, 69
    invalidating/nonoptimal attachment experiences, 72, 76, 91, 107, 167
    validating/optimal attachment experiences, 7, 20, 27, 72, 91, 167
  figures, 2, 6, 41
  generational transmission of attachment patterns, 31
  hypothesized attachment designation, 34
  loss, 2, 40
  security, 19
    balance, 21
    impact on parenthood, 21
  status in therapy
  theory. *See* Bowlby, John
  trauma, 40, 121, 168. *See also* single-event trauma
    clients with a history of, 3, 6, 183, 265
    concept of, 2
    consequences of, 2
    impact of, 12, 41, 92
    symptoms of, 3, 59
Attachment-Focused Trauma Therapy for Adults (AFTT-A) model, 1
  framework, 5, 39, 42
    differentiation, 6, 42
    integration, 7, 42
    nurturing and strengthening, 6, 42
    protection, 6, 42
    reconnection, 7, 42
  goals, 43, 61
  integration, 287
  rationale, 40
  protocols, 45
    Brainstorming Internal Resource Team Members protocol, 133–136
    Corrective Attachment Experiences Between the Child/Adolescent and True Parent Parts of Self protocol, 48, 143, 154, 161–164, 172
    Getting Client's Permission to Transition to EMDR Therapy Phases 3 to 8 protocol, 50, 242, 249–252
    Installing the Internal Resource Team protocol, 128, 136–139. *See also* Resource Team
    Negotiating New Roles for Parent and Adult Parts of Self protocol, 169, 178–182

    P-A-C diagrams protocols, 73, 76, 78, 80–83, 83–87, 87–88. *See also* Parent-Adult-Child (P-A-C) model
    Resource Team protocol, 47, 283
    Revising the Early Bonding Contract Rules protocol, 207, 212–215. *See also* Early Bonding Contract
    Safe/Calm Place/State protocol, 46, 92
    Safe Place and Higher Power for the Adult Part of Self protocol, 92, 102–106
    Safe Place and Higher Power for the Child/Adolescent Parts of Self protocol, 108, 116–119
    Strengthening the Competent Adult Part of Self protocol, 142, 149–152, 283
    Therapeutic Story protocol, 49, 219, 224–225. *See also* Therapeutic Story
    Transition From the AFTT-A Preparation Phase to EMDR Phases 3 to 8 protocol, 50, 255, 261–264
    Tucking the Child/Adolescent Part of Self Into the Safe Place protocol, 49, 186, 198–203, 254
  touchstone, 109
attachment trauma, 40, 121, 168. *See also* single-event trauma
  clients with a history of, 3, 6, 183, 265
  concept of, 2
  consequences of, 2
  impact of, 12, 41, 92
  symptoms of, 3, 59
Attitudes, Skills, Knowledge (ASK) model, 40
autonomic nervous system (ANS), 11, 170, 233
ASK model. *See* Attitudes, Skills, and Knowledge model

BASIS-32. *See* Behavior and Symptom Identification Scale
Behavior and Symptom Identification Scale (BASIS-32), 58
Berne, Eric. *See* Parent-Adult-Child (P-A-C) model
bilateral stimulation (BLS), 42, 47, 92, 111, 142, 157, 171, 174, 208, 281
butterfly hug, 155
BLS. *See* bilateral stimulation
Bonding Contract
  Early Bonding Contract, 42, 49, 205, 266, 286
    revising rules, 208–211, 266, 286
  True Bonding Contract, 51
boundaries, 5, 6
Bowlby, John, 19, 25, 27. *See also* internal working model

brain
  "Adult Brain," 5, 9, 45, 49, 51, 72, 170, 239, 280. *See also* adaptive information processing (AIP)
  "Kid Brain," 5, 9, 49, 51, 143, 194, 239
  "Thinking Brain," 45, 170. *See also* adaptive information processing (AIP)
Brainstorming Internal Resource Team Members protocol, 133–136

Child/Adolescent parts of Self. *See* Self
clients
  with a history of attachment trauma, 39, 46
  with secure attachment, 22–23
complex posttraumatic stress disorder (C-PTSD), 59, 121
complex trauma. *See* attachment trauma
containment. *See* Safe/Calm State
cognitive interweaves, 271–273
co-occurring conditions, 275
Corrective Attachment Experiences Between the Child/Adolescent and True Parent Parts of Self protocol, 48, 143, 154, 161–164, 172
corroborative information, 59
countertransference. *See* therapist
C-PTSD. *See* complex posttraumatic stress disorder
cue word, 145
cultural considerations, 8, 39, 53, 107, 265
  humility, 43, 64, 265

DAPS. *See* Detailed Assessment of Posttraumatic Stress
DBT. *See* Dialectical Behavioral Therapy
Depression Checklist and Anxiety Inventory, 58
DES. *See* disorders of extreme stress
DES-II. *See* Dissociative Experiences Scale
Detailed Assessment of Posttraumatic Stress (DAPS), 61
developmental trauma. *See* attachment trauma
diagnosis, 59
Diagnostic and Statistical Manual of Mental Disorders (DSM-5), Fifth Edition, 59
diagrams
  Developing Adult Behaviors chart, 71
  P-A-C diagrams. *See* Parent-Adult-Child model
Dialectical Behavioral Therapy (DBT), 15, 61, 62
  phone call protocol, 55
  Styles of Coping Word-Pairs checklist, 63, 325. *See also* assessments
disorders of extreme stress (DES), 59, 122

dissociative disorders, 59, 277
  adaptations for, 280
  awareness of disorganization, 34
Dissociative Experiences Scale (DES-II), 61
dissociation, 277
  patterns, 279
  Structural Dissociation model, 278
DSM-5. *See Diagnostic and Statistical Manual of Mental Disorders*, Fifth Edition

Early Bonding Contract, 42, 49, 205, 266, 286
  revising rules, 208–211, 266, 286
eavesdropping, 189, 243
ECR scale. *See* Experiences in Close Relationships scale
ego states, 154. *See* Self
EMD. *See* Eye Movement Desensitization and Restricted Reprocessing
EMDR. *See* Eye Movement Desensitization and Reprocessing therapy
EMDR International Association (EMDRIA), 9
EMDR Readiness Questionnaire (ERQ), 60, 314
EMDRIA. *See* EMDR International Association
Emotion Controller-Regulator. *See* Self
emotionally corrective therapeutic relationship, 227, 285
ERQ. *See* EMDR Readiness Questionnaire
Experiences in Close Relationships (ECR) scale, 61
Eye Movement Desensitization and Reprocessing (EMDR) therapy, 253
  adaptations for, 264
  assessment of readiness. *See* assessments
  goals, 255
  origin, 3
  past-present-future sequence, 267
  phases
    phase 1. *See* assessments
    phase 2. *See* preparation phase
    phases 3–8, 50, 239, 254, 289
    phase 4, 270
    phase 5–8, 272
    preparation phase (phase 2), 4, 39, 62, 121
      outcomes, 4, 253
      purpose, 40
  protocols
    Inverted Protocol, 268
    Reverse Protocol, 268
  touchstone event, 109, 267

Eye Movement Desensitization (EMD) and Restricted Reprocessing, 243, 254, 271

fight/flight/freeze, 11
float back method, 17, 266
forms
   Checklist for AFTT-A Steps, 46, 293
   client medical history, 307
   current and past medication list, 311
   informed consent, 54
   Release of Information, 59
   Therapist Disclosure Statement, 54, 300
   treatment goals and concerns, 321
   treatment plan template, 322
Freud, Sigmund, 70, 193
Future Rehearsal, 50, 130, 147, 207, 209, 247, 259, 268
   template, 259, 267, 274

Getting Client's Permission to Transition to EMDR Therapy Phases 3 to 8 protocol, 50, 242, 249–252
golden joinery. *See* Kintsugi
grief, 25

Higher Power, 7, 46, 95–100, 109, 156, 243
   anchoring, 99
   brainstorming, 97, 111–112
   for clients with dissociative identity disorder, 282
   installation, 99, 112

IASC. *See* Inventory of Altered Self-Concept
informed consent, 54, 280
inner child, 70
inner personality system. *See* internal personality system
Installing the Internal Resource Team protocol, 128, 136–139. *See also* Resource Team
internal personality system, 20, 42, 46
   origin, 70
   parts, 73
   structure, 48
Internal Resource Team. *See* Resource Team
internal working model (IWM), 20, 27. *See also* Bowlby
Inventory of Altered Self-Concept (IASC), 61
IWM. *See* internal working model

Kintsugi, 3, 40, 93, 228, 253

Meeting Place, 93, 128, 285. *See also* Resource Team

mental disorientation/disorganization, 2, 206, 217
Mental Status Examination (MSE), 57, 303
MID. *See* Multidimensional Inventory of Dissociation
mindful attunement, 13, 16, 29, 33, 43, 233, 248
MSE. *See* Mental Status Examination
multidimensional complex, 69
Multidimensional Inventory of Dissociation (MID), 61
Multiscale Dissociation Inventory, 61

NCQ-IF. *See* Negative Cognitions Questionnaire–Initial Form
negative cognitions, 7, 27, 29, 42, 44, 76, 109, 230
Negative Cognitions Questionnaire–Initial Form (NCQ-IF), 61, 319
Negotiating New Roles for Parent and Adult Parts of Self protocol, 169, 178–182
nesting dolls, 233
neuroception, 11

P-A-C diagrams protocols, 73, 76, 78, 80–83, 83–87, 87–88. *See also* Parent-Adult-Child (P-A-C) model
P-A-C model. *See* Parent-Adult-Child model
parallel process, 12–15
Parent-Adult-Child (P-A-C) model, 46, 70, 107
   for clients with dissociative identity disorder, 281
   protocols, 73
   scripts, 80
PAC. *See* Psychotherapy Assessment Checklist
PAI. *See* Personality Assessment Inventory
Parent part of Self. *See* Self
parts of Self. *See* Self
PBTT. *See* phase-based trauma treatment
personality. *See* internal personality system
   disorders, 59
Personality Assessment Inventory (PAI), 58
phase-based trauma treatment (PBTT), 64. *See also* Dialectical Behavioral Therapy and Radically Open Dialectical Behavioral Therapy
polyvagal system, 11
positive affect, 42, 176, 242
positive cognitions, 27–30, 96, 128, 230, 272
preparation phase. *See* Eye Movement Desensitization and Reprocessing (EMDR) therapy
psychosocial education, 45, 94, 108
Psychotherapy Assessment Checklist (PAC), 58

radical acceptance, 15
Radically Open Dialectical Behavioral Therapy (RO DBT), 62, 234
RDI. *See* Resource Development and Installation
relationships
  blended/enmeshed, 5, 141
  detached/dissociated, 5
repetition compulsion, 193, 240. *See also* Freud
reprocessing
  for clients with dissociative identity disorder, 287
  phases, 143, 242, 270
  restricted/contained, 271
Resource Development and Installation (RDI), 47, 142, 121
  Resource Map, 122
Resource Team, 47, 123, 171, 241
  anchoring, 129
  brainstorming, 125, 130
  for clients with dissociative identity disorder, 283
  goals, 124
  installation, 128–131, 257
  meeting, 48, 50, 93, 128, 171, 243, 284
  protocol, 47, 283
  subcommittee, 256
Resource Team protocol, 47, 283
Revising the Early Bonding Contract Rules protocol, 207, 212–215. *See also* Early Bonding Contract
RO DBT. *See* Radically Open Dialectical Behavioral Therapy

Safe/Calm Place/State protocol, 46, 92
Safe/Calm State (place), 46, 92, 195, 243
  boundaries, 99
  brainstorming, 95, 110
  containment, 96
  for clients with dissociative identity disorder, 282
  Inner Safe Place script, 93
  installation, 96, 110–112
Safe Place and Higher Power for the Adult Part of Self protocol, 92, 102–106
Safe Place and Higher Power for the Child/Adolescent Parts of Self protocol, 108, 116–119
sand tray, 78
SASSI-3. *See* Substance Abuse Subtle Screening Inventory 3
Self, 1
  Authentic Self, 4
    reclaiming the, 44
  continuity of Self, 27
  efficacy, 141
  harm, 62, 281
  parts of Self, 5, 70, 91
    Adult part of Self
      Competent Adult part of Self, 7, 41, 44, 47, 71, 142, 145, 170–177, 184, 283
      Emotion Controller-Regulator, 7, 48, 76, 168–177, 240
      little "a" Adult part of Self, 48, 168, 170–177, 241
    Child/Adolescent part of Self, 7, 13, 20, 25, 44, 74, 92, 107, 184, 282
      Broken-Hearted Child/Adolescent part of Self, 85
      enmeshed/"Velcro Kid," 141, 154, 186
      Essential, Creative, Adaptive aspects, 75–77, 81–84
      ingrained/"Super Glue Kid," 141, 186
      pseudo-adult, 141
      unmet needs, 109, 232
    Parent part of Self, 168
      Critical Parent part of Self, 48, 169–177, 241
      Nurturing Parent part of Self, 7
      Protective Parent part of Self, 6
      True Parent part of Self, 7, 44, 48, 160, 169
  differentiation, 6
  integration, 7
  therapist use of Self, 4, 43
  versions of, 171
Shapiro, Francine, 27, 39, 47, 61, 93, 122, 278
single-event trauma, 2
social safety zone, 13
spiritual core. *See* Spiritual Essence
Spiritual Essence, 1, 7, 40, 71, 73, 75, 77, 235
Strange Situation, 19, 26, 31, 206. *See also* assessments
Strengthening the Competent Adult Part of Self protocol, 142, 149–152, 283
Structural Dissociation model. *See also* dissociation
Styles of Coping Word-Pairs checklist, 63, 325. *See also* assessments
Subjective Units of Disturbance (SUD), 270, 272
Substance Abuse Subtle Screening Inventory 3 (SASSI-3), 59
SUD. *See* Subjective Units of Disturbance
"Super Glue Kid." *See* Self

team treatment, 63
Therapeutic Story, 49, 217, 266, 286
  Therapeutic Storytelling Outline, 327

Therapeutic Story protocol, 49, 219, 224–225. *See also* Therapeutic Story
therapist, 10
  beliefs, 229
  body language, 233
  co-regulation. *See* parallel process
  countertransference, 13
  eyebrow wag, 234
  mindfulness, 11, 235. *See also* mindful attunement
  over-function, 15
  Safe Place and Higher Power, 102, 115
  secure-based responses, 229
  self-awareness, 36, 41, 43
  team approach, 63
  transference, 13
  triggers, 14, 228, 271, 289
  with secure/earned secure status, 23
  underlying assumptions about, 41
  use of Self. *See* Self
Therapist Disclosure Statement. *See* forms
therapy
  attachment patterns and tendencies in, 33
  attachment status, 22
  commitment to, 62
  common statements, 33
  diagnostic axes, 60
  financial responsibilities, 55
  goal setting, 62, 255
  history-taking, 56
  No Surprises Act, 55–56
  screenings. *See* assessments
  termination, 55
  treatment planning, 62
time orientation, 42, 50, 156, 189, 195, 239, 242, 244, 286
touchstone. *See* Attachment-Focused Trauma Therapy for Adults (AFTT-A) model
  event. *See* Eye Movement Desensitization and Reprocessing (EMDR) therapy
transactional analysis, 70
transference. *See* therapist
Transition From the AFTT-A Preparation Phase to EMDR Phases 3 to 8 protocol, 50, 255, 261–264
transitional object, 128
trauma. *See also* attachment trauma
  descriptions of, 15
  unprocessed preverbal trauma, 218
Trauma Systems Inventory–2 (TSI-2), 61
True Bonding Contract, 51
True Essence. *See* Spiritual Essence
TSI-2. *See* Trauma Systems Inventory–2
Tucking the Child/Adolescent Part of Self Into the Safe Place protocol, 49, 186, 198–203, 254

unshakable belief, 9, 42, 44, 47, 78, 94, 103, 105, 123, 129, 235
use of Self. *See* Self

Validity of Cognition (VOC), 270
"Velcro Kid." *See* Self
visual aspect, 171
VOC. *See* Validity of Cognition

www.ingramcontent.com/pod-product-compliance
Ingram Content Group UK Ltd.
Pitfield, Milton Keynes, MK11 3LW, UK
UKHW051849210426
5322IPUK00024B/621